Markham J. Geller | Renal and Rectal Disease Texts

Die babylonisch-assyrische Medizin in Texten und Untersuchungen

Begründet von Franz Köcher

Herausgegeben von
Robert D. Biggs und Marten Stol

Band VII

Walter de Gruyter · Berlin · New York

Renal and Rectal Disease Texts

by

Markham J. Geller

⊚ Printed on acid-free paper which falls within the guidelines
of the ANSI to ensure permanence and durability.

Library of Congress Cataloging-in-Publication Data

A CIP catalogue record for this book is available from the
Library of Congress

ISBN 3-11-017964-4

Bibliographic information published by Die Deutsche Bibliothek

Die Deutsche Bibliothek lists this publication in the Deutsche Nationalbibliografie;
detailed bibliographic data is available in the Internet at <http://dnb.ddb.de>.

Printed in Germany

Table of contents

Preface

The first six volumes of the present series, *Babylonische-assyrische Medizin*, represented the monumental contribution of Franz Köcher to studies of Mesopotamian medicine. Although working mostly from photographs, Köcher was responsible for numerous identifications of new texts, as well as joins, and he remained *Großmeister* of his discipline until his death in November, 2002.

Köcher's work, nevertheless, usually consisted of copies of medical texts, with precise and detailed information about duplicate passages listed in extensive indices accompanying the copies. Rarely did he edit or translate medical texts in his published works, although he generously provided such information upon request. Köcher's plan was to publish the vast majority of medical texts in the form of autograph copies within his BAM series, to be followed later by text editions and translations.

I met with Franz Köcher frequently during the summer of 2002, during my stay at the Max-Planck-Institut für Wissenschaftsgeschichte, and I proposed a new scheme for the BAM series. The next volume would contain autograph copies of thematically selected texts. Instead of the extensive indices, the autograph copies would be accompanied by text editions and translations of the copied tablets, together with the duplicates published previously in BAM, or in Campbell Thompson's *Assyrian Medical Texts* (AMT). Köcher agreed that after publication of six volumes of copies and indices, it was now time to begin editing the medical corpus in modern transliterations and translations, to make the material accessible to non-specialists and even non-Assyriologists.

The present volume contains three sections. The first section comprises tablets dealing with diseases of the kidney and urinary tract, followed by a second group of texts dealing with diseases of the rectum and anus. A third section contains relevant texts, not specifically related to either kidney or rectal disease, but nevertheless important for studies of Mesopotamian medicine. There are good reasons for treating renal and rectal texts together in this volume. Aside from the fact that both ailments refer to the lower abdomen, a unique catalogue of medical literature from Assur lists the incipits and rubrics of renal disease texts together with incipits and rubrics of rectal disease (see Text No. 48 and Text No. 9 colophon). Furthermore, the treatments for renal and rectal diseases are often similar in comprising invasive procedures, with drugs being inserted into the urethra or anus through bronze tubes or suppositories, respectively. There are also many dissimilar features, such as different types of drugs and plants used in recipes, which are distinctive to each type of treatment. Kidney disease recipes, for instance, contain many types of mineral substances, such as ostrich-egg shell, which are not found in rectal disease recipes. More general comparisons between these two genres and other types of treatments remain to be studied.

The text editions are based upon collations and many new copies of tablets appearing in Campbell Thompson's *Assyrian Medical Texts*, and occasionally even some of Köcher's copies in BAM require collation.[1] Nevertheless, no attempt has been made to re-copy all of Campbell

[1] See the present writer's review of BAM V and VI, *Zeitschrift für Assyriologie* 74 (1984), 292–97.

Thompson's copies of tablets in AMT, except when joins have been made, or when the copy is inadequate. Campbell Thompson noted many joins to AMT tablets in his subsequent text editions and translations, but he never altered his copies to reflect the joins.

There are both institutions and individuals which deserve recognition and thanks for contributing to the completion of this volume. The bulk of the work was carried out during a research fellowship at the Netherlands Institute for Advanced Study (NIAS) in Wassenaar, where I spent the 2000–2001 academic year working with a group researching Greek and Babylonian medicine. I learned a great deal from colleagues in NIAS, but I am most indebted to Marten Stol for reading and correcting the first preliminary drafts of these transliterations and translations. I spent the following summer (2002) at the Max-Planck-Institut für Wissenschaftsgeschichte in Berlin and at the Institut für Judaistik at the Freie Universität, funded by a stipend from the Alexander von Humboldt-Stiftung, where I was able to collate many of the tablets in the Vorderasiatisches Museum. I wish to thank Peter Damerow of the Max-Planck-Institut and Peter Schäfer (then still at the Freie Universität Berlin) for their generous hospitality and support during my stay in Berlin. As always, I rely upon Irving Finkel to read and criticise my work on medicine, and his critique of the first few tablets edited here was a great help. JoAnn Scurlock was kind enough to give me her edition of text No. 49 in this corpus, which proved to be an invaluable help for copying this very difficult tablet. Barbara Böck has been very helpful and accommodating whenever I asked for information from Franz Köcher's notes on readings of various passages. In the final stages, both Marten Stol and Robert Biggs read and corrected versions of the manuscript in their capacity as editors of the BAM series, and they contributed many corrections and useful comments. Finally, I would like to thank Tzveta Pokrovska for help in mounting the plates, and to Gertrud Grünkorn and Sabine Vogt of de Gruyter for their support in bringing this volume to press.

Introductory remarks on kidney and rectal disease

Kidney disease – diagnoses

The proper diagnosis of kidney disease was not possible in antiquity, without instruments other than the naked eye. In the oldest manuscript which we have on kidney disease, the first symptom noted was simply incontinence or 'dripping of urine' (*tattīku ša šināti*).[1] A patient might have blood or pus discharging from his penis, or blisters and sores could be detected on the penis which might indicate venereal disease or urethritis, and pain occurs during urination or ejaculation. The colour of the urine was also carefully noted, and whether there was blood in the urine, although there is no suggestion that the urine was tasted for sweetness. The consistency of the urine, compared to that of an ass, clear paint, wine or beer dregs, was noted as well. All of these symptoms were associated with a condition known as 'discharge' (*mūṣu*).[2] Kidney and bladder stones were obvious symptoms to detect, but one text refers to a patient's constant itching due to a dissolved stone.[3] The patient might suffer from either premature ejaculation or inability to ejaculate.[4] Other colours and consistency in the patient's urine were also noted, in particular yellow, white, and perhaps red.[5] Symptoms associate with 'stricture of the bladder' (*ḫiniqtu*) are both physical (flaccid limbs, pain in the shoulders) and psychic (insomnia, exhaustion, forgetfulness, anxiety, and nightmares).[6] Another unidentifiable disease, *šašituna*, has symptoms consisting of frequent urination and a 'depressed' bladder (perhaps a blockage).

Nevertheless, chronic renal failure would have been almost impossible to detect in antiquity, since symptoms include lethargy, breathlessness on exertion, swollen ankles, itching and progressive darkening of the skin, loss of appetite, vomiting, numbness in the feet, aching bones, epileptic convulsions, chest pain, and difficulty in concentrating.[7] Impaired renal function does not appear as a symptom in this list because chronic renal failure is associated with hypertension, which then produces the adverse symptoms cited above. It is therefore difficult to imagine how a Babylonian healer could have diagnosed renal failure correctly.

Other conditions of the urinary tract are less frequently mentioned in the present corpus. These include isolated references to 'wind' or flatulence in the kidneys, stiffness (*mungu*)

---

1 See text No. 1: 10′.

2 See M. J. Geller and S. L. Cohen, 'Kidney and urinary tract disease in ancient Babylonia, with translations of the cuneiform sources', *Kidney International* 47 (1995), 1811–1815, and see texts 4, 5, and 9 in the present corpus.

3 Text No. 13.

4 See Text No. 2, Ms. B_1. Ejaculating while 'walking' is a euphemism for having sex, i.e., he cannot control his ejaculation or he ejaculates prematurely.

5 See text No. 5.

6 See text No. 2.

7 This information is courtesy of Charles George, and see his 'Development of the idea of Chronic Renal Failure', *American Journal of Nephrology* 22 (2002), 231–239.

or pus in the testicles, or 'collapse of the intestines' (*miqit irrī*),[8] which might be a prolapse.[9] Renal *šimertu*-disease cannot be identified since no associated symptoms are described in the text.[10]

Rectal disease

The incipits of rectal disease texts often use the phrase *ina lā simānišu*, 'at an inappropriate time for (the patient)', probably indicating that the patient's age or state of health is not consistent with the expected appearance of this disease. The usual symptoms in the texts are 'strangury' (*hiniqtu*), constipation, haemorrhoids and anal lesions, bleeding from the anus and the drying up of faecal matter within the rectum. There is no specific reference to blood in the stools themselves, but occasional reference is also made to stools which are abnormally putrid. Stinging pain in the anus (presumably during defecation) is frequently mentioned as a symptom. Some symptoms in the texts are more general in referring to other parts of the anatomy as well, e. g., weakness in the limbs, pain in the shoulders, and bloating.[11] Rectal disease is also associated with 'loin' disease (murub$_4$ gig), which may also refer to the general region of the hips (*qablā*), perhaps because renal, rectal, and 'groin' disease all occur in the lower torso. The Assur Catalogue of medical incipits from Yale also preserves the same sequence of diseases as in the texts themselves, namely renal disease (éllag.gig), rectal disease (dúr.gig), and 'groin'-disease (murub$_4$.gig).[12]

It is somewhat surprising that we find no general theory of medicine or disease within Babylonian medicine, and this is even more surprising in relation to rectal disease. By way of contrast, Egyptian medicine embraced a fundamental theory of disease based primarily upon faecal matter (*wekhedu*) circulating within the body's arteries and veins (*metu*), and this theory persisted in Ptolemaic period medicine as well.[13] Disease was caused by such faecal matter circulating through the body before being excreted through the anus. Although there are two references in our corpus to the intestines discharging putrid matter (see text No. 24 iii 21 and duplicates, text No. 50: 4), this in no way suggests a comprehensive theory of disease based upon putrid matter in the body, as in Egypt. Furthermore, although the colour and consistency (but not the taste) of urine was carefully examined as part of diagnosis, little attention was paid to the appearance or characteristics of stools within therapeutic texts.

One difficulty in analysing types of rectal disease is to distinguish between haemorrhoids and other types of anal sores or lesions (cf. *umṣatu* and *uršu*).[14] We have made a guess based upon rather sparse evidence in these texts, and the translations given here are open to question.

---

[8] Dropsy might be an alternative possibility for this disease.

[9] See text No. 9 col. iv.

[10] The disease only occurs once in this corpus, in text No. 9 iv 10′.

[11] See text No. 32.

[12] See text No. 48.

[13] See H. von Staden, *Herophilus, the Art of Medicine in Early Alexandria* (Cambridge, 1989), 11–12, 23.

[14] As Dr. Morris Greenberg has informed me:

> The "pile" proper arises internally as a varicose vein in the mucosa of the rectum and on a stalk it may emerge through the anus like a grape, sometimes being associated with varying degrees (mild to gross) of prolapse of the rectal mucosa. When a whole bunch of purple grapes emerges they are very uncomfortable and the old physicians learnt how to return them pro tem into the rectum. The internal/prolapsed pile may lead to itching and may bleed.

Finally, the unidentified disease *maškadu* is referred to several times in this corpus,[15] although the illness may be associated with both renal and rectal disease.

Drugs to treat urinary tract disease

The types of materia medica used to treat kidney and urinary-tract disease are not the same, in many instances, as those used to treat diseases of the anus and rectum. This important information may be useful to indicate that even long compound recipes were not merely concocted as a general cure-all but were specifically designed to treat a particular ailment.

One of the remarkable features of renal texts is the high proportion of *materia medica* consisting of minerals rather than plant products. Many of these minerals are found in the present corpus in texts dealing with renal disease rather than with rectal disease. Only the most commonly mentioned minerals are listed below:

renal disease:

ajartu(na$_4$.pa = pseudo-logogram *ia$_4$-artu*)	mussel shell
anzaḫḫu(an.zaḫ)	frit
biṣṣūr atāni(^{na4}peš$_4$.anše)	(a type of shell), lit. 'donkey-vulva'
gabû(^{im}saḫar.na$_4$.kur.ra)	alum, see *qitmu*
ḫaṣab(šika) *pel$_5$*(nunuz) *lurmi*(gá.nu$_{11}$^{mušen})	ostrich-egg shell
imbu' tâmti(ka.a.ab.ba)	coral
iānibu(^{na4}ni.bu/ba = *ia$_4$-ni-bu*)	(stone)
kutpû(an.zaḫ.ge$_6$)	black frit
misis tâmti	(mineral)
pallišu($^{na4.ú}$níg.bùr.bùr)	'bore'-stone (also listed as a plant)
qitmu(^{im}saḫar.ge$_6$.kur.ra)	black dye
zalāqu(^{na4}zálag)	(stone)

rectal disease:

kalû(im.kal.la)	(mineral of yellow colour)
qadūt šikāni([im].gú.en.na)	river mud

common to both:

uḫūlu qarnānu(naga.si)	horned alkali
šadânu(^{na4}ka.gi.na)	haematite

A separate condition of different origin is the "external pile" arising at the margins of the anus which can be painful under tension: a racket shaped incision in the skin at the anal margin will release the tension and dramatically relieve the pain.

There is a condition at the anus that is "sore", and that is the anal fissure. Associated with it may be a skin tag looking like a guardian pile. The treatments of the fissure are barbaric surgery, relatively gentle surgery, or time, the great healer.

There are various abscesses ("pustules") pointing in the perineum arising more or less locally or tracking down from higher up, but they are not to be plucked or cut off.

[15] See texts No. 31, 45, and 50.

The distribution of the mineral content of the *materia medica* is an indication of general differences in types of prescriptions for renal and rectal diseases, although no criteria are given to us regarding how these recipes were conceived and developed.

oils

No. 26 ii 5–8 shows a high percentage of oil being used in rectal disease preparations, which is not the case with renal disease.

> Wrap up into a wad: fat of ox kidney, fat of male sheep kidney, lion-fat, shee, oil of creeping myrtle, bird oil, oil of myrtle, oil of ..., myrrh, cedar, ..., resin of ***baluhhu***, resin of ***abukkatu***, white plant, madder, opopanax, fat of cucumber and ***kasû***, smear and put it into his anus.

Similar recipes can be found in Nos. 21 and 42, a salve for a sore anus. These are cases of special preparations for rectal disease which are not found in kidney-disease recipes. One surprise is that animal kidney as an ingredient of *material medica* occurs only in rectal disease texts, rather than in renal-disease recipes, indicating that kidney organs were not administered in recipes as a type of sympathetic magic. The following cases can be found in 'anus' texts:

ì.udu éllag udu.níta	21: 8; 21: 11; 21: 30; 21: 32; 21: 34 (= 42); 22: 11 (= No. 26); 24 ii 24; 24 (Y_2): 4 and 9; 26: 5; 28: 101; 30:21; 37 ii 5; 42: 4 (= No. 21); 58 ii 15;

plants in *materia medica*:

It is more difficult to identify plants used exclusively for one ailment. Drugs extracted from plants were apparently applied more generally, with some recipes including large numbers of plants (e. g., 75 plants in one recipe, or 93 in another).[16] One possibility might be that the recipe included many different drugs in the hope that some would be effective, although such a theory is never stated in the text. In fact, no explanation is ever provided of how recipes are made up, although ancient physicians may have relied upon a placebo effect for any drugs which they prescribed.

It is difficult to isolate plants which were used exclusively for either renal or rectal disease, although at least two examples can be found in the present corpus. The plant $^{\text{giš.ú}}$gír-*uh-ha-ah* ('thorny plant') only appears in recipes for kidney and urinary-tract disease, while the plant *pizzer* / *pinziru* occurs only in rectal disease recipes.

Simples

The main distinction between recipes is whether they consist of 'simples' or 'compounds'. 'Simples' or 'simplicia' consist of one drug (usually plant or mineral) for one disease, and such recipes can potentially supply useful information for identifying drugs. Arabic pharmacology used 'simples' predominantly rather than compound drug preparations, but this has a long

[16] See text Nos. 58 and 11.

history.[17] Dioscurides, for instance, listed many simples, while Galen himself wrote a treatise on the subject, and Mesopotamian pharmacopoeia used both simples and compounds, although the use of simples is much less common than compound recipes. We have noted instances of simplicia in the footnotes to the texts.

It is more difficult to isolate plants used uniquely for either renal or rectal disease, but specialised preparations were certainly recorded. One text, for instance, provides lists of drugs specifically for kidney problems (No. 18), while another text (No. 42) provides the ingredients for a salve to be used for a sore anus. However, the oldest renal text in the present corpus, dating from the Middle Babylonian period, contains many simplicia amongst its recipes. In fact, the majority of the simplicia occur in the MB Philadelphia tablet (Ms. A), although others are found in the partially duplicating text No. 2 as well, a later tablet from Nineveh. Most other tablets dealing with similar ailments used compound recipes consisting of numerous drugs. Nevertheless, there is insufficient evidence to suggest that, at least in the case of renal disease, recipes initially consisted of simplicia and were later expanded into more elaborate recipes. We simply have the end products of the exercise without being able to reconstruct the stages of development.

In some cases, recipes having the same incipits or symptoms provide a completely different set of drugs. A good example are several texts in the present corpus, Nos. 23, 27, and 32, all of which share the same symptoms referring to general pain in the limbs, chest, and shoulders, as well as specific pain in either the right or left testicle, but two different sets of drugs are prescribed, one of which is also found in a standard drug list (text No. 18). We do not know on what basis these traditional recipes were constructed.

mineral ingredients (simplicia):

qitmu	black dye
gabû	alum

plant ingredients (simplicia):

ajar-kaspi	silver-rosette plant
baluhhu	(aromatic tree) (mixed with pressed oil)
imhur-līm	'it confronted a thousand(diseases)'-plant
hašû	thyme(?)
irrû	cucumber
karān šēlibi	fox-vine
kasû and *mê kasî*	juice of a (garden plant) or the plant itself
kurkānû	(plant)
lišān kalbi	'dog's-tongue' plant
maštakal	(used in beer in rectal disease texts)
murru	myrrh (mixed in tavern beer)
uhhahu	thorn
zēr bīni	tamarisk seed

[17] See Martin Levey, *Early Arabic Pharmacology* (Leiden, 1973), in his chapter on 'Lists of Simples', 100–117. Simplicia will be noted when they appear in this corpus.

zēr kitî	flax seed
šaman erēni	cedar oil (mixed with vinegar)
šammu peṣû	'white plant'

animal matter (simplicia):

ḫallulāja	(insect)
zuqaqīpu	scorpion
uppat timbutti	mole cricket

Some of the simplicia mentioned above are standard ingredients of compound recipes as well, such as the *imḫur-līm* plant, with no other remarkable features. However, the simplicia are predominantly from renal disease texts, and only exceptionally from rectal-disease texts (see No. 35). Furthermore, some of the simplicia represent exotic ingredients not usually found among the *materia medica* of these texts, such as the three insects, flax seed, or the *uḫḫaḫu*-thorn.

Compound recipes

There are plants which occur in sequences which are common to both renal and rectal disease prescriptions, and these probably originated from some type of vademecum or general panacea.

Examples are as follows:

^{ú}*tara-mušₓ* ^{ú}*imḫur-līm* ^{ú}*imḫur-ešra*[18] No. 4: 4; 9: ii 31; 18: 11 (in a list of plants for kidney disease, which shows the sequence); 23: 20 (anus);
ḫašû urnû: 2 ii 7; 18: 26; 25: 2; 25: 9; 26 iii 16; 27: 15;
ḫašû nuḫurtu: 5: 16; 27: 6; 27: 15; 21; 30: 24; 34: 3; 34: 12; 34: 46 (juices);
kukru burāšu 3 ii 30; 5: 13; 9 ii 32; 9 iv 10–11; 21: 8′ (with giš); 21: 29 (giš); 21: 31; 21: 36; 21: 38(with giš); 22: 14; 23: 7; 26 ii 9–10; 27: 26; 28: 23; 28: 30; 30 rev. 23; 32: 14; 32 rev 1; 33: 9; 34: 55; 34: 67 (with giš); 35: 2 (with giš); 38: 4; 38 ii 4; 43: 9; 44: 4; 46: 17; 47: 4; 52: 1; 58: 16; 58 rev. 6; rev. 11; lower edge 22;
burāšu kukru ṣumlalû 2 (B_5): 7; 27: 11; 27: 22; 32: 10; 34:4.
sīḫu argannu barīrātu 34: 7–8; 58: 11. (cf. CAD S 242, ref. courtesy J. Tavernier)
erēnu, šurmēnu, daprānu, asu 34: 33; 54; (CAD Š/3 352, ref. courtesy J. Tavernier)

Such combinations of plants, occurring together in a particular sequence, are characteristic of renal and rectal disease texts (as well as many other genres) and hence they appear to be of more general use, rather than targeted towards any particular ailment or condition. The formulaic nature of the listing of drugs suggests that they were listed in a fixed order for literary rather than pharmacological reasons. In other words, scribes may have simply learned and copied traditional listings of drugs. Since we have no evidence of experimentation or trial-and-error investigation, it is unlikely that drugs were grouped together because of specific chemical properties they possessed or because the combination of drugs produced some desired effect in the patient.

Such compound drug preparations are not unique to Mesopotamia but were also known to the Greek-speaking world. One case was an antidote recipe consisting of more than 170 drugs

[18] lit. 'it confronted 20 (diseases)'-plant, often occurring together with the *imḫur-līm*. lit. 'it confronted a thousand (diseases)'-plant.

ascribed to Mithridates,[19] and Galen himself wrote a treatise on the *Composition of Medicines according to Places*. Comparisons between these recipes and those from Mesopotamia have never been attempted.

Nevertheless, something might be learned from the art of the apothecary, as it used to be practised before modern medicine. It is possible that various substances are added to recipes because they were known to have a desired effect, and other substances were then added to the recipe to counteract any unwanted side-effects (such as constipation or diarrhoea). Ancient recipes, like their modern counterparts, might have included the main drug used as a remedy for a particular ailment, but with other ingredients added to increase its effectiveness. The colour, for instance, of a potion might have been therapeutic, since red liquids are thought (even today) to be toxic against fevers, while green is a more soothing colour for liquids prescribed for stomach disorders.[20]

Dreckapotheke

Franz Köcher convincingly established the fact that many unpleasant or even disgusting ingredients in Akkadian medical texts (or so-called 'Dreckapotheke') were actually secret names of plants, since recipes from Uruk provide double listing of 'Dreckapotheke' as ordinary names of plants often found in medical texts. One tablet of Uruanna, the scribal listing of plants from the school curriculum, gives both names of Dreckapotheke and the ordinary drug name that it represents.[21] Furthermore, it is worth noting that Dreckapotheke is much more common in rectal disease texts than in recipes dealing with renal disease. The following examples of Dreckapotheke occur only in rectal disease texts:

rikibti arkabi (bat guano)	21: 13; 21: 21; 22: 5; 24 ii 12; 24 iii 18; 28: 30; 30: 12;31 rev 9; 33: 5;
zê alpi (ox dung)	21: 37
zê kalbi (dog excrement)	24 ii 19; 24 iv 2; 26 iii 4; 28 43; 28: 49;
piqqannu immeri (sheep dung)	46: 8′;
piqqannu ṣabīti (gazelle dung)	21: 38; 23: 11; 25: 3; 25: 10; 26 ii 17, 26 iii 18; 28: 28; 8 ii 7
gulgul amelūti (human skull)	28: 16, 32
kammu ša aškāpi (leatherworker's fungus)	28: 16

The following example of *Dreckapotheke* occurs in renal disease texts only:

zê ṣurāri (lizard excrement)	8: 13; 16 ii 13;

[19] For the Mithridatium recipes, see Pliny, NH 29.8.24 and Celsus, *De medicina* 5.23.3, and see also G. Watson, *Theriac and Mithridatium. A Study in Therapeutics* (London, 1966) [references courtesy Laurence Totelin].

[20] As Dr. Morris Greenberg informs me (personal communication):

> Substances added to have the desired effect, substances that would augment the effect, those that would act as antidotes to the collateral unwanted effects, inert bulking materials and components to aid absorption of the active ingredient. Then of course there would be the flavouring of a fluid to make it more palatable, and the covering with gold or silver leaf to add to palatability and to impress. The colouring agent was also useful, red being perceived to be tonic and the right shade of green sedative.

[21] The *Dreckapotheke* are often referred to as *pirištu* or 'secret' names of plants, cf. F. Köcher in *Uruk die Gräber*, ed. R. M. Boehmer et al. (Mainz, 1995), 204 f.

Anatomy

The recipes themselves provide scant information regarding organs or internal anatomy of patients suffering from either renal or rectal diseases. The renal disease texts, for instance, mention the *kalītu*, 'kidney', *ellibuḫḫu*, 'bladder', *muštinnu*, 'urethra', and *maslaḫu*, which is probably the semen duct. The rectal-disease texts make no distinction between rectum and anus, since the word *šuburru* appears to apply to both. There is no word for the bowel, although the rectum/anus is distinguished from the groin (*qablu*), although this word can also apply in the dual form to the hips (*qablā*).

Manuscripts

The important manuscripts in the present corpus

One of the interesting observations about the present corpus of medical texts is how relatively little overlap there is between tablets from Assur and Nineveh, even when treating similar medical conditions, which is obvious from noting all duplicate passages within recipes. Entire compositions are not generally duplicated between medical archives in Assur and Nineveh, although isolated individual recipes tend to be duplicated or groups of recipes can appear in the same order. Also interesting is the fact that standard lists of drugs occurring within recipes, in both Assur and Nineveh, can be found in the same sequence in lists of drugs designated for either renal or rectal disease.

It seems likely that tablets from Assur and Nineveh were organised into a similar order or even reflect the similar kind of arrangement of medical literature, but the evidence is not abundant. The only 'catalogue' which we have of medical incipits is from Assur, and the occasional sequence of incipits and catchlines from Nineveh seems consistent with the sequence of the Assur catalogue. However, it is worth noting that colophons of Assur tablets do not preserve catchlines and incipits which allow us to establish an order of tablets within an organised series. This divergence of manuscript traditions may only be a reflection of the archaeological record, and that new finds from both sites could alter the picture considerably. Nevertheless, there are enough tablets and enough individual recipes represented in the present corpus to come to a preliminary conclusion that medical libraries or archives in Assur and Nineveh had many general parallels but at the same time many differences and cannot be said to have represented 'Mesopotamian' medicine as a single corpus of texts. The difference is most likely to point to independent compilations of texts in the two scribal centres, perhaps stemming from different origins. In fact, there is little overlap with the few Sultantepe medical tablets in the present corpus as well, nor are medical texts treating renal and rectal diseases well attested from Sippar or Babylon collections in the British Museum. Relatively few tablets among the present collection are in Babylonian script. Although all of these factors might be attributable to chance discoveries, the picture is quite different from the magical corpus, in which there is a much closer general adherence to textual tradition among all first-millennium tablets. The interesting question remains whether textual traditions differed between *āšipūtu* and *asûtu*.

Compared to incantation literature, the distribution of medical manuscripts among various archives is quite haphazard. Whereas incantations often seem to be well represented in both Assyrian and Babylonian tablet collections (e. g., Kuyunjik, Babylon, Assur, Sippar, Borsippa, and Uruk), the medical literature tends to have texts from one particular site which have few duplicates from other sites. Hence, medical texts from Assur are often not duplicated in Nineveh, although both archives mostly used Assyrian script, and even fewer duplicates are to be found from the Sippar and Babylon collections in the British Museum, or from Uruk tablets. The reasons are not quite clear. Assur tablets come predominantly from the *Haus des Beschwörungspriesters*, while Kuyunjik tablets most likely came from library or palace archives. The

Uruk medical texts are usually medical commentaries, while the late Babylon medical tablets seem to come from scribal schools. The divergent characteristics of these individual archives may explain why relatively little overlap is to be found within the medical corpus from different cities in Mesopotamia.

Manuscripts used in the present edition

Many of the manuscripts from the British Museum are previously known from Campbell Thompson's copies in *Assyrian Medical Texts*, although most of the relevant joins to the fragments are not reflected in Thompson's copies, nor in Ebeling's copies of the same tablets, in his *Keilschrifttafeln medizinischen Inhalts* (Berlin 1922–23).

Kidney Texts:

No. 1
Ms. A = CBS 19801 (BAM 396)

A tablet of unknown provenance in MB script with prescriptions numbered in the margin and set off by rulings.

The oldest kidney text in the present corpus,[1] some individual passages are duplicated in other manuscripts, mostly from Assur, with only two short recipes found on Nineveh tablets (see text No. 1).[2] None of the later tablets, however, adhere to the unusual format of Ms. A, in which the recipes are introduced by the logogram KI plus a number in sequential order. One might assume that the numbers cross-reference a particular order of recipes from a manual or a standard reference source, but no supporting evidence exists to support such a suggestion.

Ms. A contains many simplicia, far more than in comparable texts from later periods.

The first symptoms noted in Ms. A are dribbling urine (incontinence) and a disease (*šašituna*) causing the patient to urinate frequently (polyuria). Other symptoms are pain in the kidney and groin, and blood or protein in the urine (Hippocratic *hematuria* and *albuminuria*), both of which are given the ancient diagnosis of 'discharge' (*mūṣu*), which might reflect an inflammation (pyelonephritis) or infection from a stone.[3] Several recipes are intended for treating kidney or bladder stone (Hippocratic *lithiasis*). One group of symptoms refer to discharge from the penis in the form of excessive flow of blood (compared to a menstruating woman) or having uncontrollable ejaculations, combined with sores on the penis. Although no diagnosis is provided for the latter symptoms, venereal disease is one possibility. Finally, the text ends with symptoms of premature ejaculation, in which the patient is not aware that he is ejaculating while having sex.

The text also includes an unusual ritual-remedy for a calculus in which the patient must sit upon a heated brick (col. iii 1–3), presumably simulating birth rituals.

---

1 One other tablet in the present corpus, BAM 171, is Middle Assyrian but is only partially cited in the present corpus since the tablet is mainly concerned with ailments other than those being studied here.

2 This reflects the general picture showing little overlap between tablets from Assur and Kuyunjik in the present corpus. See the discussion above.

3 Geller and Cohen, *Kidney International* 47, 1813.

No. 2
Ms. B = K 2405 + 2449 + 8757 + S 32b + 150 + 1983 (= AMT 31,1 + 59,1 + 61,1)
Ms. B_1 = K 7230 (AMT 61,1), which probably belongs to this text.

Four column tablet from Nineveh with firing holes in a neat LA script. Reverse and bottom are missing, but several smaller fragments may belong to this tablet, judging by physical appearances. Sections are divided by rulings.

The most unusual feature of this text is the way in which bladder disease (lit. 'stricture of the bladder') is associated with a wide range of symptoms unrelated to the urinary tract, such as discomfort in the limbs and shoulders, exhaustion, forgetfulness, insomnia and disturbed sleep, and periodic anxiety. Other more usual symptoms are also noted, such as difficulty in urinating or pain in the penis and groin, pustules on the penis or premature ejaculation. Although it was unlikely that ancient physicians could diagnose chronic renal failure (see above), nevertheless whoever composed this tablet was an astute observer of symptoms.

Treatments consisted of either potions or drugs to be blown into the urethra through a bronze tube.

Most of the duplicated passages occur in Assur tablets.

No. 3
Ms. C = VAT 9871 + 10397 (BAM 111). Assur, from the prince's palace archive, see Pedersén, *Archives*, II, 76–77 (N5 4).

The tablet has relatively short lines, duplicating text No. 1. It provides details of treatments for bladder disease, and allows for the possibility of a separate condition (*silīšu*) to be diagnosed among the symptoms. The recipes instruct the drugs to be taken 'without delay' for a period of three days. A further recipe appears to call for a tourniquet (*sûrtu*) to be tied to the patient's leg for three days.

No. 4
Ms. D = VAT 9870 + 10095 (BAM 112). Assur. There is no provenance, but it may be the same as above.

No. 5
Ms. E = VAT 13734 (BAM 114). Assur, exorcists' house, see Pedersén, *Archives*, II, 53, 67 (N4 354).

Mss. D and E are similar in contact and share a common feature, namely describing the colour and texture of the patient's urine with reference to the urine of an ass, wine, beer, or paint, as well as with a stone (*duhšu*) and the plant *kasû*.[4] The colours of urine are white and yellow-green, and we would argue that *kasû* gives a red colour, as in textile dying recipes.[5] The unusual feature of these descriptions is that each entry begins with the word *šum$_4$-ma* 'if', written out syllabically, rather than the usual logogram **diš** 'if' which usually occurs in therapeutic texts. The word *šumma* written out is more typical of omens rather than medical texts. In this particular case, however, there is surprisingly little similarity between the descriptions of urine in these recipes and in the *Diagnostic Handbook* (see below, text No. 49), which describes urine as being either red, yellow(-green), or black.

[4] For the latest comment on the identification on *kasû*, see N. Heeßel and F. al-Rawi, Iraq 55 (2003), 236.
[5] See M. J. Geller, *Orientalistische Literaturzeitung* 95, 4/5 (July–October 2000), 409–412.

No. 6
Ms. F = VAT 8693 (BAM 115). Assur, no provenance.

No. 7
Ms. G = A 267 + VAT 13743 (BAM 116)

The tablet is joined to a fragment known only from an Assur photo. Assur, exorcists' house, see Pedersén, *Archives,* 53, 68 (N4 378). The colophon appears in Hunger, BAK No. 286.

The duplicates to this Assur tablet come from both Assur and Nineveh, although the two Assur duplicates are lines extracted from tablets dealing with other ailments (Mss. ZZ and YY); at least one of the tablets (Ms. ZZ) comes from the exorcists' house. One Nineveh duplicate (MM) consist of a sequence of plants extracted from a long list of healing drugs, while the other Nineveh exemplar (Ms. B) duplicates only three lines from a lengthy text dealing with renal disease (see Text No. 2).

One remarkable feature of this tablet is the comment that the drugs have been 'checked' (*latkūtu*), as effective for discharge. Unfortunately, we have no information regarding this process, but the likelihood is that the notation refers to the listing of the plants in correct order or form, rather than to any experimentation with plants.

No. 8
Ms. H = S 261 (AMT 66,7)

The right top corner of a 4-column tablet, with firing holes, and sections divided by rulings.

This Nineveh fragmentary text has duplicates from Assur, although only consisting of isolated lines of text, and it also duplicates the MB renal text Ms. A (see Text No. 1).

No. 9
Ms. I = K 4957 + 11742 + S 110 + 679 + 516 + 761 + 2058 (= AMT 82,1 + unpub. + unpub. + OECT 6 pl 16 + AMT 58,4 + AMT 61,5 + AMT 39,9)

The bottom left-hand corner of a four-column tablet, of reddish clay. Sections are divided by rulings. The tablet has very few firing holes, but the edge of the tablet has an uneven surface caused by baking in antiquity.

No. 9b
Ms. J = K 2960 + 14977 (AMT 58,3) + 10268 + Rm. II, 315 (AMT 62,1)

A four-column tablet in a large hand with firing holes symmetrically placed on the tablet, and on both edges. The left corner of much of col. i is preserved, with only part of the middle of col. ii and iii, and col. iv ends in a colophon (Hunger BAK No. 329), which is the same colophon appearing in rectal disease texts No. 22 and 24 below. The column rulings were made with string rather than with the stylus.

The colophon of this tablet informs us that it is Tablet 3 of the series 'diš na éllag-*su* gu$_7$-*šú*', to be followed by anus disease recipes. The text has two main characteristics. It incorporates a long list of 90 *materia medica*, prescribed with the same dosage of two shekels per item, although a later recipe in the text partially duplicates a sequence of *materia medica* from two Nineveh lists of medicinal drugs (Mss. MM and NN). Furthermore, the tablet duplicates several Akkadian and bilingual incantations to Gula known from an Assur tablet, which includes a ritual appended to these same incantations (KAR 73, see text No. 10). The present text also includes the list of *šumma*-clauses describing the appearance of urine, duplicated in Mss. D and E above (see Text No. 4 and 5). Col. iii consists of a list of short recipes which appear to be simplicia.

No. 10
Ms. K = VAT 9024 (= KAR 73)

A one-column tablet in NA script. Assur, exorcists' house, see Pedersén, *Archives,* II 61 (N4 95).

No. 11
Ms. L = K 6493 + 6811 + Bu 91-5-9, 52 (+) K 10676

A single column tablet of reddish clay with sections divided by rulings, in a rather large crude LA script, although not cursive. Only the bottom and top half of the reverse are preserved, and a grey-coloured fragment, K 10676, has the same rather distinctive ductus, assumed to belong to the larger piece without being a physical join.

The text is similar but not an exact duplicate to the opening section of Text No. 9. This text records an extensive recipe consisting of 93 drugs, administered in dosages of one and two shekels in weight. Like text No. 9, the recipe was used together with the recitation of Gula incantations, and this text also includes a sacrificial ritual.

Ms. L_2 = K 10676, probably belongs to the same tablet.

No. 12
Ms. M = K 11829

A fragment of reddish clay consisting of the ends of lines of a left-hand column. The only remaining traces of the right-hand column are column divisions, which were made with string rather than with the stylus. Sections are divided by rulings.

No. 13
Ms. N = Rm II, 375 (AMT 39,6)

Fragment from a large tablet with no edges preserved. The script shows a library hand with rulings between sections, and the gray clay shows signs of burning.

No. 14
Ms. O = K13405 + S 804 + 926 + 2160 (AMT 53,8 + 89,4)

A single-column tablet written in a rather large cursive LB script, with sections divided by rulings. Parts of both edges and the bottom edge are preserved, but the top of the tablet is missing.

No. 15
Ms. P = K 1847 (AMT 2, 7)

Fragment on reddish soft clay, with sections divided by rulings. No tablet edges are preserved.

No. 16
Ms. Q = K 11230 + 11280 (AMT 66,11) + 16437 + S. 126

Probably from the obverse of a four column tablet, with parts of col. i and ii preserved. Sections are divided by asymmetric rulings.

The tablet is partially duplicated in an Assur tablet (Ms. C, see Text No. 3) as well as by the MB tablet (Ms. A, see Text No. 1). The second column preserves a list of drugs administered in dosages designated as a 'handful'.

No. 17
Ms. R = VAT 10818 (BAM 113). Assur, no provenance.

No. 18
Ms. MM = K 9684 + 9999 + S 341 + Rm 328 (BAM 431 v 11′–25′). List of drugs. This is the same tablet as No. 39 below, although the different extracts refer to plants for renal and rectal disease, respectively. For this reason, they have been listed separately. The plants for kidneys are duplicated in BAM 164 5–9 and 18–21.

No. 19
Ms. T = VAT 8903 (KADP no. 36 vi 14–26)

This text represents an extract from a longer list. Assur, exorcists' house, see Pedersén, *Archives,* II 62 f. (N4 136).

Rectal disease:

No. 20
Ms. U = HS 1883 rev. 15–18 (BAM 393)

This is an extract from the oldest manuscript in the present corpus, an OB tablet from Nippur.

No. 21
Ms. V = VAT 13752 + (BAM 95)

Assur, exorcists' house, see Pedersén, *Archives,* II 45, 71 (N4 496), copied by the exorcist Nabû-bēsunu.

This 7th century BC. tablet belonged to one of the early members of an important family of exorcists possessing a large archive of incantation and ritual tablets. Most of the duplicate passages are from other Assur tablets, although some lines appear on tablets from Nineveh and Sultantepe, including one Nineveh tablet in Babylonian script. Even though the tablet is described by Franz Köcher as containing recipes which were later incorporated into the *ina lā simānišu* series (see ll. 16–18), nevertheless it is not possible to place this particular composition within the series, partly because the tablet does not begin or end with an identifiable incipit or catchline. The tablet deals with anal blisters or sores and bleeding from the anus.

No. 22
Ms. W = S. 36 + 215 + 449 + 1245 + 1372 + 1452 + 1628 + 1646 + K 7925 + K 9091 (+) K 3453 (+) K 5955 + 14453 (AMT 43,1 + 43,2 + 57,6 (+) AMT 53,9 (+) 56,3 + 84,7)

A distinctive black colour with some firing holes and sections divided by asymmetrical rulings. Several fragments are assumed to belong to the upper left corner of the obv. and the bottom of col. iii and iv, based upon physical appearance, although these are not physical joins. Col. iv ends in a colophon (see Hunger, BAK No. 329), which is the same colophon of No. 9b and No. 24 in this corpus.

The incipit of this tablet identifies it as part of the *ina lā simānišu* series, and the catchline of the tablet can be found in the Assur Catalogue from Yale (see Text No. 48). Some of the recipes were intended to treat rectal disease specifically occurring 'at an inappropriate time', and a clue to what this means appears in an incipit referring to the patient suffering from rectal disease 'in his youth' (l. 19).

No. 23
Ms. X = K 6545 + 8355 + 9030 (AMT 40,5)

Only the reverse preserved of a 4-column tablet, with a much-damaged surface. Col. iv ends in a colophon (see Hunger, BAK No. 318), which was not copied by Thompson in AMT 40, 5. Sections are divided by rulings, and the few holes in the surface were probably not firing holes.

This tablet can be identified as representing the third tablet of *ina lā simānišu*. The catchline appears in the Assur Catalogue from Yale (Text No. 48 below) and as the incipit of Text No. 24 (Ms. Y), showing the sequence between tablets 3 and 4 of the series. The text has no duplicates from Assur and one recipe is partially duplicated in a Nineveh tablet in Babylonian script (Ms. ff). One feature of this tablet is the partial overlap with a list of drugs from Nineveh for kidney disease (BAM 431 = Text No. 18). The point is that although the tablet mostly deals with rectal disease, this particular recipe also deals with renal disease, since it refers to the kidneys and urethra, and the relevant drugs are taken from kidney-disease drug lists. The tablet treats, *inter alia*, the symptoms of constipation, strangury, and general rectal problems, associated with pain in the extremities and blood in the urine.

No. 24
Ms. Y = K 2433 + 3989 + 14019 + 7818 + 8172 + 14216 + 14772 + 15762 + 16409 + S 357 (AMT 47,1)

A four column tablet on reddish clay preserving the top of col. i and ii, also preserving parts of both edges of the tablet, and the bottom parts of col. iii and iv. Col. iv ends in an Assurbanipal colophon (Hunger, BAK No. 329), which is the same colophon in No. 9b and No. 22 in this corpus. According to the catchline, this is the 4th tablet in the series *ina lā simānišu*. Sections are divided by asymmetrical rulings. Firing holes are distributed unevenly, and the surface edges have buckled due to baking in antiquity. One fragment (No. 25) probably belongs to the top of col. iv, without joining physically.

The following fragments are probably components of K 2433 + (Ms. Y)
Ms. Y_2 = S 1563 (AMT 31,3) + 2061 (AMT 96,6)
Ms. Y_3 = K 15453

This compendium of recipes from Nineveh (with a standard colophon) has few duplicated passages in other tablets, except for two brief passages from Assur and Sultantepe. The tablet treats symptoms occurring after the patient awakes from sleep, as well as constipation, colic, and internal and external anal lesions (perhaps haemorrhoids). One interesting feature of this tablet is the reference to painful ankles, which is a common symptom associated with hypertension and chronic renal failure.

No. 25
Ms. Z = K 4104 (AMT 58,2) (*ina lā simānišu* V)

Top left hand corner of what was probably a four-column tablet somewhat asymmetrical in layout, with sections divided by rulings. Written in a small script on reddish clay, the surface is uneven from firing.

Judging by its physical appearance, this smallish fragment probably belongs to the previous tablet, No. 24, as the top left hand corner of the rev. (the beginning of col. iv). It has two partial Assur duplicates, which unfortunately provide no clues as to how the text continues in the break or its possible connection to No. 24. The symptoms refer to a suppurating anus.

No. 26
Ms. AA = EHE 331 + VAT 8694 + 14118 (BAM 96)

Assur, exorcists' house, see Pedersén, *Archives*, II 53, 72 (N4 524).
Ms. AA_2 = Ass. 13955/r* (BAM 102)

This Assur tablet contains three recipes duplicated in Nineveh, and the same recipes are duplicated in Assur tablets. The text deals with general rectal illness.

No. 27
Ms. BB = VAT 10723 (BAM 88)

Assur, no provenance.

This Assur tablet is duplicated in recipes from both Assur and Nineveh, although the recipes are found in compositions dealing with other types of illness, such as 'Hand of the Ghost'-disease and *sūalu* (cough). This explains why in one recipe in this compendia, bowel disease is ascribed to the 'Hand of the Ghost', probably reflecting the fact that the recipe was originally copied from a different therapeutic text.

No. 28
Ms. CC = VAT 10092 (BAM 104)

Assur, from the prince's palace archive, see Pedersén, *Archives*, II, 77, 79 (N5 6).

A damaged Assur text with few duplicated passages, with only one fully preserved incipit which records treatment for an 'inflamed anus' with sores (l. 42).

No. 29
Ms. CD = S 1587 (AMT 44,5)

Small flake in a small script in a library hand, with sections divided by rulings. No edges are preserved.

The main feature of this fragment from Nineveh is the symptom that 'his stools are dried out' (*šittašu ītanabbal*), and the same expression occurs in the following text (No. 30) as well.

No. 30
Ms. dd = S 1283 + 1947 (AMT 40,4 + 57,5)

One of the few tablets in LB script in this corpus, the single column tablet is written in a large script, with rulings dividing the sections. Bottom of the obv. and top half of the rev. are missing.

This Nineveh tablet deals with constipation. The symptoms refer to passing blood from the anus, having dried stools blocking the anus (see No. 29), and rectal sores. The last preserved recipes concern the diseased windpipe (gi.gíd mur.meš // *embūb hašê*), but it is not easy to see why lung disease would be associated with rectal disease symptoms. On the other hand, some of the recipes from rectal disease texts are duplicated in tablets dealing primarily with *suālu* (lit. cough).

No. 31
Ms. EE = O 194 (BAM 182)

Assur, no provenance.

This Assur tablet has one recipe duplicated in another Assur tablet, but other duplicates are all from Nineveh. The tablet is unusual in containing recipes for both renal and rectal disease, divided between obverse and reverse of the tablet, but this reflects the sequence of renal disease and rectal disease incipits in the Assur Catalogue from Yale (text No. 48). The tablet also includes an incantation against *maškadu*-disease, which appears in two other texts in this corpus (see No. 45 and 58). All three of these tablets have a common characteristic of being relevant to renal disease as well as rectal disease, although there is no formal connection (of catchlines and incipits) grouping these tablets together. Renal symptoms include strangury, stinging pain in the penis, bleeding from the penis, while rectal disease symptoms include haemorrhoids (or abscesses) and moles on the anus, bleeding from the anus, stinging pain and bloating in the rectum.

No. 32
Ms. ff = K 8248 (AMT 56,1), cf. JRAS 1937, 276 f., see RA 26, 73.

Another LB script tablet, with the top half only of this single column tablet being preserved, although the surface of the left edge has eroded. Sections are divided by rulings. The ductus appears to be the same hand as K 3550 (AMT 22,2 = text No. 50), also in LB script.

A Nineveh tablet, with duplicated recipes from both Assur and Nineveh, the text opens with a recipe for stricture of the rectum, which includes symptoms drawn from other parts of the body: weakness in the limbs, pain in the shoulders and either the right or left kidney, and passing blood in the urine. Other symptoms refer to stinging pain and cramps in the anus, bloating, and putrid discharge from the anus. The symptoms on the reverse of the tablet all refer to stiffness in the groin or hips, which might be included because they refer to a close part of the anatomy, but otherwise have no obvious connection with the rectal ailments of the obverse. This sequence of incipits, however, reflects the order of incipits in the Assur Catalogue from Yale (see text No. 48: 16′).

No. 33
Ms. GG = K 9441 (AMT 43,5), cf. RA 26, 72

Top left hand corner of a reddish tablet, and the ductus resembles K 4104 and K 2433.

Although most of the recipes are duplicated in Nineveh, the one recipe duplicated in Assur was popular, since it also appears in two other Nineveh tablets. The symptoms refer mainly to constipation, described as the anus being stopped up. Other symptoms include cramps, spitting up phlegm, and passing abnormal stools.

No. 34
Ms. HH = VAT 9138 (BAM 168)

(also duplicates Suālu Tablet V, edited Cadelli, *Recherche*, p. 258 ff.)

Assur, exorcists' house, see Pedersén, *Archives,* II 53, 62 (N4 131).

This tablet has many duplicated passages, mostly from Assur, although three of the recipes are also found in Sultantepe, in the same sequence. The text includes recipes from a variety of different ailments. In addition to the usual format, the second recipe for Hand of the Ghost-disease includes a lengthy list of drugs, with dosages prescribed for each drug. The symptoms given in the first recipe refer to bloating and flatulence, combined with 'sun-fever' (an unidentified type of fever), ascribed to the 'Hand of the Ghost-disease' (see No. 27 above). Other symptoms include stricture of the bladder, rectal sores, and constipation. In addition to one recipe for fever, the final recipes concern painful groin (or hips) 'at an inappropriate time' (*ina lā simānišu*), which has duplicates from both Assur and Nineveh. This sequence of incipits reflects the order of incipits in the Assur Catalogue from Yale (see text No. 48: 16′).

No. 35
Ms. II = VAT 13726 (BAM 99)

Assur, exorcists' house, see Pedersén, *Archives,* II, 53, 63 (N4 161). For the colophon, cf. Hunger, BAK No. 202.

This tablet contains a series of treatments for bleeding from the anus, with the final recipes being duplicated in Nineveh. Lines 38–39 are simplicia.

No. 36
Ms. JJ = A 254 (BAM 100)

Assur, exorcists' house, see Pedersén, *Archives,* II 53, 60 (N4 35). The layout of the recipes in short lines suggests that the individual phrases comprising the recipe may originally have been a collection of simplicia.

See above, No. 35.

No. 37
Ms. KK = K 8182 + 11102 + 13404 (AMT 50,6 + 53,11 + 95,3)

Fragment from the bottom of the obv. of a four column tablet, with sections divided by asymmetrical lines, and few firing holes. A small part of the bottom edge is preserved.

This Nineveh tablet has no identified duplicates in the present corpus. One symptom refers to incontinence, but another diagnosis (ii 4) clearly refers to rectal disease.

No. 38
Ms. LL = K 8369 (AMT 101,3)

Fragment of the obv. of a four column tablet in a neat hand, with firing holes and rulings dividing sections. The edges of the tablet are not preserved.

Another (so far) unduplicated tablet from Nineveh, the recipes treat various types of anal sores. Two remarkable aspects of this tablet is the use of a sharp pointed flint instrument to scrape away a type of anal *lamṣatu*-sore (l. 8); this sore may have been thought to be caused by a fly or flea of the same name. The end of the tablet refers to a 'lead pessary' (lit. 'lead finger'), although the broken passage gives no clues as to its usage.

No. 39
Ms. MM = K 9684 + 9999 + S 341 + Rm 328 (BAM 431) v 7′–10′

This is an extract from a plant list.

No. 40
Ms. NN = K 4164 + 11691 + Rm 352 (+) K 4176 (BAM 430) v 3′–8′

This is an extract from a plant list.

No. 41
Ms. OO = A 223 (BAM 98)

Assur, exorcists' house, see Pedersén, *Archives,* II 66 (N4 301).

No. 42
Ms. PP = Ass. 13955/k* (BAM 101)

Assur, exorcists' house, see Pedersén, *Archives,* II 53, 59 (N4 14). For the colophon, cf. Hunger, BAK No. 208.

No. 43
Ms. QQ = STT 100 and 100A

Sultantepe.

The tablet has no identified duplicates in the present corpus. It is included because of the diagnosis that the patient suffers from rectal disease.

No. 44
Ms. rr = K 10567 + 13901 (AMT 58,9 + 81,9)

Written in a rather large cursive LB script, with the right edge preserved. The top edge appears to be preserved, although the first line of the obv. is mostly eroded. This same edge forms the bottom of the rev. although the last line is eroded. Lines on the rev. carry over onto the right edge, and sections are divided by rulings.

No. 45
Ms. SS = K 2428 + 2548 + 6728

This previously unpublished single column tablet is written in a large rather poor hand and does not have the appearance of a library text. The obv. preserves part of the right and left edges, but neither the top or bottom of the tablet is preserved. The reverse is better preserved, and sections are divided by rulings.

See above, text No. 31.

No. 46
Ms. TT = K 6056 (= AMT 69,8)

Much more of the clay is preserved than drawn by Thompson, although most of the surface is worn away. Sections are divided by rulings and a few firing holes remain. The surface of the tablet is uneven due to firing. The clay has a yellowish tinge.

No. 47
Ms. UU = 81-7-27, 72 (AMT 57,1)

More uninscribed clay is preserved than shown by Thompson. The fragment is the bottom left hand corner of what probably was a four-column tablet, and a small part of the top left corner of the rev. is preserved as well. Sections are divided by rulings, and the script shows a library hand.

No. 48
Ms. VV

YBC 7123+ and 7126 (+) 7139, see *Abraham Sachs Memorial Volume*, 11–14.

This is the only catalogue of medical texts which is currently known, consisting of a group of fragments from Assur which belong to the same tablet although do not physically join. The author has had the benefit of Franz Köcher's notes and transliteration of these fragments, made from both the published copies and photos of the tablets. The sequence of incipits shows that rectal disease followed kidney disease in a fixed order, often reflected in the tablets of the present corpus.

No. 49
Ms. ww = (VAT 303+)

A large 4-column tablet in a very late Babylonian script was partially copied by Reisner (SBH 148). The new copy here includes a join to the tablet and a copy of the reverse, which was previously left uncopied. The tablet preserves the right and left edges and bottom of the tablet. A new edition of the tablet is being prepared by J. Scurlock and independently by N. Heeßel.

Ms. ww_2 = BM 38655 (see Heeßel, *BAD*, 145)

This late copy of the *Diagnostic Handbook* is included in the present corpus since the text gives symptoms for both renal and rectal disease, although the relevant passages are still not completely preserved. Nevertheless, the technical vocabulary describing symptoms is not the same as the language of the therapeutic recipes, indicating that these two genres were composed in different workshops.

No. 50
Ms. AC = K 3550 (AMT 22,2)

The tablet includes symptoms of both rectal and renal disease, with duplicates from both Nineveh and Assur.

No. 54
Ms. AB = Ass. 13955bu (BAM 89)
From Assur, exorcist's house, see Pedersén, *Archives*, II, 53, 60 (N4 61).

Additional tablets in this edition:

Ms. XX = A 198 (BAM 159)
This large 6-column tablet is a collection of recipes dealing with many types of ailments, including illnesses affecting urination, general 'internal sickness', eye and tooth disease, illnesses caused by ghosts, and finally veterinary medicine dealing with horses. Only sections dealing with urinary tract disease are treated in the present corpus.

Ms. YY= A 239 (BAM 161)
A large 8-column tablet dealing with various diseases, among which are recipes against kidney disease, which are edited in the present corpus.

Ms. ZZ = A 234 (BAM 164)
Collection of recipes for unspecified ailments, from Assur, exorcists' house, see Pedersén, *Archives*, II, 68 (N4 367). For the colophon, cf. Hunger, BAK No. 201.

Ms. AAA = A 199 + VAT 9586 (BAM 171)
Middle Assyrian, from Assur temple archive, see Pedersén, *Archives*, II 18, 26 (N1 119).

Ms. BBB = VAT 13789 (BAM 158)
Assur, exorcists' house, see Pedersén, *Archives*, II, 75 (N4 611).

Ms. AD = VAT 10170 (BAM 152)
Assur, no provenance.

Ms. AE = STT 197

Ms. AF = VAT 8027 (BAM 54)
From Assur, exorcist's house, see Pedersén, *Archives*, II, 53 and 59 (N4 22)

Ms. AG = A 250 (BAM 108)
From Assur, exorcist's house, see Pedersén, *Archives*, II (N4 145)

Ms. AH = VAT 16449 (BAM 97)
Assur, no provenance.

Ms. AI = K 2477+ (AMT 94,2) = BAM 471 i 9′–11′; ii 3′–6′

Ms. AJ = VAT 10649 (BAM 94)
Assur, no provenance.

Ms. AK = K 2417 (AMT 31, 4: 7–9)

Ms. AL = CT 23 10 26 ff.

Ms. AM = John Rylands Library 10, 74

Ms. AN = VAT 8269 (BAM 253)
From Assur, exorcist's house, see Pedersén, *Archives,* II, 59 (N4 10).

Ms. AO = K 5834 + 6703 + 7055 + 8049 + 8441 + 8760 + 9843 + 10501 + 13931 + S 1517 + 81-2-4, 195 (= BAM 579)

Ms. AP = VAT 13733 + 13738 BAM 52 (*suālu*)
From Assur, exorcist's house, see Pedersén, *Archives,* II, 46, 48, 70f. (N4 474), and for the colophon, cf. Hunger, BAK No. 212 (copied from a writing board and an exemplar from Uruk, by Kiṣir-Assur).

Ms. AQ = VAT 7822 (BAM 49)
Assur, no provenance.

Ms. AR = VAT 14082 (BAM 50)
From Assur, exorcist's house, see Pedersén, *Archives,* II, 72 (N4 520). For the colophon, cf. Hunger, BAK No. 191.

Ms. AS = VAT 11203 (BAM 53)
Assur, no provenance.

References

Beckman, G., and Foster, B. 'Assyrian Scholarly Texts in the Yale Babylonian Collection', apud *A Scientific Humanist, Studies in Memory of Abraham Sachs,* ed. E. Leichty et al. (Philadelphia, 1988), 1–26.

Cadelli, D. S., *Recherche sur la médecine mésopotamienne* (unpubl. Ph.D dissertation, Paris I, 2000).

Collins, T., *Natural Illness in Babylonian Medical Incantations* (unpubl. Ph.D dissertation, Chicago, 1999).

Goltz, D., *Studien zur altorientalischen und griechischen Heilkunde, Therapie – Arzneibereitung- Rezeptstruktur* (Wiesbaden, 1974).

Heeßel, N., *Babylonisch-assyrische Diagnostik* (Münster, 2000)

Herréro, P., *Thérapeutique mésoptamienne* (Paris, 1984)

Hunger, H., *Babylonische-assyrische Kolophone* (Neukirchen-Vluyn, 1968)

Küchler, F., *Beiträge zur Kenntnis der assyrisch-babylonischen Medizin* (Leipzig, 1904)

Labat, R., *Traité akkadien de diagnostics et pronostics médicaux* (Paris and Leiden, 1951).

Pedersén, O., *Archives and Libraries in the City of Assur* (Uppsala, 1985–1986).

Stol, M., *Birth in Babylonia and the Bible* (Groningen, 2000).

Stol, M., *Epilepsy in Babylonia* (Groningen, 1993)

Thompson, R. C., *Assyrian Medical Texts* (Oxford, 1923).

idem., 'Assyrian Medical Prescriptions for Diseases of the Stomach', *Revue d'Assyriologie* 26 (1929), 47–92.

idem., 'Assyrian Prescriptions for the "Hand of the Ghost"', *Journal of the Royal Asiatic Society* 1929, 801–823.

idem., 'Assyrian Prescriptions for Diseases of the Urine', *Babyloniaca* 14 (1934), 57–151.

idem., *A Dictionary of Assyrian Botany* (London, 1949).

Catalogue of tablets for BAM VII

Texts 1–20 = kidney disease (also No. 56 and 57)
Texts 21–49 = anus disease
numbers in **bold** = primary publication

A 54*	BAM 105	42	
A 198	BAM 159	1, 3, 4, 31	
A 199	BAM 171	9	
A 216	BAM 258	55	
A 223	BAM 98	**41**, 42	
A 234	BAM 164	7, 18	
A 239	BAM 161	5, 7, 8, 9, 18, 35, 36	
A 250	BAM 108	22, 34	
A 254	BAM 100	35, **36**	
A 267	BAM 116	2, 7	
Ass. 13955/bu	BAM 89	24, 54	
Ass. 13955/k*	BAM 101	24, **42**	
Ass. 13955/r*	BAM 102	26a	
Bab Excav. No 47097		51	pl. 36–37
CBS 19801	BAM 396	1, 2, 3, 4, 6, 8	
EHE 331 + VAT8694 + 14118	BAM 96	21, 22, 24, 25, **26**, 27, 28	
JRL 10		35	
K 1847	AMT 2,7	15	pl. 13
K 2160 (to K 13405)	AMT 53,8		
K 2405 + 2449 + 8757 + S 32b + 150 + 1983 (+) 7230 (+) S 467	AMT 31,1+	**2**, 6,7	pl. 1–3
K 2417	AMT 31,4	29	collated
K 2428 + 2458 + 6728	AMT 82,2	31, **45**	pl. 29–30
K 2433 + 3989 + 4019 + 7818 + 8172 + 14216 + 14772 + 15762 +16409 + S 357	AMT 47,1+	**24**, 26, 28, 30, 31, 32, 33	pl. 21–24
K 2449 (to 2405)	AMT 59,1		
K 2458 (to K 2428)	AMT 82,2		
K 2477 + (AMT 94,2)	BAM 471	27, 32, 34	
K 2960 + 14977 + 10268 + Rm. II, 315	AMT 58,3+	9	pl. 6–8
K 3453 (to S 36+)	AMT 53,9	**22**	

K 3550	AMT 22,2	21, **50**	
K 3989 (to K 2433)	AMT 56,5		
K 4019 (to K 2433)			
K 4104	AMT 58,2	**25**, 26, 27	
K 4164 + 11691 + Rm 352 (+) K 4176	BAM 430	5, 9, 39, **40**	
K 4176 (to 4164)			
K 4957 +11742 + S 110 + 679 +516 + 761 + 2058	AMT 82,1+	5, **9**	pl. 4–5
K 5834 +	BAM 579	34, 58	
K 5864	AMT 58,6	2, 3, 4	pl. 3
K 5955 + 14453 (to S 36+)	AMT 84,7 + 56,3	**22**, 35	
K 6056	AMT 69,8	32, **46**	
K 6493 + 6811 + Bu 91-5-9, 52 (+) K 10676		**11**	pl. 11–12
K 6545 + 8355 + 9030	AMT 40,5	**23**, 24, 27, 32	pl. 19–20
K 6728 (to K 2428)	AMT 82,2		
K 6811 (to K 6493)9			
K 7230 (to K 2405)	AMT 61, 1	1, 2	pl. 3
K 7818 (to K 2433)	AMT 53,1		
K 7925 (to S 36)	AMT 43,2	**22**	
K 8172 (to K 2433)	AMT 58,1		
K 8182 + 11102 + 13404	AMT 95,3 + 50,6 + 53,11	37	pl. 27
K 8248	AMT 56,1	23, 27, 31, **32**, 46	
K 8355 (to K 6545)			
K 8369	AMT 101,3	38	
K 8757 (to 2405)	AMT 59,1		
K 9030 (to K 6545)			
K 9091 (to S 36+)	AMT 57,6	**22**	
K 9441	AMT 43,5	30, 31, 32, **33**	
K 9684 + 9999 + S 341 + Rm 328	BAM 431	5, 7, 9, **18**, 39, 47	
K 9999 (to 9684)			
K 10268 (to K 2960)	unpub.	9	
K 10567 + 13901	AMT 58,9 + 81,9	44	pl. 28
K 10676 (to K 6493)			pl. 12
K 11102 (to K 8182)	AMT 50,6		
K 11230 + 11280 + 16437 + S 126	AMT 66,11 +	1, 3, **16**	pl. 14
K 11280 (to 11230)	AMT 66,11		
K 11691 (to 4164)			
K 11742 (to K 4957)	unpub.		
K 11829	unpub.	12	pl. 11
K 13403	AMT 40,3	2	pl. 3
K 13404 (to K 8182)	AMT 53,11		
K 13405 + S 804 + 926 + 2160	AMT 89,4 + 53,8	14	pl. 13
K 13901 (to K 10567)	AMT 81,9		
K 14216 (to K 2433)	Oppenh. Dreams 364		

K 14453 (to K 5955)	AMT 56,3		
K 14772 (to K 2433)	AMT 56,2		
K 14977 (to K 2960)			
K 15453			pl. 24
K 15762 (to K 2433)			
K 16409 (to K 2433)			
K 16437 (to 11230)	AMT 65,6		
K 16453	AMT 70,6	2	pl. 3
S 32b (to K 2405)	AMT 59,1		
S 36 + 215 + 449 + 1245 + 1372 + 1452 + 1628 + 1646 +K 7925 + 9091 (+) 3453 (+) 5955 + 14453	AMT 43,1 + 57,6 (+) 53,9 (+) 87,4 + 56,3	21, 22, 26, 34, 35	pl. 15–18
S 110 (to K 4957)	unpub.		
S 126 (to K 11230)	unpub.		
S 150 (to K 2405)	AMT 59,1		
S 215 (to S 36)			
S 261	AMT 66,7	4, 8	
S 341 (to 9684)			
S 357 (to K 2433)	AMT 7,7		
S 449 (to S 36)			
S 467	AMT 58,5	2	pl. 3
S 516 (to K 4957)	AMT 58,4		
S 679 (to K 4957)	OECT 6 16		
S 761 (to K 4957)	AMT 61,5		
S 804 (to K 13405)	AMT 89,4		
S 926 (to K 13405)	AMT 89,4		
S 1245 (to S 36)	AMT 43,1		
S 1283 + 1947	AMT 40,4 + 57,5	21, 30, 31, 33	pl. 25–26
S 1372 (to S 36)	AMT 43,1		
S 1452 (to S 36	AMT 43,1		
S 1563 + 2061	AMT 31,3 + 96,6	24	pl. 24
S 1587	AMT 44,5	29	collated
S 1628 (to S 36)	AMT 43,1		
S 1646 (to S 36)	AMT 43,1		
S 1947 (to S 1283)	AMT 57,5		
S 1983 (to K 2405)	AMT 59,1		
S 2058 (to K 2433)	AMT 39,9	9	
S 2061 (to 1563)	AMT 96,6		
S 2160 (to K 13405)			
S 9091 (to S 36)	AMT 57,6		
Rm 328 (to 9684)			
Rm. 352 (to 4164)			
Rm. II, 315 (to K 2960)	AMT 62,1	9	
Rm. II 375	AMT 39,6	13	
81-7-27, 72	AMT 57,1	47	
Bu 91-5-9, 52 (to K 6493)			
BM 38655		49	pl. 35
BM 42576 + 43546 + 43589		52	
HS 1883		20	

STT 97		34	
STT 100		43	
STT 100A		24	
STT 197		21, 28	
O. 194	BAM 182	30, **31**, 32, 33, 45	
VAT 303 + 404 + 579 + 589 + 1751	SBH 148	49	pl. 31–34
VAT 404 (to 303)			
VAT 579 (to 303)			
VAT 589 (to 303)			
VAT 1751 (to 303)			
VAT 7822	BAM 49	34	
VAT 8027	BAM 54	21	
VAT 8693	BAM 115	1, 2, **6**, 8	
VAT 8903	KADP 36	19	
VAT 9024	KAR 73	9, 10	pl. 9–10
VAT 9138	BAM 168	21, 22, 27, **34**	
VAT 9467 + 10300 + 10414	BAM 165	18	
VAT 9586	BAM 171	9	
VAT 9870 + 10095	BAM 112	1, 3, **4**, 5, 8, 9	
VAT 9871 + 10397	BAM 111	1, **3**, 4	
VAT 10092	BAM 104	21, 24, 26, **28**	
VAT 10095 (to 9870)			
VAT 10170	BAM 152	21, 35,	
VAT 10300 (to 9467)			
VAT 10397 (to 9871)			
VAT 10414 (to 9467)			
VAT 10649	BAM 94	28	
VAT 10723	BAM 88	25, 26, **27**, 33, 32, 34	
VAT 10818	BAM 113	17	
VAT 11203	BAM 53	37	
VAT 11819	BAM 162	18	
VAT 13726	BAM 99	21, 22, **35**, 36	
VAT 13733 + 13738	BAM 52	34	
VAT 13734	BAM 114	4, **5**, 9	
VAT 13743	BAM 116	2, **7**, 8	
VAT 13752 + 13791 + 14190 + 14373	BAM 95	**21**, 22, 28, 34, 35, 42	
VAT 13789	BAM 158	9	
VAT 13791 (to 13752)			
VAT 13908	BAM 118	57	
VAT 13910	BAM 117	56	
VAT 13913	BAM 163	18	
VAT 14082	BAM 50	34	
VAT 14118 (to 8694)			
VAT 14190 (to 13752)			
VAT 14373 (to 13752)			
VAT 16449	BAM 97	26, 34	
YBC 7123 +	Sachs Mem. Vol.	9, **47**	
YBC 7126 (+) 7139	Ibid. no. 9c–d	22, 24, 25, **47**	

Bibliography of sources

AMT 2,7	K 1847	15	pl. 13
AMT 7,7	S 357		
AMT 22,2	K 3550	21, **50**	
AMT 31,1 +	K 2405 + 2449 + 8757 + S 32b + 150 + 1983 (+) 7230 (+) S 467	**2**, 6, 7	pl. 1–3
AMT 31, 3 + 96,6	S 1563 + 2061	24	pl. 24
AMT 31,4	K 2417	29	collated
AMT 39,9	S 2058	**9**	
AMT 39,6	Rm. II 375	13	
AMT 40,3	K 13403	2	
AMT 40,4 + 57,5	S 1283 + 1947	21, **30**, 31, 33	pl. 25–26
AMT 40,5	K 6545 + 8355 + 9030	**23**, 24, 27, 32	pl. 19–20
AMT 43,2	K 7925 (to S 36)		
AMT 43,1	S 1245 (to S 36)		
AMT 43,1	S 1372 (to S 36)		
AMT 43,1	S 1452 (to S 36)		
AMT 43,1	S 1628 (to S 36)		
AMT 43,1	S 1646 (to S 36)		
AMT 43,1 +	S 36 + 215 + 449 + 1245 + 1372 + 1452 + 1628 + 1646 + K 7925 + 9091 (+) 3453 (+) 5955 + 14453	21, **22**, 26, 34, 35	pl. 15–18
AMT 43,2	K 7925 (to S 36)		
AMT 43,5	K 9441	24, 30, 31, 32, **33**	
AMT 44,5	S 1587	29	collated
AMT 47,1 +	K 2433 + 3989 + 4019 + 7818 + 8172 + 14216 + 14772 + 15762 + 16409 + S 357 (+) K 3453	**24**, 26, 28, 30, 31, 32, 33	pl. 21–24
AMT 50,6	K 11102 (to K 8182)		
AMT 53,11	K 13404 (to K 8182)		
AMT 53,1	K 7818 (to K 2433)		
AMT 53,8	K 2160 (to K 13405)		
AMT 53,9	K 3453 (to S 36)		
AMT 56,1	K 8248	23, 27, 31, **32**, 46	
AMT 56,2	K 14772 (to K 2433+)		
AMT 56,3	K 14453 (to K S 36)		
AMT 56,5	K 3989 (to K 2433)		

AMT 57,1	81-7-27, 72	47	
AMT 57,5	S 1947 (to S 1283)		
AMT 57,6	S 9091 (to S 36)		
AMT 58,1	K 8172 (to K 2433)		
AMT 58,2	K 4104	**25**, 26, 27	
AMT 58,3 +	K 2960 + 14977 + 10268 + Rm. II, 315	9	pl. 6–8
AMT 58,4	S 516 (to K 4957)		
AMT 58,5	S 467	2	pl. 3
AMT 58,6	K 5864	2, 3, 4	pl. 3
AMT 58,9 + 81,9	K 10567 + 13901	44	pl. 28
AMT 59,1	K 2449 (to 2405)		
AMT 59,1	K 8757 (to 2405)		
AMT 59,1	S 32b (to K 2405)		
AMT 59,1	S 150 (to K 240)		
AMT 59,1	S 1983 (to K 2405)		
AMT 61,1	K 7230 (to K 2405)	1, 2	pl. 3
AMT 61,5	S 761 (to K 4957)		
AMT 62,1	Rm. II, 315 (to K 2960)	9	
AMT 65,6	K 16437 (to 11230)		
AMT 66,11	K 11280 (to 11230)		
AMT 66,11 +	K 11230 + 11280 + 16437+ S 126	1, 3, **16**	pl. 14
AMT 66,7	S 261	4, **8**	
AMT 69,8	K 6056	32, **46**	
AMT 70,6	K 16453	2	pl. 3
AMT 81,9	K 13901 (to K 10567)		
AMT 82,1 +	K 4957 + 11742 + S 110 + 679 + 516 + 761 + 2058	5, **9**	pl. 4–5
AMT 82,2	K 2428 + 2458 + 6728	31, **45**	pl. 29–30
AMT 82,2	K 2458 (to K 2428)		
AMT 84,7	K 5955 (to S 36)		
AMT 89,4	S 804 (to K 13405)		
AMT 89,4	S 926 (to K 13405)		
AMT 89,4 + 53,8	K 13405 + S 804 + 926 + 2160	14	pl. 13
AMT 95,3 + 50, 6 + 53,11	K 8182 + 11102 + 13404	37	pl. 27
AMT 96,6	S 2061 (to 1563)		
AMT 101,3	K 8369	38	
BAM 49	VAT 7822	34	
BAM 50	VAT 14082	34	
BAM 52	VAT 13733 + 13738	34, 46	
BAM 53	VAT 11203	37	
BAM 54	VAT 8027	21	
BAM 88	VAT 10723	25, 26, **27**, 33, 32, 34	
BAM 89	Ass. 13955/bu	24, 54	
BAM 94	VAT 10649	28	
BAM 95	VAT 13752 + 13791 + 14190 + 14373	**21**, 22, 28, 34, 35, 42	

BAM 96	EHE 331 + VAT 8694 + 14118	21, 22, 24, 25,**26**, 27, 28	
BAM 97	VAT 16449	26, 34	
BAM 98	A 223	**41**, 42	
BAM 99	VAT 13726	21, 22, **35**, 36	
BAM 100	A 254	35, **36**	
BAM 101	Ass. 13955/k*	24, **42**	
BAM 102	Ass. 13955/r*	26a	
BAM 104	VAT 10092	21, 24, 26, **28**	
BAM 105	A 54*	42	
BAM 108	A 250	22, 34	
BAM 111	VAT 9871 + 10397	1, **3**, 4	
BAM 112	VAT 9870 + 10095	1, 3, **4**, 5, 8, 9	
BAM 113	VAT 10818	17	
BAM 114	VAT 13734	4, **5**, 9	
BAM 115	VAT 8693	1, 2, **6**, 8	
BAM 116	A 267 VAT 13743	2, **7**, 8	
BAM 117	VAT 13910	56	
BAM 118	VAT 13908	57	
BAM 152	VAT 10170	21, 35,	
BAM 158	VAT 13789	9	
BAM 159	A 198	1, 3, 4, 31	
BAM 161	A 239	5, 7, 8 , 9, 20, 35, 36	
BAM 162	VAT 11819	18	
BAM 163	VAT 13913	18	
BAM 164	A 234	7, 18	
BAM 165	VAT 9467 + 10300 + 10414	18	
BAM 168	VAT 9138	21, 22, 27, **34**	
BAM 171	A 199	9	
BAM 171	VAT 9586	9	
BAM 182	O. 194	30, **31**, 32, 33, 45	
BAM 258	A 216	55	
BAM 396	CBS 19801	1, 2, 3, 4, 6, 8	
BAM 430	K 4164 + 11691 + Rm 352 (+) K 4176	5, 9, 39, **40**	
BAM 431	K 9684 + 9999 + S 341 + Rm 328	5, 7, 9, **18**, 39	
BAM 471	K 2477 + (AMT 94,2)	27, 32, 34, 46	
BAM 579	K 5834 +	34, 58	
Sachs Mem. Vol. no. 9c–d	YBC 7126 (+) 7139	22, 24, 25, **48**	
Sachs Mem. Vol.	YBC 7123 +	9, **48**	
FsWGL 159	BM 42576 + 43546 + 43589	52	
FsWGL 163 f.	BM 42342 (81-7-1, 102)	53	
HS 1883		20	
KADP 36	VAT 8903	19	
KAR 73	VAT 9024	9, 10	pl. 9–10
OECT 6 16	S 679 (to K 4957)		
Oppenh. Dreams 364	K 14216 (to K 2433)		

SBH 148	VAT 303 + 404 + 579 + 589 + 1751	49	pl. 31–34
STT 97		34	
STT 100		43	
STT 100A		24	
STT 197		21, 28	

Kidney disease texts

No. 1 = BAM 396 Middle Babylonian

A	=	CBS 19801 (BAM 396), cf. Lutz, AJSL 36 (1920), 67–83, see JCS 31 231 (collated)
XX	=	A 198 (BAM 159 ii 10ff.) = i 14′; iv 3′–6′
C	=	VAT 9871 + 10397 (BAM 111 ii 19–20; iii 8–12, 15–18) [text no. 3] = i 14′; 20′–22′; ii 1′–12′
F	=	VAT 8693 (BAM 115 2′–4′) [text no. 6] = ii 26′–30′; iii 21′–32′
Q	=	K 11230 + 11280 + 16437 + S 126 (AMT 66,11+ 19′–20′) [text no. 16] = ii 5′–12′; 22′
B_1	=	K 7230 (AMT 61,1) [Text no. 2a] = iv 6′–12′
D	=	VAT 9870 + 10095 (BAM 112 i 9ff.) [text no. 4] = iv 1–5

col. i

0′	A	[ki 15: ....] x ⸢ki a nag⸣-[*ma i-ne-eš*][1]
1′	A	ki 16: ^{im}sahar.ge$_6$.kur.ra *ina* a nag-*ma i-ne-eš*
2′	A	ki 17: zì ^{ú}nam.tal nita zì ^{ú}gír-*uh-ha-ah*
3′	A	*ina* kaš *ba-lum pa-tan* nag-*ma i-ne-eš*
4′	A	ki 18: dabin(zì.da.še) zì ^{ú}gír *ina* kaš nag-*ma i-ne-eš*
5′	A	ki 19[2]: *im-hur-lim* ki.min
6′	A	ki 20: ^{ú}geštin.ka$_5$.a hád.du *ta-sàk ana* a kaš *u* ì.giš šub
7′	A	*ina* mul$_4$ *tuš-bat* nag-*ma i-ne-eš*
8′	A	ki 21: ^{ú}*a-ar*-kù.babbar *ina* kaš *u* ga hi.hi
9′	A	*ba-lu pa-tan* nag-*ma i-ne-eš*

10′	A	diš na[3] *ta-at-ti-kam ša* kàš gig 1 sìla dè *ṣú-pur* udu.níta
11′	A	1 sìla dè nam.tal nita
12′	A	*ba-lum pa-tan* ki a nag.nag ud.5.kám
13′	A	*ka-la u$_4$-mi* nag.nag-*ma i-ne-eš*

14′	A	diš na *ša-a-ši-tu-nam un-nu-ut ù ma-gal* zi.zi-*bi*
	XX	diš na *ša-a-ši-tu-na un-nu-⸢ut⸣u ma-gal* zi.meš
	C	diš na *ša-a-ši-ta-na un-nu-un-ta u ma-gal* zi.zi-*bi* uzu.bun-*šu he-sa-at*
15′	A	numun ^{giš}šinig numun ^{ú}eme.ur.gi$_7$
16′	A	^{šim}šeš *ta-sàk ana* kaš.sag šub
17′	A	*ina* mul$_4$ *tuš-bat ina* á.gú.zi.ga
18′	A	*ba-lum pa-tan* nag-*ma i-ne-eš*

19′	A	ki.min ^{ú}sikil ^{ú}hab ^{šim}im.di[4] ^{ú}eme.ur.gi$_7$
20′	A	hád.du *t*[*a*]-*sàk šum-ma i+na*[5] geštin *šum-ma i+na* ga
	C	diš-*niš* súd *lu ina* geštin *lu ina* ga
21′	A	*šum-ma ina* kaš nag.nag *la i-sà-dar*[6]
	C	*lu ina* kaš.sag *la ú-sa-dar*
22′	A	*ina* ud.3.kám ud.1.kám nag-*ma i-ne-eš*
	C	*ina* ud.3.kám ud.1.kám nag.meš

1 The traces on the tablet do not appear in Köcher's copy in BAM 396.
2 Köcher's copy of this sign is incomplete.
3 It is worth noting the use of the logogram na for *amīlu* in a MB text [courtesy R. D. Biggs].
4 usual is^{šim}im.man.du
5 This sign is written as a ligature.
6 see CAD S 11f. 'do regularly'.

0′ [Prescription No. 15: ....] drink [....] with water [and he will get better.]

1′ Prescription No. 16: He drinks black *qitmu*-dye in water and he will get better.[1]

2′–3′ Prescription No. 17: He drinks the flour of male mandrake and flour of *uhhahu*-thorn in beer on an empty stomach, and he will get better.

4′ Prescription No. 18: He drinks *tappinnu*-flour and flour of *acacia*-thorn in beer and he will get better.

5′ Prescription No. 19: Ditto (= he drinks) *imhur-lim* and ditto (= he will get better).[2]

6′–7′ Prescription No. 20: Dry out and you crush[3] fox-vine and put it into water, beer, or oil, leave it out overnight (lit. you keep it overnight under a star), and he drinks it and he will get better.[4]

8′–9′ Prescription No. 21: Mix 'silver-rosette'(-plant) in beer or milk, he drinks it on an empty stomach, and he will get better.[5]

10′ If a man suffers from dribbling (*tattīku*) urine, he should keep drinking one *sila*-measure of ash of the hoof of a spring lamb,

11′ one *sila* of ash of male mandrake,

12′ on an empty stomach in water for five days;

13′ he should keep drinking throughout the day and he will get better.

14′ If a man is laid low by *šāšituna*-disease and constantly gets up (at night), (var. and his bladder is swollen),

15′ you crush seed of tamarisk, seed of 'dog's tongue',

16′ and myrrh, put it into premium beer,

17′ keep it out over night and in the morning

18′ he drinks it on an empty stomach and he will get better.

19′ Ditto. Dry out and you crush (var. together) 'pure'-plant, madder, *suādu*, 'dog's tongue',

20′ have him keep drinking it, either in wine or in milk,

21′ or in (premium) beer, and not let any time elapse,

22′ he drinks it each day for 3 days and he will get better.

---

[1] Simplicium.

[2] Simplicium.

[3] It is difficult to distinguish between *tasâk* and *tahaššal*, translated here as 'you crush' and 'you pound', although 'you grind' might also be possible. The present translation opts for pounding as a translation of *hašālu* because it is the verb most closely associated with the use of mortar and pestle.

[4] Simplicium.

[5] Simplicium.

23′	A	diš na ^{uzu}éllag-*su* gu$_7$-*šu* murub$_4$-*šú* tag.tag-*šú ù* kàš-*šú* gim kàš anše babbar
24′	A	egir kàš-*šu* múd *ú-kal-la-ma* na.bi *mu-ṣa-am* gig
25′	A	2 gín ^{šim}šeš 2 gín illu *ba-lu-hi-im*
26′	A	2 sìla a.geštin.na téš.bi *ina* ^{dug}kam *tu-šab-šal*
27′	A	šed$_7$ ì.giš bára.ga *ma-al-ma-liš* hi.hi
28′	A	*mi-iš-lam ina* mud zabar
29′	A	[š]è[1] *mùš-tin-ni-su*[2] *ta-ša-pak*
30′	A	[*mi-i*]*š-lam ina* kaš.sag hi.hi
31′	A	[*ina* mul$_4$] *tuš-bat ba-lum pa-tan* nag-*ma i-ne-eš*

col. ii

1′	A	[diš].⌜na x *na ša*? *mu*?⌝ [...
	C	[............................... k]àš-*šú* na$_4$ šub-*a* na.bi [..........................]
2′	A	^{ú}numun.eme.ur.gi$_7$ hád.d[u *ta-sàk*....
	C	x numun ^{ú}eme.ur.gi$_7$ [.........
3′	A	*ina* kaš.sag *tara-sà-an* ki nu tag.g[e ....
	C	[......................] x nu kù kaš nu tag.ga
4′	A	*ba-lum pa-tan* nag-*ma i-*[*ne-eš*]
	C	[............................-*m*]*a* ti

5′	A	ki 2: ^{šim}šeš $^{na4.ú}$níg.bùr.bùr[3] ^{ú}*a-ar*-kù.babbar
	Q	[........ gi]g *ana* ti-*šú* ^{šim}šeš ^{šim}buluh [............
6′	A	numun ^{ú}eme.ur.gi$_7$ numun ^{ú}gír-*uh-ha*-[*ah*]
	C	[n]umun ^{ú}eme.ur.gi$_7$ [.............................]
	Q	[n]umun ^{ú}eme.ur.gi$_7$ numun ^{ú}gír.hab
7′	A	^{na4}peš$_4$.anše šika nunuz ga.nu$_{11}$$^{m⌜ušen⌝}$
	C	[.. p]eš$_4$.anše šika nunuz gá.nu$_{11}$^{mušen}
	Q	[................... nun]uz ⌜ga⌝.nu$_{11}$^{mušen}
8′	A	ú.hi.a *an-nu-ti* téš.bi *ta-sàk*
	Q	téš.bi gaz sim
9′	A	*ina* kaš.sag *ba-lu pa-tan* nag-*šu*[4]
	C	[...] kaš nu *pa-tan* nag-*ma*
	Q	[..........................] x x
10′	A	*ina* mud zabar *ana*(šè)[5] *mùš-tin-ni-su* mú-[*ah*]
	C	[....................] *ana* gìš-*šú* mú-*ah*
	Q	*ina* mud zabar *ana* gìš-*šú* mú
11′	A	*ina* a kúm *ir-ta-na-haṣ*
	Q	[.......................................sah]ar munu$_4$ *ki-šú-ma* ti
	C	[.............................] x e$_{11}$-*šú* sahar munu$_4$
12′	A	*ù i-ra-am tu-ba-har-ma i-n*[*e-eš*][6]
	C	[.....................................] *ina-eš*

---

[1] There is more of this sign visible on the tablet than in Köcher's copy.

[2] The *-su* at the end is puzzling, since it occurs elsewhere in this same text with the same word (see ii 10′), although in iv 10 the same word appears with the suffix *-šu*.

[3] The term is used in this text for both a plant and mineral name; one might translate *pallišu* as 'bore'-stone, but this does not help in the identification.

[4] Köcher's copy shows *-ma*.

[5] See M. Stol, SEL 8 (1991), 193[21].

[6] *iri'u*, 'beer dregs'; see RLA 7 328b s. v. Malz, and cf. MSL 10 24 n. 1.

23′ If a man has pain in his kidney, his groin constantly hurts him, and his urine is white like donkey-urine,
24′ and later on his urine shows blood, that man suffers from 'discharge' (*mūṣu*-disease),
25′ you boil 2 shekels of myrrh, 2 shekels of *baluhhu*,
26′ (and) 2 *sila*-measures of vinegar together in a jug;
27′ cool it and mix it in equal measure in pressed oil.
28′–29′ You pour half into his uretha in a copper tube,
30′ mix half in beer,
31′ you leave it out [over night] and he drinks it on an empty stomach and he will get better.

---

col. ii

[Prescription No. 1: ....]
1′ [If] a man [.......] and his urine discharges a calculus, that man [suffers from ....]
2′ dry out [and you crush] seed of 'dog's tongue', [.............]
3′ and steep it in premium beer, not touching the ground...,[1]
4′ and he drinks it on an empty stomach and he [will get better].

5′ Prescription No. 2: (Take) myrrh, *pallišu*-plant/stone, 'silver-rosette',
6′ seed of 'dog's tongue', seed of *uhhahu*-thorn,
7′ 'donkey-vulva'-shell, shell of ostrich-egg,
8′ you crush together all of these drugs,
9′ and he drinks it in premium beer on an empty stomach.
10′ Blow it into his urethra through a bronze tube,
11′ he keeps bathing in hot water (see variants below)
12′ and you heat up beer dregs and he will [get better].

---

[1] I.e. before he gets out of bed; see Text No. 2 (K 2405+): 8.

13′ A ki 3: ^{ú}eme.ur.gi$_{7}$ hád.du *ta-sàk*
14′ A *ina* kaš.sag *tara-sà-an ina* mul$_{4}$ *tuš-bat*
15′ A *ba-lu pa-tan* nag-*ma i-n*[*e-eš*]

16′ A ki 4: ì ^{giš}eren a.geštin.na hi.hi níg.bùr.bùr[1]
17′ A *ina* mud zabar *ana*(šè) *mùš-tin-ni*-SU d[ub-*ak*][2]
18′ A *ina* ud.3.kám *ú-ga-am-ma-ra-am-ma i*-[*ne-eš*]

19′ A ki 5:<...>-*ma ù* kàš-*šú ú-ṣa-nu* ^{šim}šeš *ta-s*[*àk*]
20′ A ki *ku-ru-un* kaš.ú.sa *ù* ga kúm hi.h[i][3]
21′ A *ša-ap-ti-šu* šéš-*ma* kéš.d[a]
22′ A na$_{4}$ *i-ša-ah-hu-uh*
Q na$_{4}$ *i-šah-hu-uh*

23′ A ki 6: ^{šim}šeš *ta-sàk ana* kaš {3.kam}[4] *sa-bi-*⌜*i*⌝
24′ A *ina* mul$_{4}$ *tuš-bat ina še-ri* nag-*ma né-e*[*š*]

25′ A diš na na$_{4}$ gig a ^{giš}eren ^{giš}*šu-ur-min* ^{šim}l[i][5]
26′ A gi.du$_{10}$.ga šim.hi.a *ka-li-šu-nu* hi.[hi]
F gi.du$_{10}$.ga šim.hi.a [..........................]
27′ A *ina ka-li*$^{!}$(text *at*)-*tu* bún[6]-*ma i-na a-h*[*e-e*]
F [..]
28′ A igi *mùš-tin-ni-su* nu dab-*bat*
F [..........................] dab-*bat*
29′ A *ru-ub-ṣu i-de-ek-ke-e-m*[*a*$^{?}$]
F *ru-ub-ṣa i-de-ka-a* [........
30′ A gig nu zu *ú-ṭa-ab-šu*
31′ A úr ^{ú}eme.ur.gi$_{7}$ gu$_{7}$-*ma i-ne-*[*eš*]
F [..............................] *i-tab-ba-ka ul* tag-*su ni*$^{?}$ [........................]

---

rev. col. iii

1 A ki 2: ú giš ^{ú}gír-*uh-ha-a*[*h* ....[7]
2 A sig$_{4}$.a[l.ur$_{5}$.r]a[8] *tu-u*[*m-ma-am*][9]
3 A *ina* ugu dúr-*ma*[10] [*i-ne-eš*]

---

4 A ki 3: numun ^{ú}eme.ur.gi$_{7}$ ^{ú}ukuš *t*[*i-gi-lu*]
5 A hád.du *ta-sàk ina* ì.giš š[ub-*ma i-ne-eš*]

---

6 A ki 4: ^{ú}ukuš.lagab *ina* kaš nag-*ma* [*i-ne-eš*]

---

1 Reading from collation.
2 Following Lutz' copy.
3 A similar simplicium occurs below, No. 3 ii 6–9, in which myrrh is mixed in beer and given as a potion.
4 These signs are corrupt. The scribe probably intended to write kaš lú, but instead his eye skipped and he wrote tab(!) ud.3.kam.
5 collated.
6 *napāhu*, see CAD N/1, 264, citing KAR 384: 20.
7 See below, l. 15.
8 The signs al.ur$_{5}$.ra are erased on the tablet.
9 For the restoration, see CAD A/1 163 and E 148.
10 The idea of sitting on a brick is reminiscent of the brick of birth mentioned very occasionally in myths and hemerologies; see M. Stol, *Birth*, 118ff. The idea may be here that just as a brick is useful in childbirth to produce the baby, the same brick will help 'give birth' to the calculus.

13′ Prescription No. 3: Dry out and you crush 'dog's tongue',
14′ steep it in premium beer, leave it out over night,
15′ and he drinks it on an empty stomach and he will [get better].[1]

16′ Prescription No. 4: Mix oil of cedar with vinegar,
17′ blow *pallišu* into his urethra through a copper tube,
18′ and have him finish the treatment on the third day and he [will get better].[2]

19′ Prescription No. 5: <...> and his urine smells, crush myrrh,
20′ mix it with *kurunnu*-beer, *billatu*-beer and warm milk,
21′ you anoint the lip (of his penis) and bind it, and
22′ the (kidney) stone will dissolve.[3]

23′

24′ Prescription No. 6: You crush myrrh into tavern-beer
25′ leave it out over night, he drinks it in the morning and it is better.[4]

25′ If a man suffers from a calculus, mix sap of cedar, *šurminu*, juniper,
26′ 'sweet' reed, all of the aromatics,
27′ blow (them) into the kidney, but
28′ the opening of his urethra should not be grasped on the sides.
29′ He shall remove the flux and
30′ it will make him better (in respect to) the undiagnosed disease,
31′ he eats root of 'dog's tongue'-plant and he will get better (var. he pours [........], it should not affect him .. [....]).

rev. col. iii

1 [Prescription No. 2]: [You crush] the plant and wood of (*uhhahu*)-thorn, ...
2 you heat up the brick,
3 make him sit upon (it) and [he will get better].

---

4 Prescription No. 3: Dry out and you crush seed of 'dog's tongue' and gourd, ...
5 put (it) in oil [and he will get better].

---

6 Prescription No. 4: He drinks cucumber (*irrû*) in beer, and [he will get better].[5]

---

[1] Simplicium.
[2] Simplicium.
[3] Simplicium, see similarly No. 3 ii 6–9.
[4] Simplicium.
[5] Simplicium.

7	A	ki 5: ^{ú}eme.ur.gi$_7$ *ša ina* zi-*ka* ^{d}utu [nu igi][1]
8	A	hád.du *ta-sàk ana* kaš.lú.tin.na [šub]
9	A	*ina* mul$_4$ *tuš-bat ba-lum pa-tan* [nag-*ma i-ne-eš*]
10	A	ki 6: ^{ú}geštin.ka$_5$.a *ana* kaš.lú.⸢tin.na⸣ [šub][2]
11	A	*ina* mul$_4$ *tuš-bat* [nag-*ma i-ne-eš*]
12	A	ki 7: *ha-lu-la-a*[3] hád.du *ta-sàk ina* m[ul$_4$ *tuš-bat*]
13	A	nu sikil nu igi[4] nag-[*ma i-ne-eš*]
14	A	ki 8: šika nunuz ga.nu$_{11}$^{mušen} ^{ú}[.................
15	A	^{ú}*nu-ṣa-ba* giš ^{ú}gír-*uh-ha-ah* ⸢^{ú}⸣[...........
16	A	^{ú}a.zal.lá ud.7.kam ú.hi.[a *an-nu-ti*]
17	A	*ina* a zú.lum *ù* kaš.sag hi.hi
18	A	nag-*ma i-ne-*[*eš*]
19	A	ki 9: numun ^{ú}gír<*uh-*>*ha-ah* ^{ú}níg.bùr.bùr téš.bi *ta-sà*[*k*]
20	A	*ana* geštin šub *i+na* mul$_4$ *tuš-bat* nag-*ma né-e*[*š*]
21	A	ki 10: ^{na4}*za-la-qu* ^{na4}ka.gi.na *mu-ṣa-am*
	F	^{na4}zálag ^{na4}kur.nu.dib ^{na4}*mu-ṣu*
22	A	an.záh ^{na4}peš$_4$.anše ^{šim}šeš
	F	an.záh ^{na4}peš$_4$.anše [........]
23	A	šika ^{giš}nu.úr.ma šika nunuz ga. n[u$_{11}$^{mušen}]
	F	[.........................] šika nunuz ga.nu$_{11}$^{mušen}
24	A	an.záh.ge$_6$ nita *ù* munus
	F	an.záh níta *u* munus
25	A	^{ú}*a-ar*-kù.babbar numun ^{giš}šinig ka.a.ab.[ba]
	F	^{ú}*a-a-*[...] ka.a.ab.ba
26	A	^{ú}níg.bùr.bùr ^{ú}*tara-muš* ^{ú}gír-*uh-ha-a*[*h*]
	F	^{na4}níg.bùr.bùr ^{giš}*tara-muš* ^{ú}gír-*h*[*a*-..]
27	A	numun ^{ú}eme.ur.gi$_7$ ^{ú}eme.ur.gi$_7$
28	A	numun ^{ú}dili téš.bi *ta-ša-*[*qa*]*-a*[*l*]
	F	numun ^{ú}dili *mal-ma-liš ta-šá-qàl*
29	A	*ta-sàk ina* ì.giš *ù* ì.giš bára.ga hi.hi
	F	súd *ina* kaš.sag [....................
30	A	*ana* igi ⸢mul.ùz⸣ *tuš-bat ina še-ri* nag.na[g]
	F	[.....................] *tuš-bat ina še-rim* nag
31	A	*la i-sa-a-dar ù* a kúm
	F	*la i-sa-dir ina* a kúm
32	A	*ir-ta-na-*⸢*haṣ-ma i-ne-eš*⸣
	F	(broken)

col. iv

1	A	[ki.m]in pa ^{giš}šinig sig$_7$ ^{ú}*in-uš* gú.níg.àr.ra
	D	diš ki.min pa ^{giš}*bi-ni* si[g$_7$ ....]
2	A	téš.bi gaz lá-*ma i-ne-eš*

[1] See CAD N/2 6, citing Küchler *Beiträge* pl. 10 iii 25, '... which was not exposed to the sun when you pulled (it) out'. See also below, text No. B$_2$.

[2] This recipe is a simplicium.

[3] see W. Farber in Fs. Reiner, 103 f.

[4] Reading with Lutz, not Köcher.

7 Prescription No. 5: Dry out and you crush 'dog's tongue' when you pluck it [when not exposed to] the sun,
8 and [put it] into brewer's-beer,
9 you leave it out over night and [he drinks it] on an empty stomach [and he will get better].[1]

10 Prescription No. 6: [Mix] fox-vine into brewer's-beer,
11 you leave it out over night and [he drinks it and he will get better].[2]

12 Prescription No. 7: Dry out and you crush *halulaja*-insect, [you leave it out] over night,
13 he drinks it, not exposed to anything impure, [and he will get better].[3]

14 Prescription No. 8: [You crush] shell of ostrich egg, [.........]
15 *nuṣabu*-plant, wood of *uhhahu*-thorn, [.......]
16 *azallû*-plant, for 7 days mix [these] drugs
17 in date-juice and premium beer,
18 he drinks it and he will [get] better.

19 Prescription No. 9: You crush together seed of *uhhahu*-thorn, and *pallišu*-plant,
20 put it into wine and you leave it out over night, he drinks it and [he] is better.

21 Prescription No. 10: you weigh out together: (minerals:) *zalāqu*, hematite, *muṣanu*
22 frit, 'donkey-vulva'(-shell), myrrh,
23 pomegranate-rind, shell of ostrich egg,
24′ male' and 'female' black frit,
25′ silver-rosette'-plant, seed of tamarisk, 'sea-fruit',
26 *pallišu*-plant/stone, *taramuš*, *uhhahu*-thorn,
27 seed of 'dog's tongue', 'dog's tongue', and
28 seed of 'single'-plant.
29 You crush and mix them in oil and in pressed oil (var. premium beer),
30 you leave them out over night before the appearance of the Goat-star[4] and he keeps drinking it in the morning,
31 do not let any time elapse and he should bathe
32 in hot water and he will get better.

col. iv

1 Ditto: Pound together green tamarisk leaf, *maštakal*, and legumes,
2 bind it on and he will get better.

[1] Simplicium.
[2] Simplicium.
[3] Simplicium. An alternative is to take igi as a logogram for *mahāru*, 'not receiving (what) is not pure'.
[4] See E. Reiner, *Astral Magic in Babylonia* (Philadelphia, 1995), 52, stating that the Goat-star corresponds to the constellation Lyra which represents Gula, the goddess of healing.

3	A	[diš n]a *ina* gìš-*šú* múd *ú-tab-ba-kam* gim dam ^{giš}tukul *ma-h*[*i-i*]*ṣ*
	XX	diš na *ina* gìš-*šú* múd *ú-tab-ba-ka* gim munus ^{giš}tukul *ma-hi-iṣ*
	D	diš na *ina* gìš-*šú* múd *ú-tab*-[*ba-ka* ....]
4	A	gú.níg.àr.ra ^{ú}nu.luh.ha naga.si
	XX	*ana* [t]i-*šú* gú.gal ^{ú}nu.luh.ha naga.si diš-*niš* súd
	D	*ana* ti-šú gú.gal ⸢^{ú}⸣[...............................
5	A	*ina* kaš *si-bi* nag.nag-*ma i-ne-eš*
	XX	[.............] *ina* mul$_4$ *tuš-bat ina še-rim* nu *pa-tan* nag-*ma* ti
	D	*ina* ⸢gi.sag.kud gíd-*ád u*⸣[.................
6	A	diš na *i+na-aṭ*-⸢*ma*⸣ *i+na* gin-*šu re-hu-us-su* gin-*ma* nu zu
	B$_1$	[...........-*n*]*a-aṭ-ma i-na* gin-*šú re-hu-su* gin-*ma* nu zu
7	A	[gim *š*]*a* gal$_4$.la-*šu* gin-*ma ma-as-ra-ah*
	B$_1$	gim *šá ana* munus gin-*m*[*a* ....]
8	A	⸢gìš⸣-*šu* ù.bu.bu.ul *ma-li*
	B$_1$	[...............b]ú.bú.ul *šiq-ta* diri
9	A	^{im}sahar.na$_4$.kur.ra naga.si *ina* ì.giš hi.hi
	B$_1$	^{im}sahar.na$_4$.kur.ra naga.si súd *ina* ì$^{?}$.g[iš$^{?}$......]
10	A	*ina* mud zabar *ana*(šè) *mùš-tin-ni-šu* dub
	B$_1$	[...]
11	A	*ù ina* ì.giš *ù* kaš hi.hi
	B$_1$	x *ina* ì *hal-ṣi u* kaš.sag nu *pa-tan* na[g-............
12	A	nag-*ma i-ne-eš*
	B$_1$	[..] x hi.a ra-*su-ma* [ti]
13	A	diš na šir-*šú* gig gír.tab hád.du *ta-sàk*
14	A	*ina* kaš nag-*ma i-ne-eš*
15	A	diš ⸢na⸣ šir.dili <gig>[1]gír.tab ti.la ^{dug}kal ì.giš diri
16	A	[.. *ina* š]à šub ud.14.kám *ina* ⸢giš⸣.i.dub[2] *te-tem-me-er*
17	A	e$_{11}$-*ma* ⸢kaš⸣ nag-*šu-m*[*a*]$^{?}$ *in-du-hal-la-ta-am*[3]
18	A	hád.du *ta-sàk ana* šà hi.hi lú *šu-ù ša-pu-li-šu* šéš
19	A	*ù* íb.tag$_4$ nag-*ma i-ne-eš*
20	A	ki 2: eme.šid *ša* edin *tur-ár ta-sàk ina* ì.giš šéš
21	A	*i+na* kaš nag-*ma i-ne-eš*
22	A	ki 3:mu.ùr.ra^{ku6} ti.la dab-*bat* kàš-*šu*
23	A	*ana* ugu-*ša iš-tan ana* íd bar-*ši-ma i-ne-eš*
24	A	ki 4: é.gi$_4$.a-^{d}utu sa$_5$ *in-du-hal-la-ta ša eqli*(a.šà)
25	A	*ina* ga *ù* a$^{!}$ kúm *tu-šab-šal* nag-*ma né-eš*
26	A	ki 5: *ia-ra-ra qá-ta-an-tú ša* a.šà
27	A	[*ina*] ì.giš$^{?}$ ⸢*tu-šab-šal*⸣ nag-*ma i-ne-eš*

[1] Lutz' copy reads uzu.dili, but the signs appear to be šir.dili.

[2] an erroneous Sumerogram for *askuppu*? Alternatively, the logogram could be an error for é.ì.dub, for *našpaku*, 'storehouse'.

[3] *anduhallatu*-lizzard

3 [If a] man drips blood from his penis and is 'struck by the weapon' like a (menstruating) woman:
4 (var. to cure him crush together) legumes, *nuhurtu*, and horned alkali,
5 he should keep drinking it in *sibu*-beer and he will get better (var. you leave it out over night and in the morning he drinks it on an empty stomach and he will recover). (2nd var. he will suck it up via a pipette).

---

6 If a man has a *urinary complaint* and ejaculates while 'going' (i. e. having sex) without being aware of it,[1]
7 as one who has sex with his 'vagina' (var. a woman), and his semen duct
8 is full of pustules/boils (var. and scales);
9 (var. crush and) mix alum and horned alkali in oil,
10 pour it into his urethra via a copper tube,
11 and mix it in (var. pressed) oil or (var. premium) beer,
12 he drinks it (var. on an empty stomach) and he will get better (var. bathe him in ... and [he will recover]).

---

13 If a man's testicles are diseased, dry and you crush a scorpion,
14 and he drinks it in beer and he will get better.[2]

---

15 If a man <is ill in> one testicle, you fill a living scorpion in an *urrubbu*-vessel (with) oil,
16 put [..] into it, on day 14 you bury it in the *threshold*,
17 (then) you take it out and have him drink beer. Dry out and crush a lizard,
18 mix it in, and rub it on that man's hips,
19 and he drinks the rest and he will get better.

---

20 Prescription No. 2: You dry out and you crush a desert lizard, anoint (the patient) with oil,
21 he drinks it in beer and he will get better.

---

22 Prescription No. 3: Seize a live *girītu*-fish,[3] (the patient)
23 will urinate onto its head, you will release it into the canal and he will get better.

---

24 Prescription No. 4: Boil a red dragonfly (and) a field lizard
25 in milk and warm water and he drinks it and will get better.

---

26 Prescription No. 5: You boil a thin *iarara*-(insect) of the field,
27 [in] oil[?], he drinks it and he will get better.

---

1 Presumably this symptom describes premature ejaculation, assuming that the verb *alāku* here is used as a euphemism for sex. The alternative translation that the man ejaculates while 'walking' seems unlikely and unrealistic as a symptom.

2 Simplicium.

3 See CAD Š/1 409.

No. 2 AMT 31,1 + 59,1 + 61,1 (plates 1–3)

B	=	K 2405 + 2449 + 8757 + S 32b + 150 + 1983 [= AMT 31,1 + 59,1 + 61,1]
G	=	A 267 + VAT 13743 (BAM 116 rev. 10′–14′) [text no. 7] = ii 19–20
A	=	CBS 19801 [= text no. 1] (BAM 396 iv 6–12) = B$_1$ 5′–7′
F	=	VAT 8693 (BAM 115 10′–12′) = ll. 11′–12′
B$_1$	=	K 7230 [text no. 2a] (AMT 61, 1), probably belongs here, based upon appearance and similar text
B$_2$	=	K 13403 (AMT 40,3), probably belongs here, based upon appearance and similar text
B$_3$	=	K 16453 (AMT 70, 6), probably belongs here, based upon appearance and similar text
B$_4$	=	S 467 (AMT 58,5), probably belongs here, based upon appearance and similar text
B$_5$	=	K 5864 (AMT 58, 6), probably belongs here, based upon appearance and similar text
MM	=	K 9684 + (BAM 431 v 26–31), a list of kidney-disease drugs[1] = ii 7–8

col. i

1 B [diš na] *mi-na-tu-šú* dub.dub á^2-*šú kim-ṣa-a-šú ù bir-ka-šú* [gu$_7$.meš *ana* ti-*šú*][2]
2 B [x g]ín im.gá.li 1 gín ^{šim}šeš 5 gín ^{ú}nu.luh.ha *ṭe-ri-tú* 3 ú.hi.⸢a⸣ [.........................]

---

3 B [diš] na maš.sìla^2-*šú* gu$_7$.meš-*šú i-ta-an-na-ah im-ta-na-aš-ši* ní *ṭe$_4$-en-*⸢*šú*⸣ *i*[*š-ta-na-an-ni*][3]
4 B [má]š.gi$_6$.meš-*šú par-da* síg ugu-*šú* gub.gub-*az* šà-*šú pi-qam là pi-qam i-par-r*[*u-ud-ma*]
5 B [*ur-r*]*a u* ge$_6$ *la i-ṣal-lal* na.bi *hi-niq-ti* bun gig *ana* ti-*šú* im.gá.li ^{giš}n[am.tar$^?$]
6 B [....... n]íta ^{ú}*kur-ka-nam* šika nunuz gá.nu$_{11}$^{mušen} ^{ú}ku$_6$ ^{ú}eme.ur.gi$_7$ ^{ú}igi-*lim* ^{ú}[.........]
7 B [^{ú}*i*]*r-kul-*⸢*la*⸣ ^{ú}ugu-*kul-la* ^{ú}dili ^{ú}har.lum.ba.šir ^{ú}hab 16 ú.hi.a *an-*[*nu-ti* ....]
8 B [...] ⸢x x gaz *ina* ge$_6$ *ina* šà⸣ *šu-tuk-ki* x x x x [...] ud *a-na lìb-bi a*[*l-*............ *la-a*]*m* gìri-*šú ana* ki gar-*nu* nag-*m*[*a ina-eš*]

---

9 B [é]n ìr.gìri.ma hi.hi *áš-ni-ma ma-al-*[*ma-al* suhuš-*su ṣa*]*-ri-ih pa-al-gu ṣa-ri-ih* ul.bi silim *er-b*[*i*]
10 B silim *er-bi* ka.du$_8$.a *ina qí-bit* ^{d}*ma*[*rduk* en .....*-r*]*e-ti* én *an-ni-tu$_4$* 3-*šú* šid-*nu* nag-*ma ina-eš*

---

11 B ì.giš bára.ga *u* kaš.sag *ina* m[ud.zabar *ina* gìš-*šú* du]b-*ak* illu ^{šim}buluh *ina* izi šeg$_6$-*šal ta-šá-hal*
F ì.giš bára.ga *ù* kaš.sag *ina* mud zabar *ana* [.................... i]llu ^{šim}buluh *ina* izi šeg$_6$-*šal ta-šá-hal*
12 B *ana* gìš-*šú* dub ^{ú}babbar *ina* ì.giš [bára.ga *u* kaš.šag ki.mi]n ^{im}sahar.na$_4$.kur.ra *ina* ì.giš *u* kaš.sag ki.min
F *ana* [.............. ^{ú}]babbar *ina* ì.bára.ga *u* kaš.sag ki.min ^{im}sahar.na$_4$.kur.r[a] x

---

[1] The lines from Ms. MM which duplicate Ms. B is a composite of relevant lines from Text No. 18 below, including from Ms. ZZ (BAM 164), another listing of medicinal plants.
[2] Restored after the incipit of text No. 32 below.
[3] For the restoration, cf. AMT 21, 2 10.

TRANSLATION

1 [If a man's] limbs are constantly flaccid and his (pairs of) arms, shins, and knees [hurt him, in order to cure him,]

2 [x] shekel(s) of yellow *kalû*-ochre, 1 shekel myrrh, 5 shekels of beaten *nuhurtu*, 3 drugs [......]

---

3 [If] a man's shoulders hurt him and he is frequently exhausted, forgetful, and he himself [keeps changing] his mind,

4 his dreams are disturbing, the hair of his scalp stands on end, his heart is frightened from time to time,

5 he cannot sleep day and night, that man suffers from 'stricture of the bladder'.[1] To heal him, (take) yellow *kalû*-ochre, mandrake?,

6 male [........], *kurkānû*-tree, ostrich-egg shell, *urânu*, dog's tongue-plant, *imhur-līm*-plant [..]-plant,

7 *irkulla, elikulla*, 'single'-plant, *harmunu*, madder, pound these 16 drugs [.....]

8 [....]..... at night within the reed hut ...., *when* into the .. [.....] before he gets out of bed (lit. before he puts his foot on the ground), he drinks it and [he will be better].

---

9 Incantation. Mix ...... I repeated each one: [its 'root' is] hot, the 'canal' is hot,[2] ..., come in, well-being!

10 come in, well-being! ..... By the command of Marduk [lord of] *exorcism*, recite this incantation 3 times, he drinks it and he will get better.

---

11 You pour pressed oil and premium beer via a bronze tube [into his penis]. You boil over a fire and filter *baluhhu*-resin,

12 you pour (it) into his penis. Ditto (= he drinks) 'white'-plant in pressed oil and premium beer, or ditto (= he drinks) alum in oil and premium beer (and he will get better).

---

[1] See P. Adamson, 'Anatomical and pathological terms in Akkadian: part ii', JRAS (1979), 5f., suggesting that this condition is likely to be a stricture in the male urethra, caused by trauma or gonorrhea.

[2] The arcane language here presumably refers to the penis.

13	B	numun ^{ú}eme.ur.gi$_{7}$ ^{ú}n[u .... ^{ú}*t*]*i-ia-tu* ^{šim}šeš numun ^{giš}kiši$_{16}$.hab numun ^{ú}gazi^{s}[^{ar}]
14	B	numun ^{giš}šinig [.........] 7 ú.hi-a *hi-niq-*[*ti* bun]
15	B	^{ú}igi-*lim u* ^{ú}*nu-ṣa-bu* ^{ú}kur.[ra ^{ú}ní]g.bùr.bùr ^{ú}eme.ur.gi$_{7}$ ^{šim}šeš šika nunuz ga.nu$_{11}$^{mušen} 7 ú.[hi.a *hi-niq-ti* bun]
16	B	diš na *hi-niq-ti* bun gig šika nu[nuz gá.nu$_{11}$^{m}]^{ušen} ka.a.ab.ba súd *ina* ì kaš [na]g
17	B	^{ú}*šá-šú-gim* ^{na4}da-x [...............] súd *ina* ka[š] nag
18	B	diš na *ana* kàš-*šú aš-ṭu-*⸢*ú-tì*⸣ x [*hi-ni*]*q-ti* bun gig numun ^{ú}úkuš.hab^{s}[^{ar} k]aš nag[1]
19	B	^{šim}šeš súd *ina* ì.giš hi.hi *ina* mud zabar *ana mùš-tin-ni-šú* mú ⸢^{ú}*nu-ṣa-ba*⸣ [*ina* k]ašbir (KAŠ.A.SÙ) nag
20	B	numun ^{giš}šinig súd *ina* kaš nag[2]
21	B	a gazi^{sar} a ^{giš}zú.lum.ma ì.giš bára.ga al.ús.sa buru$_{5}$.íd.da ú babbar súd *ina* ga nag
22	B	illu ^{šim}buluh ì bára.ga *tu-šab-šal ta-šá-hal ina* mud zabar *ana mùš-tin-ni-šú* mú[3]
23	B	ú babbar *ta-sàk ina* ì.giš hi.hi *ina* mud zabar *ana mùš-tin-ni-šú* mú[4]
24	B	^{im}sahar.na$_{4}$.kur.ra súd *ina* kaš nag : še.li![5] suhuš giš ^{ú}gír súd *ina* kaš nag
25	B	^{giš}nim *ta-sàk ina* kaš suhuš ^{giš}kiši$_{16}$ súd *ina* kaš : ga usduha(u$_{8}$.udu.hi.a) *ina* kaš hi.hi *la pa-tan* ud.3.kám nag.meš
26	B	^{ú}igi-*lim* an.zah.ge$_{6}$ šika nunuz ga.nu$_{11}$^{mušen} ^{šim}še.li súd *ina* geštin.šur nag al.ús.sa ku$_{6}$ *ina* a nu *pa-tan* nag
27	B	al.ús.sa buru$_{5}$ *ina* a ^{giš}nu.úr.ma nag 10 <gín> ì.giš a gazi^{sar} 10 gín ì.giš bára.ga 2/3 sìla kaš hi.hi 15 gín numun ^{ú}eme.ur.gi$_{7}$
28	B	*ina* ge$_{6}$ *ana* igi mul ud$_{5}$ gar-*an ina šèr-ti la-am* ^{d}utu.è *la-am* gìri-*šú ana* ki gar-*nu* nag
29	B	^{im}sahar.ge$_{6}$.kur.ra súd *ina* kaš nu *pa-tan* nag[6]
30	B	zì! ^{giš}nam.tar níta zì ^{giš}kiši$_{16}$.hab *ina* kaš nag : *im-hur-lim* súd *ina* kaš nag

1 Simplicium.
2 Simplicium.
3 Simplicium.
4 Simplicium.
5 text: šen.ša. The signs are likely to be a mistake for še.li = *kikkirânu*, which occurs in l. 26, and the /ša/-sign looks like the end of /li/.
6 Simplicium.

13 Seed of 'dog's tongue', [...]-plant, *tijātu*-plant, myrrh, *dadānu*-seed, *kasû*-seed,
14 tamarisk-seed, [........], 7 drugs for 'stricture of the [bladder]'.

15 *imhur-lim, nuṣābu, nīnû, pallišu*, 'dog's tongue', myrrh, shell of ostrich egg, 7 drugs [for 'stricture of the bladder'].

16 If a man suffers from 'stricture of the bladder', crush shell of ostrich egg and coral, he drinks it in oil (and) beer.

17 Crush *šaššūgu* .... [....], and he drinks it in beer.

18 If a man has *difficulty* with urine ... he suffers from stricture of the bladder, he drinks cucumber seed in beer.

19 Crush myrrh, mix it in oil, blow it through a bronze tube into his urethra, he drinks *nuṣābu* [in] thin beer.

20 Crush seed of tamarisk and he drinks it in beer.

21 Crush *kasû*-juice, date-tree juice, pressed oil, fish sauce, river locust and 'white' plant, and he drinks it in milk.

22 You boil and filter resin of *baluhhu*(-aromatic) and pressed oil, you blow it through a copper tube into his urethra.

23 You crush 'white'-plant and mix it in oil and blow it through a copper tube into his urethra.

24 Crush alum and drink it in beer. Crush *kikkirânu* and root of acacia, and he drinks it in beer.

25 Crush *baltu*-thorn, crush root of acacia in beer, mix (them) in beer (alternative: mix sheep and goat milk in beer), and he keeps drinking them on an empty stomach (for) three days.

26 Crush *imhur-lim*, black frit, shell of ostrich-egg, *kikkirânu*(-aromatic), he drinks it in drawn wine. He drinks fish-sauce in water on an empty stomach.
27 He drinks locust-sauce in pomegranate-juice. Mix 10 <shekels> oil (and) *kasû*-juice, 10 shekels of pressed oil, two-thirds *sila* of beer; put 15 shekels of seed of 'dog's tongue'
28 at night under the Goat-Star, and he drinks it in the morning before sunrise before he gets out of bed (lit. before he puts his foot on the ground).

29 Crush *qitmu*-dye in beer and he drinks it on an empty stomach.

30 He drinks flour of 'male' mandrake, and flour of *dadānu* in beer : (alternatively) crush *imhur lim* in beer and he drinks it.

31 B ^{giš}geštin.ka$_5$.a hád.du súd *ana* a kaš *u* ì.giš šub *ina* mul$_4$ *tuš-bat* nu *pa-tan* nag

---

32 B pa *a-a-ár* kù.babbar *ša* ^{ú}*nu-ṣa-bu* mu.ni súd *ina* kaš nag : illu ^{šim}buluh *ina* kaš hi.hi nu *pa-tan* nag[1]

---

33 B diš na *hi-niq* bun gig *ana* ti-*šú* ^{ú}igi-*lim* ^{ú}igi-*ešra* ^{ú}*tara-muš* numun ^{ú}*pu-qut-tú* ^{ú}*ár-zal-lu$_4$* ^{ú}*nu-ṣa-bu*
34 B ^{giš}lum.ha ^{šim}šeš illu ^{šim}buluh šika nunuz ga.nu$_{11}$^{mušen} 10 ú.hi.a šeš 1-*niš* súd *lu ina* geštin *lu ina* kaš nu *pa-tan* nag-*ma* ti

---

35 B diš na gig *hi-niq* bun gig *ana* ti-*šú* ^{ú}*tara-muš* ^{ú}igi-*lim* ^{ú}igi-*ešra* illu *ṣar-ba-te* ^{ú}kur.kur ^{ú}har.har
36 B ^{ú}*ṣi-bu-ra* ^{ú}kur.gi.rín.na ^{ú}hab ^{ú}*šá-mi*-giš.gi[2] ^{ú}sumun.dar ^{ú}*šá-ka-be-gal-zu* ^{ú}*ti-gi-lat* KUR-*i*
37 B ^{ú}*nu-ṣa-ba* ^{ú}lag.a.šà ^{giš}geštin.ka$_5$.a ^{ú}sikil ^{ú}*an-ki-nu-te* ^{ú}sig.meš *šá* kur-*i*
38 B ^{ú}dumu.mí.a.šà ^{ú}*el-kul-la* ^{ú}*eli-kul-la* numun ^{giš}šinig numun ^{ú}dili numun ^{ú}*šu-nim* su-huš ^{ú}ku$_6$
39 B numun ^{ú}*pu-qut-tú* numun ^{giš}esi ^{ú}*šib-bur-ra-tú* ^{šim}šeš ^{šim}gúr.gúr ⸢^{ú}⸣*ár-zal-la* ^{šim}g[am ..]
40 B numun ^{ú}eme.ur.gi$_7$ numun ^{ú}ki.^{d}iškur ^{ú}*šuq-da-na* ^{ú}*al-la-an* [numun$^?$] ⸢^{ú}*ha-zal-lu*⸣-[*na*]
41 B illu ^{šim}buluh buru$_5$.en.me.li a.šà.ga šika nunuz g[a.nu$_{11}$^{mušen} ....]
42 B téš.bi *ta-sàk lu ina* geštin.kala.ga [*ina* kaš nu *pa-tan* nag-*ma* ti]

---

43 B numun ^{ú}dili numun ^{giš}geštin.ka$_5$.a numun ^{giš}kiši$_{16}$.hab ⸢ú⸣[......................]
44 B ^{ú}hab ^{ú}kur.gi.rín.na ^{ú}*bu-uṭ-*⸢*nu*⸣ [......................]
45 B ^{im}sahar.babbar.kur.ra ^{šim}šeš il[lu ....x ú.hi.a *an-nu-ti*]
46 B *hi-niq-ti* bun *ma-al-m*[*a-liš* ....ti]

---

47 B (traces)

col. ii

1 B [^{ú}nu.luh.h]a naga.si [...................]

---

2 B [^{giš}]kiši$_{16}$.hab ^{ú}nu.luh.ha 3 ú.meš *hi-niq-ti u šim-m*[*a$^?$-ti* ....]

---

3 B [diš na *hi*]-*niq-ti* gig naga.si gú.níg.àr.ra *ina* kaš.s[ag nag-*ma* ti]

---

4 B [^{ú}i]gi-*lim* ^{ú}igi-*ešra* ^{ú}*tara-muš* numun ^{ú}eme.ur.gi$_7$ ^{ú}*pu-qut-tu* ka.ab.ba *kar-* x x
5 B [ní]g.na$_4$.gú.tur naga.si $^{\text{na4}}$*ga-bi-i* ^{šim}šeš šika nunuz ga.nu$_{11}$^{mušen} ^{ú}nu.luh.ha ^{giš}šin[ig]
6 B ^{ú}*nu-ṣa-bu* ^{ú}geštin.ka$_5$.a 17 ú.hi.a níg.lá sag.[ki][3]

---

[1] Simplicium.
[2] For this plant name, see CAD A/2 199, citing Uruanna II 327.
[3] KADP 36 vi 25 [ref. courtesy M.Stol], and see Text No. 19, reading *naṣmattu* (as CAD N/2), and not *ṣimdu*, as Goltz, *Heilkunde* 328.

31 Dry out and crush fox-vine and put it into water, beer, or oil, leave it out over night and he drinks it on an empty stomach.

---

32 Crush the leaf of 'silver-rosette', (and that) which is called *nuṣābu*, he drinks it in beer : (alternatively) mix resin of *baluhhu* in beer, and he drinks it on an empty stomach.

---

33 If a man suffers from 'stricture of the bladder', to cure him, (plants:) *imhur-lim, imhur-ešra, taramuš,* seed of *puquttu, arzallu, nuṣābu,*
34 *barīrātu*, myrrh, resin of *baluhhu*(-aromatic), shell of ostrich-egg; crush together these 10 drugs, either in wine or in beer, he drinks it on an empty stomach, and he will recover.

---

35 If a man suffers from 'stricture of the bladder', to cure him: crush together *taramuš, imhur-lim, imhur-ešra,* resin of Euphrates poplar, *ata'išu, hašû,*
36 *ṣibaru, kurkānû,* madder, *šami-api, šumuttu, šagabigalzu,* mountain cucumber,
37 *nuṣābu*, 'clod of the field'(-plant), fox-vine, 'pure'-plant, *ankinutu*-plant,[1] 'thin-ones of the mountain'-plant.
38 Crush together 'daughter of the field'-plant, *elkulla, elikulla,* seed of tamarisk, seed of the 'single' plant, seed of *šunim*?, root of *šimru* / *urânu*[2]
39 seed of *puquttu*, seed of *ušû*-wood, rue, myrrh, *kukru*(-aromatic), *arzallu*, .[...]
40 seed of 'dog's tongue', seed of *qudru*-plant, *šiqdu*-plant, *allanu*, [seed? of] *hazallūnu*,
41 *baluhhu*-resin, praying mantis, shell of ostrich-egg, [...............].
42 [He drinks it] either in strong wine [or in beer on an empty stomach, and he will improve].

---

43 Seed of 'single'-plant, seed of fox-vine, seed of *dadānu*, [......]
44 madder, *kurkanû*, pistachio, [..............................]
45 *alluharu*(-mineral), myrrh, resin [of ....these x drugs for],
46 stricture of the bladder, equally [................, and he will recover].

---

col. ii

1 *nuhurtu*, horned alkali, [....................................].

---

2 *dadānu, nuhurtu,* 3 drugs for 'stricture' and *paralysis* [..........].

---

3 [If a man] suffers from 'stricture' , [he drinks] horned alkali and legumes in premium beer [and he will recover].

---

4 *imhur-lim, imhur-ešra, taramuš,* seed of 'dog's tongue', *puquttu,* coral, ...
5 pea-pod(?), horned alkali, alum, myrrh, shell of ostrich-egg, *nuhurtu,* tamarisk,
6 *nuṣābu*, fox-vine: 17 drugs for the binding of the head.

---

[1] lit.'plant 'not approaching heaven and earth,' see CAD A/2 124.
[2] See CAD Š/3 8–9, both readings are possible for this logogram.

7 B [^{š}]^{im}šeš ^{ú}*nu-ṣa-bu* šika nunuz ga.nu$_{11}$^{mušen} *pu-qut-tú* ^{ú}har.har ^{ú}*úr-nu-u* ^{ú}kur.kur ú babbar ⸢ú⸣[x]
MM ^{ú}har.har ^{ú}*úr-nu-u* ^{ú}kur.kur ^{ú}*ti-ia-tú*[1] *sah-lé-e*
8 B [n]umun ^{ú}si.sá ^{ú}*zi-bu-u* ^{ú}*šu-un-'u* gazi^{sar} ^{ú}*an-nu-ha-ra* 14. ú.meš *hi-níq-ti lu ina* geštin *lu ina* kaš n[ag-*ma* ti]
MM numun ^{ú}si.sá ^{ú}*zi-bu-u* gazi^{sar} $^{\text{na4.im}}$sahar.na$_4$.kur.ra ^{ú}*šu-un-hu-'u*

---

9 B [^{š}]^{im}šeš ^{ú}*nu-ṣa-bu* šika nunuz ga.nu$_{11}$^{mušen} ^{giš}kiši$_{16}$.hab ^{ú}igi-*lim* ^{ú}igi-*ešra* [....]
10 B [7] ⸢ú⸣.hi.a *hi-niq-ti lu ina* kaš *lu ina* gešti[n nag-*ma* ti]

---

11 B ⸢ú⸣igi-[*lim*] ⸢ú⸣igi-*ešra* ^{ú}*tara-muš* ^{šim}šeš $^{\text{na4}}$*ga-bi-i* ^{giš}hab numun ^{ú}eme.ur.gi$_7$ ^{giš}[......]
12 B ⸢ú⸣níg.bùr.bùr[2] ⸢ú⸣níg.sì.sì⸣^{sar} ^{ú}*nu-ṣa-bu* šika nunuz ga.nu$_{11}$^{mušen} peš$_4$.anše 14 [ú.hi.a *hi-niq-ti*]

---

13 B ^{ú}*pu-qut-tú* ^{ú}*nu-ṣa-bu* $^{\text{na4}}$*ga-bi-i* ^{ú}*tara-muš* ^{ú}igi-*lim* ⸢ú⸣[igi-*ešra* ... ^{ú}*nu-ṣa-bu*]
14 B [š]ika nunuz ga.nu$_{11}$^{mušen} 9 ú.hi.a *hi-ni*[*q-ti* ...]

---

15 B [^{š}]^{im}li ^{ú}nu.luh.ha *ṭe-ri-tú* ^{šim}šeš ^{ú}*pu-qut-tu$_4$* níg [....................................]

---

16 B én ìr gìri.ma hi-hi *aš-ni-ma ma-al-ma-al* : suhuš-*su ṣa-ri-*[*ih* ....]
17 B *šu-ul-mu* silim *er-bi*[3] silim *er-bi* dug$_8$.a[4] [........................]

---

18 B ka.inim.ma [................]

---

19 B dù.dù.bi ^{ú}igi-*lim* ^{šim}šeš šika nunuz ga.nu$_{11}$^{mušen} an.záh.ge$_6$ 1-*niš* s[úd ....]
G ^{ú}igi-*lim* ^{šim}šeš šika nunuz gá.nu$_{11}$^{mušen} $^{\text{na4}}$an.zah.ge$_6$ diš-*niš* súd *ina* 3 *u$_4$-me ina šiqqi*
20 B 3 *u$_4$-mi ina* geštin.šur.ra 3 *u$_4$-mi ina* a ^{giš}nu.úr.ma nag.meš-*ma* t[i]
G 2 *u$_4$-me ina* geštin.šur.ra 3 *u$_4$-me ina* a.meš $^{\text{[gi]š}}$*nu-ur-m*[*i*]-*i* nag.meš-*ma*

---

21 B diš ki.min ^{šim}li ^{šim}šeš ^{ú}nu.luh.ha ^{giš}kiši$_{16}$.hab [..........]

---

22 B diš na murub$_4$.meš-*šú lu ina* gen-*šú lu ina* ki.ná-*šú* tag.ga.meš-*šú* g[ìš-*šú* ....]
23 B [t]áb.táb-*su ú-ha-ma-at-su i-tar-rak-šú* egir kàš.meš-*šú iš-t*[*i-nu* ....]
24 B [*ana* t]i-*šú* ^{ú}*ha-bi-in* numun ^{ú}dili ^{giš}geštin.ka$_5$.a ⸢geštin.šur⸣.[ra ....]
25 B ⸢ú⸣[*nu-ṣ*]*a-bu* ^{ú}kur.kur ú babbar ^{ú}hab [...]
26 B ^{n}[$^{\text{a4}}$pe]š$_4$.anše $^{\text{na4}}$p[eš$_4$...]
27 B *u* [.................h]a a [..]
28 B *ina* [..

---

[1] The correspondence might indicate that *tiātu* is used to translate ^{ú}babbar. See AHw 1357, giving the logogram for *tījātu* (from Ugarit) as ù.luh^{sar}.

[2] Although usually a stone name, *pallišu* is also a plant name in text No. 5: 13 below (see duplicates). The same difficulty arises with the following drug, since *sāpinu* is usually a stone name (na$_4$.sì.sì), but may be listed here as a plant.

[3] See above, l. 9–10, where the incantation has been rendered as di.ir.bi (mumbo-jumbo), but in this case the word *šulmu* may suggest a gloss or interpretation of an otherwise meaningless phrase. We have left both versions as possible interpretations of this incantation.

[4] See above, l. 10, ka.dug$_8$.a, 'open-mouthed'.

7 Myrrh, *nuṣābu*, shell of ostrich-egg, *puquttu*, *hašû*, *urnû*, *kurkānû*, 'white'-plant, [...]
8 seed of *šurdunû*, black cumin, *šun'u*, *kasû*, and *annuhara*: 14 drugs for 'stricture', [he drinks them] either in wine or in beer [and he will improve].

---

9 Myrrh, *nuṣābu*, shell of ostrich-egg, *dadānu*, *imhur-lim*, *imhur-ešra*, [........]
10 [7] drugs for 'stricture', [he drinks them] either in beer or wine [and he will recover].

---

11 *imhur*-[*lim*], *imhur-ešra*, *tara-muš*, myrrh, alum, madder, seed of 'dog's tongue', ..[...]
12 *pallišu*-plant, *sāpinu*[?], *nuṣābu*, shell of ostrich-egg, and 'donkey-vulva'(-shell); 14 [drugs for stricture].

---

13 *puquttu*, *nuṣābu*, alum, *taramuš*, *imhur-lim*, [*imhur-ešra* ..., *nuṣābu*]
14 shell of ostrich-egg, 9 drugs for 'stricture' [...].

---

15 Juniper, beaten[?] *nuhurtu*, myrrh, *puquttu*, ..[....].

---

16 Incantation. Mix .... I repeated each one: its 'root' is hot ...[.....
17 come in, well-being! come in, well-being! ... [.....................]

---

18 Incantation [for ....]

---

19 Its ritual: pound together *imhur-lim*, myrrh, shell of ostrich-egg, and black frit, he keeps drinking them in three days in (fish) brine,
20 (and) for 3 (var. 2) days in drawn-wine and for 3 days in pomegranate juice, and he will improve.

---

21 If ditto: juniper, myrhh, *nuhurtu*, *dadānu*, [..........]

---

22 If a man's hips (groin) afflict him either when he walks or lies down, [his] penis [................]
23 stings him, burns him, and throbs;[1] after he urinates, he passes [blood ....]
24 [To cure] him: *hahin*-plant, seed of 'single'-plant, fox-vine, drawn-wine, [..................],
25 *nuṣābu*, *ata'išu*, 'white'-plant, madder, [................]
26 donkey-vulva(-shell), ... [............]
27 ff......

---

[1] lit. hits him.

No. 2a additional fragments which may belong to K 2405+

B_1	=	K 7230 [text no. 2a](AMT 61,1)
A	=	CBS 19801 [text No. 1] (BAM 396 iv 6–12) = ll. 5′–8′

1′	B_1	(traces)
2′	B_1	[diš na....................] x dab.meš-*ta*[1] *i-na-a* [............................]
3′	B_1	[.............. *a*]*na* ti-*šú* mud zabar *ana* gìš-[*šú* mú-*ah* ....]
4′	B_1	[..................] *ana* gìš-*šú* mú-*ah-ma* ⸢*i*?⸣-[*ne-eš*]
5′	B_1	[diš na *i-n*]*a-a*[2] *ina* gin-*šú re-hu-su* gin-*ma* nu zu gim *šá ana* munus gin-*m*[*a*.....]
	A	[d]iš na *i-na-a-ma ina* gin-*šu re-hu-us-su* gin-*ma* nu zu [... *š*]*a* gal$_4$.la-*šu* gin-*ma ma-as-ra-ah*[3]
6′	B_1	[....... ù.b]ú.bú.ul *šiq-ta* diri ^{im}sahar.na$_4$.kur.ra naga.si súd *ina* ì?.g[iš? ..]
	A	gìš-*šu* ù.bu.bu.ul *ma-li* ^{im}sahar.na$_4$.kur.ra naga.si *ina* ì.giš hi.hi
7′	B_1	[.. du]b *ina* ì *hal-ṣi u* kaš.sag nu *pa-tan* na[g ...]
	A	*ina* mud zabar *ana*(šè) *mùš-tin-ni-šu* dub *ù ina* ì.giš *ù* kaš hi.hi nag-*ma i-ne-eš*
8′	B_1	[*ina* a giš.še.n]á.a ra-*su-ma* [.........]
9′	B_1	[diš na *ina* gen-*šú r*]*e-hu-su* gen-*ma* nu zu *ka-la ú-ri-šú* [................................]
10′	B_1	[ù.b]ú.bú.ul tur.meš diri ^{im}sahar.na$_4$.kur.ra naga.[si súd ....]
11′	B_1	[*ina* mud zaba]r *ana muš-tin-ni-šú* dub *ina* ì *u* kaš hi.hi nag-*ma* geštin.ka$_5$.[a ....]
12′	B_1	[diš na *iš-tu*] gìš-*šú* múd lugud è.meš-*šú* gim *ṣi-bit* ur.bar.ra *lu* x [....................]
13′	B_1	[........] šéš *rib-ki ina* a gazi^{sar} kúm šid *ina* [.......... nag ....]
14′	B_1	[diš na ...... *t*]*as-li-a-te-šú*[4] tag.ga-*šú*[5] kàš.meš-*šú* dab.meš-*t*[*a* ....]
15′	B_1	[......... egi]r? kaš *u* ga šeg$_6$-*šal iš-tu e-la-an ú-r*[*i-šú* ....]
16′	B_1	[..............] x lál ^{šim}šeš súd *ina* kaš *u* [ga hi.hi ....]
17′	B_1	[..............] x x *kal* 7 ud.me nag-*m*[*a* ....]
18′	B_1	[..] x *šá* x [..................]

[1] Read *ṣubbuta*, see AMT 48,1 10 + 78,3:7, dib.dib-*at*, and TDP 138 ii 70.

[2] see CAD N/2 133 'to have a urinary or bowel disease'

[3] see text No. 3 (BAM 111) ii 23.

[4] see AHw 1337, s. v. *taslītu*, 'abwertende Rede', but the noun is likely to be related to *salā'u* (to be ill).

[5] CAD L 89 restores [*iškāšu*] ... tag.ga-*šú*, 'his testicles hurt him'.

TRANSLATION

2′ [If a man's ....] are affected (and) *he has a urinary complaint* [.....................]
3′ [.... in] order to cure him: [blow ......] through a bronze tube into [his] penis,
4′ blow [...] into his penis, and he [will get better].

5′ If a man *has a urinary complaint* (and) ejaculates while 'going' but he does not know it and when he has sex with a woman, the semen duct of
6′ his penis is full of pustules (and) scales, crush alum and horned alkali and mix it in oil,
7′ pour it via a copper tube into his urethra and (var. mix it and) he drinks (it) in pressed oil or premium beer on an empty stomach and he will get better.
8′ Bathe him [in sap] of *šunû*(-wood), and [he will get better].

9′ [If a man while 'going'] ejaculates but does not know it, and his whole pubic region [......................]
10′ is filled with small pustules, [crush] alum and horned alkali [............................]
11′ and pour it [via a copper tube] into his urethra. Mix it in oil or beer and he drinks it and [...........] fox-vine.

12′ [If from a man's] penis blood and pus are discharged, like the attack of a wolf or [......],
13′ anoint (it) [in oil], knead the decoction into hot *kasû*(-beet) juice (and) [he drinks it] in [.......].

14′ [If a man's ... and] his ... is affected, his urine is affected, ..[....],
15′ [......] *afterwards* heat up beer or milk, and from the upper part of his pubic region [...]
16′ bind on [....], crush myrrh, [mix it] in beer or [milk ...][1]
17′ he drinks it [................].. each of 7 days [and he will recover].

18′ (traces)

[1] Simplicium, see also No. 3 ii 6–9.

B$_2$ = **K 13403 (AMT 40,3)**, cf. Thompson, RA 26, 85 (plate 3)

1′ (Traces)

2′ [..............] ud.3.kám [............

3′ [.........] *ina* kaš nu *pa-tan* [nag ......

4′ [...............] súd *ina* kaš.sag [............

5′ [..........] x na dir illu *a-bu-ka-*[*tu* ....
6′ [......... n]u *pa-tan* n[ag ....]

7′ [.............zi-*a*]*h* nu igi.du$_8$ nu *pa-tan* n[ag.........[1]

8′ [......... nu ig]i.du$_8$ *ina* mul$_4$ *tuš-bat* nu *pa-tan* [nag ....

9′ [diš na.....mú.m]ú-*ma* šà-*šú ṣa-bit-m*[*a* ....
10′ [........] x *ina* mud zab[ar ....
11′ [........h]i.hi ì.giš šeg$_6$-*šal* [.................
12′ [..........-*m*]*a ina* x [.....................

13′ (traces)

B$_3$ = **K 16453** (AMT 70,6) (plate 3)

1′ [.................] x *iš-tu* im [........................

2′ [.............] a súd *ina* ì.giš r[a$^?$ ....

3′ [..........].ga *ina* mud zabar [.........

4′ [........ -*t*]*u$_4$* súd *ina* ka[š ....

B$_4$ = **S 467** (AMT 58,5) (plate 3)

1′ x [....................................

2′ diš *en* mu [...............................

3′ diš na sa tùm[2] [.....................
4′ *ina mar-ha-ṣi* x [................
5′ kàš.meš-*šú lu šá* [.................

6′ diš na *ina* kàš.meš-*šú* m[úd *ú-tab-ba-kam* ......
7′ *ina* a.meš gazi^{sar} ra [.......
8′ mud zabar *ana* k[a gìš-*šú* dub-*ak* .....

9′ diš na *kis* šà-*šú* sìg-[*su* ....
10′ *iš-ta-an* lú x [.........

11′ ⸢diš na *lu* x⸣ [..................

[1] Cf. Text No. 1 iii 7.
[2] coll.

TRANSLATION (B_2)

2′ [.............] on the 3rd day [..................

3′ [.............he drinks it] in beer on an empty stomach

4′ Crush [...............] in premium beer [................

5′ [.................].... *abukkatu*-resin [...........
6′ [....... he drinks it] in [....] on an empty stomach [..............

7′ [...........] extracted (while) not exposed (to the sun, i.e., before sunrise), he drinks (it) on an empty stomach [.........

8′ [............ before] sunrise, you leave it out over night [and he drinks it] on an empty stomach [......

9′ [If a man's ...] is swollen and his innards are affected and [..
10′ [......, blow it] through a bronze tube [into the opening of his penis ....
11′ mix [..........] heat (it) in oil [..
12′ [...............] in [...

(broken)

TRANSLATION (B_4)

1′–2′ broken

3′ If a man [suffers from] .... [............
4′ you [.....] in a lotion ..[.........................
5′ His urine is either of [..........................

6′ If a man [passes] blood in his urine [........
7′ bathe him in *kasû*-juice [................
8′ blow [.....] (through) a bronze tube into the opening [of his penis....]

9′ If a man's belly has been struck by colic (i.e., *kīs libbi*-disease) [..............
10′ the patient urinates, [...

11′ If a man either ...[................................

(broken)

B_5 = **K 5864 (AMT 58,6)** (plate 3)
restored after text No. 4 17′–27′, and see below for the complete *Partitur*

1′ [$^{\check{s}im}$]li 2 gín ú babbar *ina* kaš.lú.tin.n[a] x x x [..........................

2′ [diš.na gì]š-*šú* gír.gír-*su* u_4*-ma* kàš.meš-*šú i-šá-ti-nu re-*[*hu-su* šub-*a ina* šà-*šú ṣa-bit-ma*]
3′ [*ana* munus gin-*ka* lá lugud g]*i-na-a ina* gìš-*šú* gin na.bi *mu-ṣa* gig *ana* ti-*šú* [^{ú}babbar *ina* ì.giš]
4′ [mud urudu *ana* gìš-*šú ina* ka-*ka*] mú-*ah-ma* ^{giš}geštin.ka_5.⌜a⌝ súd *ina* kaš.lú$^!$.t[in.na nag-*ma*]
5′ [kaš *u* ì.giš $šeg_6$-*šal* šub.šub-*šú* ^{šim}]]i ^{šim}gúr.gúr pa $^{giš}gi_6$.pàr diš-*niš* súd *ina* ì.udu h[i.hi sag gìš-*šú* lá-*ma* ti]

6′ [ki.min$^?$ numun ^{ú}*pu-qut-te* súd *ina* ì.giš *ina* m]ud zabar *ana* šà gìš-*šú ina* ka-*ka* m[ú-*ah* ^{ú}eme.ur.gir_7 súd *ina* kaš nag]
7′ [*ina* a *u* ì.giš šub.šub-*šú* ^{šim}li ^{šim}gúr.gú]r ^{šim}gam.ma pa ^{giš}*bi-ni* pa ^{giš}⌜*šu*⌝-[*še* diš-*niš* súd *ina* ì.udu hi.hi min]

8′ [ki.min u_5.gar.ib^{mušen} súd *ina* ì.giš *ina* mud zabar *ana* š]à ⌜gìš⌝-*šú ina* ka-*ka* mú-*a*[*h-ma* ^{ú}babbar súd *ina* ì.giš nag *ina* a gazi^{sar}]
9′ [*sek-ru-ti* ra-*su* .....^{ú}kur.kur ^{š}]^{im}hab pa ^{giš}g[i zú.lum.ma zú.lum.ma diš-*niš* súd *ina* ì.udu hi.hi]

TRANSLATION

1′ Juniper, 2 shekels of 'white'-plant, in tavern-beer ... [............

2′ [If a man's] penis stings him when he passes urine (or) ejaculates, [he is affected in his innards and]

3′ [is 'diminished' (i. e., cannot get erect) when he has sex with a woman, pus] flows constantly from his penis, that man suffers from 'discharge'. To cure him:

4′ you blow ['white'-plant in oil with your mouth in a copper tube into his penis] and you crush fox-[vine], and give it to him to drink in tavern-beer.

5′ [You heat the beer and oil and keep applying them to him], you crush together juniper, ***kukru***, leaf of *lipāru*-wood, mix them in fat [and bind them on his corona, and he will recover].

6′ [Ditto?: you crush seed of *puquttu*-plant, (mix) it in oil, and you blow it with your mouth into the shank of his penis [via] a copper tube. [You crush 'dog's-tongue', he drinks it in beer],

7′ [keep applying it in water and oil. Crush together juniper], ***kukru***, ***ṣumlalu***, leaf of tamarisk, and leaf of *šūšu*-wood, [mix them in fat, ditto (= and he will recover)].

8′ [Ditto. Crush bat guano in oil], you blow (it) with your mouth [into] the shank of his penis [via a copper tube],

9′ [and you crush 'white'-plant, he drinks it in oil, [bathe him in heated *kasû*-juice]. You crush together [...., *ata'išu*], *ṭurû*, leaf of ***kūru*** [(and) dates and mix it in fat].

No. 3 = BAM 111

C	=	VAT 9871 + 10397 (BAM 111) (collated)
XX	=	A 198 (BAM 159) i 15–20; ii 15′–20′
A	=	CBS 19801 (BAM 396) [= text no. 1] = ii 5 ff., 15′–16′; iii 8′–18′
B_5	=	K 5864 (AMT 58,6) [see text no. 2] = i 16′–20′
Q	=	K 11230 + 11280 + 16437 + S 126 (AMT 66, 11 +) [text no. 16] = iii 8′–14′
D	=	VAT 9870 + 10095 (BAM 112, 17′–21′ = bottom of col. i) [text no. 4] = i 16′–20′

NB: According to F. Köcher, BAM I xxiv (note to BAM 111), K 7230 [text no. 2a](Ms. B_1) duplicates ii 23′–26′, but the texts are not close enough to be considered parallels.

col. i

1′	C	[..] x
2′	C	[......................................] x kàš.meš-*šú*
3′	C	[...................................... *ina* kà]š.meš-*šú* múd.meš
4′	C	[..................................] x *ana* ti-*šú*
5′	C	[..................................] x -*tu* ì *hal-ṣa*
6′	C	[..................................] gìš-*šú* dub-*ma* *ina-eš*
7′	C	[........................] gazi^{sar} *ina* ì.nun.⸢na⸣ eš.meš-*su* *ina-eš*
8′	C	[......................*t*]*ur-ár* šà gìš-*šú* diri
9′	C	[........................] x ì *ina* dílim.a.bár súd *te-qí-šú*
10′	C	[...........................]-*e* ki.min
11′	C	[...................................š]à? gìš-*šú* diri ki.min
12′	C	[.............................s]úd šéš-*su*
13′	C	[......................................] x súd ki.min
14′	C	[....................................] *ina* a gazi^{sar}
15′	C	[.............................sag gìš-*š*]*ú* lá (see l. 20′ below)
16′	D	[diš n]a gìš-*šú* *ú-zaq-qa-su* u_4-*ma* kàš.meš-*šú* *i-šá-ti-nu* *re-hu-su* šub-*a*[1]
	B_5	[..........gì]š-*šú* gír.gír-*su* u_4-*ma* kàš.meš-*šú* *i-šá-ti-nu* *re*-[.................]
	C	[.........................gí]r.gír-*su* u_4-*ma* kàš-*šú* [..]
17′	D	[*ina*] šà-*šú* *ṣa-bit-ma* *ana* munus gin-*ka* lá[2] lugud *gi-na-a* *ina* gìš-*šú* gen-*ak* [na.b]i *mu-ṣa* gig *ana* ti-*šú*
	B_5	[.. *g*]*i-na-a* *ina* gìš-*šú* gen na.bi *mu-ṣa* gig *ana* ti-*šú*
	C	(traces)
18′	D	ú babbar *ina* ì.giš *ina* mud urudu *ana* gìš-*šú* *ina* ka-*ka* mú[3]-*ma*
	B_5	[..] mú-*ah-ma*
19′	D	[^{giš}gešt]in.ka$_5$.a súd *ina* kaš.lú!.tin.na nag-*ma* kaš *u* ì.giš šeg$_6$-*šal* šub.šub-*šú*
	B_5	^{giš}geštin.ka$_5$.a súd *ina* kaš.lú.t[in.na ....]
20′	D	[^{ú}*tara*]-*muš$_8$* ^{šim}gúr.gúr pa ^{giš}gi$_6$.pàr!(text: na$_4$) diš-*niš* súd *ina* ì.udu hi.hi sag[4] gìš-*šú* lá-*ma* ti
	B_5	[^{šim}l]i ^{šim}gúr.gúr pa ^{giš}gi$_6$.pàr diš-*niš* súd *ina* ì.udu h[i.hi ....]

1 See text No. 48. 7′ (YBC 7123+), for a possible parallel.

2 *muṭṭu* < *maṭû*

3 coll.

4 coll.

TRANSLATION

1′ [...................................]

2′ [If a man ....] his urine,
3′ [..............................] haemorrhage [in] his urine,
4′ [.............he suffers from ....-disease], to cure him:
5′ [.............................]..., and pressed oil,
6′ pour it [through a bronze/copper tube into] his penis, and he will get better.

7′ [Ditto ....], rub him with *kasû*-[juice] in ghee and he will get better.
8′ You dry out [..............] and soften the shank of his penis,
9′ [.................] you crush [....] in oil and daub him with a salve.
10′ [.............................].. ditto.

11′ [............................] soften the shank of his penis, ditto.
12′ Crush [.............................] and anoint him.
13′ Crush .. [......................], ditto.
14′ [.............................] in *kasû*-juice,
15′ bandage [............................ on] his corona.

16′ [If a man's] penis constantly stings him when he passes urine(or) ejaculates,
17′ he is affected [in] his innards and is 'diminished' (i. e. cannot get erect) when he has sex with a woman, and pus flows continually from his penis, that man suffers from 'discharge'. To cure him
18′ you blow 'white'-plant in oil with your mouth via a copper tube into his penis.
19′ You crush fox-vine, and he drinks it in tavern-beer and you heat the beer and oil, you keep applying them to him,
20′ you crush together *taramuš* (var. juniper), *kukru*, leaf of *lipāru*, mix them in fat, bind them on his corona, and he will recover.

col. ii

1′	C	[..] ⌜nag⌝-*šú-ma*
2′	C	[..............................] x x ⌜šeg$_6$⌝-*š*[*al*] igi.4.gál.⌜la⌝
3′	C	[š]im x [..........] igi.4.gál.la numun ^{ú}eme.ur.gi$_7$ súd
4′	C	[..] x kaš *u* ì *hal-ṣi* gaz *ina* mul$_4$ *tuš-bat*
5′	C	[n]u *pa-tan 7 u$_4$-me* nag.meš-*ma* ti

6′	C	[diš ki].min ^{šim}šeš súd *ana* kašbir kaš.lú.tin.na
7′	C	[šu]b-*ma ina* mul$_4$ *tuš-bat* nu *pa-tan 7 u$_4$-me* nag.meš
8′	C	[gi]m *si-li-'-šu il-tap-tu-šú* ^{šim}še.li babbar
9′	C	$^{[š]im}$li súd *ina* kaš nag-*ma* ti

10′	C	diš ki.min 15 še ^{na4}an.zah.ge$_6$ igi.4.gál.la ^{šim}⌜li⌝
11′	C	diš-*niš* súd *ina* kaš.sag nag.meš-*ma* ti

12′	C	diš ki.min ì.giš sag ì.giš bára.ga téš.bi hi.hi
13′	C	^{ú}eme.ur.gi$_7$ súd *ana* šà šub *ina* mul$_4$ *tuš-bat*
14′	C	*ina še-rim* nu *pa-tan* nag-*ma* ti

15′	C	diš ⌜na⌝ *ša-a-ši-ta-na un-nu-un-ta*
	XX	diš na *ša-a-ši-tu-na un-nu*-⌜*ut*⌝
	A	diš na *ša-a-ši-tu-nam un-nu-ut*
16′	C	*u ma-gal* zi.zi-*bi* ^{uzu}bun-*šu he-sa-at*
	XX	*u ma-gal* zi.meš b[ú]n-*šú he-sa-at*
	A	*ù ma-gal* zi.zi-*bi*
17′	C	na.bi ud.da kur-*id ana* ti-*šú* ^{ú}eme.ur gi$_7$
	XX	na.bi ud.da sá.sá *ana* ti-*šú* numun ^{ú}eme.ur.gi$_7$
18′	C	numun *bi-ni* numun *pu-qut-te* ^{šim}šeš illu ^{šim}buluh
	XX	numun ^{giš}*bi-ni* numun ^{ú}gír.hab šim.hi.a ^{šim}šeš
19′	C	diš-*niš* súd *lu ina* geštin *lu ina* ga *lu ina* kaš.sag
	XX	diš-*niš* súd *lu ina* geštin *lu ina* ga *lu ina* kaš.sag
20′	C	*la ú-sa-dir ina* ud.3.kám ud.1.kám nag.meš
	XX	nu *ú-sa-dir ina* ud.3.kám ud.1.kám nag

21′	C	diš na kàš.meš-*šú ut-ta-na-tak ka-la-a*
22′	C	*la i-la-a'* ^{uzu}bun-*šu he-sa-at*
23′	C	im diri-*ma ma-as-la-ah* kàš.meš-*šú*
24′	C	*i-bi-ta* diri *ana* ti-*šú* ^{ú}*pu-qut-tu* súd
25′	C	*ina* ì.giš *hal-ṣi* gaz *ina* mud zabar *ana* šà gìš-*šú*
26′	C	dub-*aq ina* a gazi^{sar} ^{giš}*šu-nim* ra-*su*
27′	C	*ina kim-ṣi-šu-ma su-ur-ta* šub-*di*
28′	C	lál-*su-ma* 3 *u$_4$-me* nu du$_8$ *ana* murub$_4$.meš-*šú*
29′	C	dub-*šu*[1] *ki-ma si-li-'-šu il-tap-tu-šú*
30′	C	^{šim}gúr.gúr ^{šim}li ^{šim}še.li babbar

[1] Reading *tasarraq* rather than *tašappak*, since the latter term usually indicates an invasive procedure through which drugs are introduced into the urethra via a tube; see CAD Š/1 417f.

col. ii

1′ He drinks it and [............................],
2′ heat up [..................................] crush one fourth of
3′ [...]-aromatic, ... [............] and a fourth of the seed of 'dog's tongue',
4′ pound [...........into] beer and pressed oil, and you set it out over night,
5′ he keeps drinking it for 7 days on an empty stomach, and he will recover.

6′ [If ditto], crush myrrh, put it into thin beer and tavern-beer,
7′ and leave it out over night; he keeps drinking them in 7 days on an empty stomach.[1]
8′ When (it is the case that) *sili'šu* (bladder disease) has affected the patient, crush white *kikkirânu*
9′ and juniper, he drinks it in beer and he will recover.

10′ If ditto, crush together 15 grains (*še*) of black frit, a quarter of juniper,
11′ he keeps drinking it in premium beer and he will recover.

12′ If ditto, mix together premium oil and pressed-oil,
13′ crush 'dog's tongue', and apply it to the shank (of his penis), you keep it out over night,
14′ he drinks it in the morning on an empty stomach, and he will recover.

15′ If a man is laid low by *šāšituna*-disease,
16′ and always getting up (at night),[2] and his bladder is swollen,
17′ that man is overcome by 'sun-fever'. In order to cure him, crush together 'dog's tongue',
18′ tamarisk seed, *puquttu* seed, myrrh, *balukkatu*-resin,
19′ either in wine or in milk or in premium beer;
20′ he must not delay, but over 3 days he drinks it daily.

21′ If a man constantly dribbles his urine and he is not able to hold it back,
22′ his bladder is swollen,
23′ and he is full of wind, his urethra[3]
24′ is full of blisters; in order to cure him, crush *puquttu*,
25′ pound it in pressed oil, and pour it into his penis through a bronze tube.
26′ Bathe him in the juice of *kasû* and *šunû*,
27′ put a *tourniquet*[4] on his shin
28′ bind it and do not remove it for 3 days,
29′ (and) spread (the *materia medica*) onto his groin. When (it is the case that) *sili'šu* (bladder disease) has affected him,
30′ crush together (l. 32) these 8 plants: *kukru*, juniper, white *kikkirânu*,

---

[1] simplicium
[2] or has an erection?
[3] not 'semen duct', as CAD M/1 325.
[4] See CAD S 415, 'circle'.

31′	C	numun ú dili ^{šim}šeš ^{ú}eme.ur.gi$_7$ numun *pu-qut-te*
32′	C	^{ú}*a-ši-i* 8 ú.hi.a šeš diš-*niš* súd *ina* kaš nag.meš
33′	C	[.....] x ^{ú}*ha-lu-la-ia* ^{šim}gúr.gúr
34′	C	[................ ^{šim}]šeš illu ^{šim}buluh
		(rest broken)

rev. col. iii

1′	C	(traces)
2′	C	[.......................]-*hu* ú.hi.a šeš
3′	C	[.......................] ⌜téš⌝.bi hi.hi *ina* geštin šeg$_6$-*šal*
4′	C	[.......................*h*]*a*-⌜*lu*⌝ *pa-tan* nag-*ma* ti

---

5′	C	[.....................^{ú}nu.lu]h.ha uzu ùz
6′	C	[.................... e]gir-*nu* muš ge$_6$
7′	C	[.....................]x ti

8′	C	[............. *ana* t]i-šú ^{šim}šeš
	A	ki 2: ^{šim}šeš
	Q	[...... g]ig *ana* ti-*šú*
9′	C	[.. n]umun ^{ú}eme.ur.gi$_7$
	A	$^{\text{na4.ú}}$níg.bùr.bùr ^{ú}*a-ar*-kù.babbar numun ^{ú}eme.ur.gi$_7$
	Q	^{šim}šeš ^{šim}buluh [n]umun ^{ú}eme.ur.gi$_7$
10′	C	[...................................... p]eš$_4$.anše šika nunuz gá.nu$_{11}$^{mušen}
	A	numun ^{ú}gír-*uh-ha-*[*ah*] $^{\text{na4}}$peš$_4$.anše šika nunuz gá.nu$_{11}$^{mušen}
	Q	numun ^{ú}gír.hab [.............................. nun]uz ⌜ga⌝.nu$_{11}$^{mušen}
11′	C	[..] kaš nu *pa-tan* nag-*ma*
	A	ú.hi.a *an-nu-ti* téš.bi *ta-sàk ina* kaš.sag *ba-lu pa-tan* nag-*ma*
	Q	téš.bi gaz sim [.......................] x x
12′	C	[........... zaba]r *ana* gìš-*šú* mú-*ah*
	A	*ina* mud zabar *ana*(šè) *mùš-tin-ni-su* mú-[*ah*]
	Q	*ina* mud zabar *ana* gìš-*šú* mú
13′	C	[.......................................] e$_{11}$-*šú* sahar munu$_4$
	Q	[... sah]ar munu$_4$
	A	*ina* a kúm *ir-ta-na-haṣ*
14′	C	[.......................................] *ina-eš*
	A	*ù i-ra-am tu-ba-har-ma i-*[*ne-eš*]
	Q	*ki-šú-ma* ti [............................

15′	C	[diš.na .... k]àš-*šú* na$_4$ šub-*a* na.bi
16′	C	[............................] x numun ^{ú}eme.ur.gi$_7$
	A	[..............................] ^{ú}numun.eme.ur.gi$_7$
17′	C	[.......................................] x -*nu* kù kaš nu.tag.ga
	A	hád.d[u .....] *ina* kaš.sag *tara-sà-an* ki nu.tag x
18′	C	[...] x ti
	A	[............] *ba-lum pa-tan* nag-*ma i-*[*ne-eš*]

19′	C	[...] hi.hi *ina* mu[d zab]ar
20′	C	[..] *ina-*[*eš*]
21′	C	[...] x

31′ seed of ‘single’-plant, myrrh, ‘dog’s tongue’-plant, *puquttu* seed,
32′ *ašû*, he continually drinks them in beer.
33′ [......], *halulaja*-insect, *kukru*,
34′ [..........] myrrh, and *baluhhu-resin*.

rev. col. iii

2′ [.........................], these drugs
3′ [...................] mix together and heat them in wine;
4′ he drinks [.....................] on an empty stomach and he will recover.

5′ [..........................], *nuhurtu*, goat meat,
6′ [.........................] afterwards, black snake
7′ [...............................] he will recover.

8′ [If a man ....., to] cure him, myrrh,
9′ *pallišu*-stone, silver-rosette, seed of ‘dog’s tongue’,
10′ seed of *uhhahu*-thorn, ‘donkey-vulva’(-shell), ostrich-egg shell;
11′ you crush (var. pound and sieve) these drugs together and he drinks them in premium beer on an empty stomach.
12′ Blow them into his urethra (var. penis) through a copper tube.
13′ [............] Remove it, take malt-powder in this manner (var. he keeps bathing in hot water and you heat up beer dregs)
14′ and he will get better.

15′ [If a man ....] his urine *casts out a calculus*, that man
16′ [suffers from .... In order to cure him,] dry out seed of ‘dog’s tongue’,
17′ soak [....] .... in premium beer (var. not touching the ground) ....
18′ he drinks [.........] on an empty stomach and he will get better.

19′ Mix [.........................] through a copper tube
20′ [................................. he] will get better.
21′ ....

Ms. YY = A 239 (BAM 161 v 15–20) According to the BAM index ad loc., this passage parallels BAM 111, but the parallels are not close enough to be considered a duplicate.

15 diš na *ana* kàš-*šú ma-gal* zi.meš[1]
16 ^{šim}šeš numun ^{giš}*bi-nu*
17 ^{ú}eme.ur.gi_7 numun ^{ú}gír.hab
18 illu ^{šim}buluh súd *lu ina* kaš
19 *lu ina* geštin *lu ina* ga ku_7
20 ud.1.kam nag

[1] *ittenebbi.* This incipit is also known from BAM 116: 8 and 164: 20, see text No. 7.

TRANSLATION

15 If a man constantly 'rises' because of his urine,
16 pound (l. 18) myrrh, tamarisk seed,
17' 'dog's tongue'-plant, *dadānu*,
18 *baluhhu*-resin, (and) either in beer
19 or in wine or in sweet milk,
20 he drinks (it) for one day.

No. 4 = BAM 112

D	=	VAT 9870 + 10095 (BAM 112) (collated 30-8-02)
H	=	S 261 (AMT 66,7) [text no. 8] = 9′–12′
B_5	=	K 5864 (AMT 58,6) [see text no. 2] = 17′–28′
E	=	VAT 13734 (BAM 114) [text no. 5] = 13′–16′
A	=	CBS 19801 (BAM 396) [text no. 1] = ii 10′
X	=	A 198 (BAM 159) = ii 17′–19′
C	=	VAT 9871 + 10397 [text no. 3] (BAM 111 16′–17′;) = 17′–18′

col. i

1′	D	(traces)
2′	D	[........]-*a-šú* murub$_4$.meš-*šú* gu$_7$.meš-š[*ú* ....
3′	D	[egir k]àš.meš-*šú* múd *ú-kal-lam* na.bi [*mu-ṣa* gig]
4′	D	[*ana* t]i-*šú* ^{ú}*tara-muš*$_8$ ^{ú}igi-*lim* ^{ú}igi-*ešra* ^{ú}*ir-kul*-[*lu*]
5′	D	^{ú}*ak-tam* ^{ú}kur.kur numun ^{ú}dili ^{ú}babbar numun ^{ú}eme.ur.[gi$_7$]
6′	D	numun ^{giš}esi$_4$ numun ^{giš}⸢*bi*⸣-*ni* numun ^{ú}*pu-qut-te* ^{ú}hab ⸢ú⸣[.....
7′	D	⸢ú⸣*hal-tap-pa-a-nu* ^{ú}*ṣa-ṣu-un-tú* ^{ú}sikil gú.níg.àr.r[a ....
8′	D	[n]umun ^{ú}*in*-⸢*nu-uš* ^{ú}har.lum.ba.šir ^{na4}*ga-bi-i*⸣
9′	D	$^{[n]a4}$zálag ^{na4}an.zah ^{na4}an.zah.ge$_6$ ^{na4}níg.b[ù]r.bùr ^{na4}[...]
	B	^{na4}zálag ^{na4}an.zah ^{na4}a[n.................................
10′	D	[$^{n]a4}$*mi-si-sa* ^{na4}šuba níta *u* munus ^{na4}gi.dub-*tam-tim* ^{na4}x
	B	[.......................................] munus ^{na4}gi.dub-*tam-tim* ^{n}[^{a4}.]
11′	D	na$_4$.pa ^{ú}*a-ku-ṣi-ma-na* 37 ú.hi.a šeš diš-⸢*niš*⸣ súd *mal*-[*ma-liš*]
	B	[..]-*liš*
12′	D	[*t*]*u-šam-ṣu šum*$_4$-*ma ina* geštin.šur.ra *šum*$_4$-*ma ina* kaš *u* ì.giš *hal-ṣú* gaz nag.me[š]
	B	*tu-šam-ṣa šum-ma ina* geštin.šur *šum-ma ina* [...]

13′	D	[*šum*$_4$-*ma*] kàš.meš-*šú* gim kàš anše na.bi *mu-ṣa* g[ig]
	E	[........................... g]im kàš anše na.[........................]
14′	D	[*šum*$_4$-*ma*] kàš.meš-*šú* gim *šur-šum-me* kaš na.bi *mu-ṣa* gi[g]
	E	[.................................... *šur-šu*]*m-me* kaš na.bi *m*[*u*-..........]
15′	D	[*šum*$_4$-*ma*] kàš.meš-*šú* gim *šur-šum-me* geštin na.bi *mu-ṣa* gi[g]
	E	[.. *š*]*ur.šum.me* geštin [.................]
16′	D	[*šum*$_4$-*ma*] kàš.meš-*šú* gim še.gín *he-li-ti* na.bi *mu-ṣa* gig
	E	[................................ g]im še.gín *he-li-ti* [...................]

17′	D	[diš n]a gìš-*šú ú-zaq-qa-su u*$_4$-*ma* kàš.meš-*šú i-šá-ti-nu re-hu-su* šub-*a*[1]
	B_5[2]	[..........gì]š-*šú* gír.gír-*su u*$_4$-*ma* kàš.meš-*šú i-šá-ti-nu re*-[.....................]
	C	[.......................gí]r.gír-*su u*$_4$-*ma* kàš-*šú* [..]
18′	D	[*ina*] ⸢šà-*šú* *ṣa-bit-ma ana* munus gin⸣-*ka* lá lugud *gi-na-a ina* gìš-*šú* gin-*ak*
	B_5	[.. *g*]*i-na-a ina* gìš-*šú* gin-[..]
	C	(traces)
19′	D	[na.b]i *mu-ṣa* gig *ana* ti-*šú* ú babbar *ina* ì.giš {ta´lag}[3] mud urudu *ana* gìš-*šú ina* ka-*ka* mú[4]-*ma*
	B_5	na.bi *mu-ṣa* gig *ana* ti-*šú* [..] mú-*ah-ma*

---

[1] *iddâ*.

[2] The fragment duplicates BAM 112 except for the first line: [^{šim}l]i 2 gín^{ú}babbar *ina* kaš lú.tin.n[a] x x x [.]

[3] coll.

[4] coll.

TRANSLATION

2′ ..., his groin hurts him.........

3′ [afterwards] his urine shows blood, that man [suffers from 'discharge'].

4′ [To] cure him, *taramuš, imḫur-lim, imḫur-ešra, irkullu*

5′ *aktam, ata'išu*, seed of 'single-plant', 'white'-plant, seed of 'dog's tongue'-plant,

6′ *ušû* seed, tamarisk seed, seed of *puquttu* seed, madder, ...

7′ *ḫaltappānu, ṣaṣuntu*, 'pure'-plant, pulses, ...

8′ *maštakal* seed, *ḫarmunu*, alum,

9′ *zalāqu*-stone, frit, black frit, *palliš̆u*-stone, ...

10′ *misisu*, male and female agate, 'stylus of the sea', ...

11′ *ajartu*-mussel, *akuṣīmānu*: you crush together these 37 drugs, and

12′ you use them in eqal amounts, whether in drawn wine or whether in beer, or in pressed oil, you pound them and he keeps drinking them.

13′ [If] his urine is like ass' urine, that man suffers from 'discharge'.

14′ If his urine is like beer dregs, that man suffers from 'discharge'.

15′ If his urine is like wine dregs, that man suffers from 'discharge'.

16′ If his urine is like clear paint, that man suffers from 'discharge'.

17′ If a man's penis stings him when he passes urine (or) ejaculates,

18′ he is affected [in] his innards and is 'diminished' (i. e., cannot get erect) when he has sex with a woman, and pus flows constantly from his penis,

19′ that man suffers from 'discharge'. To cure him: you blow 'white'-plant in oil with your mouth (through) a copper tube into his penis;

20′ D [^{giš}geštin]in.ka$_5$.a súd *ina* kaš.lú$^!$.tin.na nag-*ma* kaš *u* ì.giš šeg$_6$-*šal* šub.šub-*šú*

B$_5$ ^{giš}geštin.ka$_5$.a súd *ina* kaš.lú$^!$.t[in..]

21′ D [^{ú}*tara*]-*muš$_8$* ^{šim}gúr.gúr pa ^{giš}gi$_6$.pàr$^!$(text: na$_4$) diš-*niš* súd *ina* ì.udu hi.hi sag[1] gìš-*šú* lá-*ma* ti

B$_5$ [^{šim}l]i ^{šim}gúr.gúr pa ^{giš}gi$_6$.pàr diš-*niš* súd *ina* ì.udu h[i.hi ....]

22′ D [ki.min$^?$ n]umun ^{ú}*pu-qut-te* súd *ina* ì.giš *ina* mud zabar *ina* šà giš-*šú* *ina* ka-*k*[*a* mú-*ah-ma*]

B$_5$ [.. m]ud zabar *ana* šà giš-*šú* *ina* ka-*ka* m[ú-*ah-ma*]

23′ D [^{ú}em]e.ur.gir$_7$ súd *ina* kaš nag *ina* a *u* ì.giš šub.šub-*šú* ^{šim}li ^{šim}gúr.gúr

B$_5$ [..^{šim}gúr.gú]r

24′ D [^{šim}ga]m.ma pa ^{giš}*bi-ni* pa ^{giš}*šu-še* diš-*niš* súd *ina* ì.udu hi.hi min

B$_5$ ^{šim}gam.ma pa ^{giš}*bi-ni* pa ^{giš}⸢*šu*⸣-[...]

25′ D [ki.min] ⸢u$_5$⸣.gar.ib^{mušen} súd *ina* ì.giš *ina* mud zabar *ana* šà gìš-*šú* *ina* ka-*ka*

B$_5$ [... š]à ⸢gìš⸣-*šú* *ina* ka-*ka*

26′ D [..]-*ah-ma* ú babbar súd *ina* [ì.gi]š nag *ina* a gazi^{sar}*sek-ru-ti* ra-*su*

B$_5$ mú-*a*[*h* ....]

27′ D ⸢x x x ^{ú}kur.kur[2] ^{šim}⸣hab pa ^{giš}gi.zú.lum.ma zú.lum.ma diš-*niš* súd *ina* ì.udu hi.hi

B$_5$ [........................ ^{ši}]^{m}hab pa ^{giš}g[i ....]

28′ D [k]i.min ^{ú}⸢*ur-né*⸣-*e* súd *ina* ì.giš ina mud zabar *ana* šà gìš-*šú* *ina* ka-*ka*

B$_5$ (trace)

29′ D [mú-*a*]*h-ma*[3] numun ^{ú}sikil súd *ina* kaš nag *ina* a pú *sek-ru-ti* šub.šub-*šú*

30′ D [^{giš}g]i$_6$.pàr$^!$ pa ^{giš}*šu-še* ^{ú}kur.ra pa ^{giš}gi.zú.lum.ma diš-*niš* súd *ina* ì.udu *u* ga šeg$_6$-*šal* min

---

31′ D [ki.min] ⸢^{ú}⸣geštin.ka$_5$.a súd *ina* ì.giš *ina* mud zabar *ana* šà gìš-*šú* *ina* ka-*ka*

32′ D [mú-*a*]*h-ma* ^{ú}har.har súd *ina* kaš nag *ina* a šub.šub-*šú* ^{šim}li ^{šim}gúr.gúr

33′ D [.... ^{ši}]^{m}buluh pa ^{giš}gi$_6$.pàr$^!$ diš-*niš* súd *ina* ì.udu *u* ga šeg$_6$-*šal* min

---

34′ D [diš na gìš-*šú*] gír.gír-*su* *u$_4$-ma* kàš.meš-*šú* *i-šá-ti-nu re-hu-su* šub-*a*

35′ D [*ina* šà-*šú*] *ṣa-bit-ma ana* munus gin-*ki*[4] lá lugud *gi-na-a ina* gìš-*šú* gin-*ak*[5]

36′ D [na.bi *mu-ṣa*] gig *ana* ti-*šú* *ina* šen.tur a *u* kaš kalag ^{giš}*si-ha* ^{ú}*ár-gan-nu*

37′ D [..........^{ú}*š*]*u-nim* ^{ú}*at*-⸢GAM[6] ^{na4}x x⸣ šeg$_6$-*šal ta-šá-hal*

38′ D [...........] *ma* x [..................].meš-*su* ^{ú}*sa-man*

39′ D [..-*m*]*a ana*[7] gìš-*šú* dub-*ak-ma* ti

40′ D [diš na ....-*t*]*a u i-na-a*

41′ D [...] x gìš-*šú* GAM-*ma-at*

42′ D [..] x šúd[8]

---

[1] coll.

[2] coll.

[3] coll.

[4] ku is also a possible reading. An erasure follows this sign.

[5] see above ll. 17′–19′

[6] a writing of *atkam* for *aktam*.

[7] coll.

[8] coll.

20′ crush fox-vine, and he drinks it in tavern-beer. You heat the beer and oil and keep applying them to him,
21′ crush together *taramuš* (var. juniper), ***kukru***, leaf of *lipāru*-tree, mix them in fat and bind them on his corona, and he will recover.

22′ [Ditto]: Crush ***puquttu*** seed and you blow it with your mouth into the shank of his penis through oil in a bronze tube,
23′ [and] crush 'dog's-tongue', he drinks it in beer, keep applying it in water and oil.[1] Crush together (aromatics) juniper, ***kukru***,
24′ and *ṣumlalu*, leaf of tamarisk, and leaf of *šūšu*, mix them in fat, ditto (= and he will recover).

25′ [Ditto] Crush bat guano, you blow (it) with your mouth into the shank of his penis through oil in a bronze tube,
26′ and crush 'white'-plant, he drinks it in oil, and bathe him in heated *kasû*-juice.[2]
27′ Crush together [..........] *ṭurû*, leaf of ***kūru*** (and) dates and mix it in fat.

28′ Ditto. Crush *urnû*, you blow it with your mouth into the shank of his penis through oil in a bronze tube,
29′ and crush the seed of the 'pure'-plant, he drinks it in beer, and keep applying it with heated well-water.[3]
30′ Crush together *lipāru*, *šūšu*-leaf, *ninû*, leaf of ***kūru***, you heat them in fat and milk, and ditto (he will recover).

31′ [Ditto]. Crush fox-vine, [you] blow it with your mouth into the shank of his penis through oil in a bronze tube,
32′ and crush *hašû* and he drinks it in beer. Keep applying it to him in water. Crush together juniper, ***kukru***,
33′ [...], *baluhhu*, *lipāru*, and heat them in fat and milk, ditto (= he will recover).

34′ [If a man's penis] stings him when he passes urine (or) ejaculates,
35′ and he is affected [in his bowel], he is 'diminished' when he has sex with a woman, and pus flows from his penis,
36′ [that man] suffers from ['discharge']. In order to cure him: you heat and filter in a small vessel water and strong beer, *sīhu*, *argānu*,
37′ [...........] *šunû*, *atkam* (= *aktam*), ...
38′ [.........................].., *samānu*-plant,
39′ [.....................], and pour it into his penis and he will recover.

40′ [If a man ....] and he has a *urinary complaint*,
41′ [...] .. of his penis is ...,
42′ crush [..]

[1] These clauses represent the combination of two simplicia.
[2] These clauses represent the combination of two simplicia.
[3] These clauses represent the combination of two simplicia.

43′ D (traces)
44′–48′ D (broken)
49′ D [.................................... *ina* kaš *u* g]a nu *pa*-⌜*tan* nag⌝-*ma* t[i]

---

col.ii

1′–3′ D (traces)

4′ D diš na [............
5′ D [...........
6′ D diš na gìš-*šú* kúm [...............
7′ D ud.da sá.sá x [............

8′ D diš na [gì]š-*šú* im *iš-bi* [....................
9′ D ^{ú}[si]kil gú.níg.àr.ra [................

10′ D diš ki.min pa ^{giš}*bi-ni* si[g$_7$ ....]
A [diš n]a pa ^{giš}šinig sig$_7$ ^{ú}*in-uš* gú.níg.àr.ra téš.bi gaz lá-*ma i-ne-eš*

11′ D diš na gìš-*šú* im *iš-bi* [.............
12′ D u$_4$.bú!.bú!.ul! diri ì [...........
13′ D *u* kaš.sag hi.hi *ina* a [.............
14′ D ì.giš kúm eš [............................

15′ D diš na murub$_4$^{2}-*šú* gig-*m*[*a* ....
16′ D hád.a súd *ina* geštin.šur.[ra ....

17′ D diš na *ina* gìš-*šú* múd *ú-tab*-[*ba-ka* ....
Xdis ˇ na *ina* gìš-*šú* múd *ú-tab-ba-ka* gim munus ^{giš}tukul *ma-hi-iṣ*
18′ D *ana* ti-šú gú.gal ⌜ú⌝[.............
X *ana* [t]i-*šú* gú.gal ^{ú}nu.luh.ha naga.si diš-*niš* súd
19′ D *ina* ⌜gi.sag.kud gíd-*ád u*⌝ [.....................
X[................................] *ina* mul$_4$ *tuš-bat ina še-rim* nu *pa-tan* nag-*ma* ti

43′–48′ broken
49′ [...............], he drinks it [in beer or] milk on an empty stomach and he will recover.

col. ii

1′–3′ ....
4′–5′ If a man [..]
6′ If a man's penis is hot [..............................]
7′ he is overcome by 'sun-light' (disease), ..[..............

8′ If a man's penis is 'blasted' by wind [...................]
9′ 'pure'-plant, pulses, [....................................].

10′ If ditto, pound together leaf of green tamarisk, *maštakal*, pulses, and bind them (on him) and he will get better.

11′ If a man's penis is 'blasted' by wind [and his penis]
12′ is covered with boils (or pustules), mix oil [.................]
13′ and premium beer, and in water [.................].
14′ Rub on hot oil [.................................].

15′ If a man's groin is sore and [................]
16′ dry out and crush [.........] in drawn wine.

17′ If a man's penis drips blood like a menstruating woman,
18′ to cure him: crush together pea, *nuhurtu*, and horned alkali,
19′ he sucks (them) in via a pipette and [......... (var. leave it out over night and he drinks it in the morning on an empty stomach and he will recover).

No. 5 = BAM 114[1]

E	=	VAT 13734 (BAM 114)
I	=	K 4957 + 121742 + S 110 + 679 + 516 + 761 + 2058 (= AMT 82,1 + OECT 6 pl 16 + AMT 58,4 + AMT 61,5 + AMT 39,9) [text no. 9] = 5–23.
D	=	VAT 9870 + 10095 (BAM 112) [text no. 4] = 1–4
NN	=	K 4164 + (BAM 430 iv 32′ ff.) [text no. 40] = 11–23
YY	=	A 239 (BAM 161 iv) = 8–23
MM	=	K 9684 + (BAM 431 iii 27 ff.) [text no. 18] = 11–23

1	D	[*šum$_4$-ma*] kàš.meš-*šú* gim kàš anše na.bi *mu-ṣa* g[ig]
	E	[............................ g]im kàš anše na.[.........................]
2	D	[*šum$_4$-ma*] kàš.meš-*šú* gim *šur-šum-me* kaš na.bi *mu-ṣa* gi[g]
	E	[....................................... *šur-šu*]*m-me* kaš na.bi *m*[*u*-.........]
3	D	[*šum$_4$-ma*] kàš.meš-*šú* gim *šur-šum-me* geštin na.bi *mu-ṣa* gi[g]
	E	[....................................... *š*]*ur-šum-me* geštin [.......................]
4	D	[*šum$_4$-ma*] kàš.meš-*šú* gim še.gín *he-li-ti* na.bi *mu-ṣa* gig
	E	[.................................g]im še.gín *he-li-ti* [....................]
5	I	*šum$_4$-⸢ma* kàš-*šú* gim a.m[eš ....]
	E	[........................] gim a.meš gazi^{sar} na.bi ud.da k[ur-*id*]
6	E	[m]in sig$_7$ *hi-niq-ti* murub$_4$ [gig]
	I	*šum$_4$-ma* kàš-*šú* s[ig$_7$ ....]
7	I	*šum$_4$-ma* kàš-*šú* babbar-*ma e-ba-a* [.................................]
	E	min babbar-*ma e-ba-a* na.bi na$_4$ *šá-hi-h*[*u* gig]
	YY	[...] gig
8	I	*šum$_4$-ma* kàš-*šú* gim $^{na4!}$duh.ši.a[2] [.............]
	E	min gim ^{na4}duh.ši.a na$^{!}$.bi na$_4$ [gig]
	YY	*šum$_4$-ma* kàš-*š*[*ú* ....] duh.ši.a na.bi na$_4$ g[ig]
9–10	I	*šum$_4$-ma* kàš-*šú* gim *šá gi-na-a* murub$_4$^{2}-*šú u* s[ag....................] *ana* ti-*šú*
	E	min gim *šá gi-na-a* murub$_4$.meš-šú sag šà-*š*[*ú* x x] na.bi *hi-niq-ti* dúr gig *ana* [....]
	YY	*šum$_4$-ma* kàš-*šú* gim *šá gi*-[...] murub$_4$.meš-šú *u* sag šà-*šú* gu$_7$-[*šú*] na.bi *hi-niq-ti* bun gig *ana* ti-*šú*
11	E	^{ú}tara.muš ^{ú}igi-*lim* ^{ú}igi-*ešra* ka.a.ab.ba ^{š}[^{im} ...]
	I	^{ú}tara.muš ^{ú}igi-*lim* ^{ú}ig[i-*ešra* ....
	YY	^{ú}tara.muš ^{ú}igi-*lim* ^{ú}igi-*ešra* ka.a.ab.ba
	MM	om. ^{ú}tara.muš ^{ú}igi-*lim* ^{ú}igi-*ešra* ka.a.ab.ba
	NN	^{ú}tara.muš ^{ú}igi-*lim* ^{ú}igi-*ešra* [.... a]b.ba

[1] This tablet begins with a series of *šumma* clauses, noting symptoms in a way similar to the way symptoms are recorded in TDP; cf. below, VAT 303+ (Text No. 49), although the vocabulary differs considerably from that used in TDP.

[2] see M. Stol, RLA 534 s. v. Leder (industrie).

TRANSLATION

1 [If] his urine is like ass' urine, that man suffers from 'discharge'.
2 [If] his urine is like beer dregs, that man suffers from 'discharge'.
3 [If] his urine is like wine dregs, that man suffers from 'discharge'.
4 [If] his urine is like clear paint, that man suffers from 'discharge'.
5 If his urine is like *kasû*-juice, that man is overcome by 'sun-light' disease.
6 If his urine is yellow-green, that man [suffers] from stricture of the groin.
7 If his urine is white and thick, that man [suffers] from a dissolving calculus.
8 If his urine is like *dušû*-stone, that man [suffers] from a calculus.
9–10 If his urine is as normal, but his groin and epigastrium cause [him] pain, that man suffers from stricture of the rectum (var. bladder). To cure him:
11 *taramuš*, *imhur-lim*, *imhur-ešra*, coral, ...

12–13	E	^{šim}li na$_4$.pa ^{na4}ni.bu ^{na4}*ga-[bi-i]* ^{na4}peš$_4$.anše ^{ú}kur.kur ^{ú}níg.sù.s[ù]
	I	^{na4}*ga-bi-i* na$_4$.pa ^{na4}n[i.bu ....]
	YY	^{šim}gúr.gúr ^{giš}li ^{na4}*ga-bi-e* na$_4$.pa ^{na4}*iá-ni-ba* ^{na4}peš$_4$.anše ^{ú}kur.kur ^{ú}níg.sù.sù
	MM	^{šim}gúr.gúr ^{šim}li ^{na4}*ga-be-e* na$_4$.pa ^{na4}ni.bu ^{na4}peš$_4$.anše ^{ú}kur.kur $^{na4.ú}$níg.bùr.bùr
	NN	^{šim}gúr.gúr [...l]i ^{na4}*ga-be-e* na$_4$.pa [....].bu ^{na4}peš$_4$.anše [......k]ur ^{ú}níg.bùr.bùr
14	E	^{ú}níg.bùr.bùr ba.ba.za.^{d}íd numun ^{ú}eme.ur.g[i$_7$]
	I	^{na4ú}níg.bùr.bùr ba.ba.za.^{d}í[d ....]
	YY	$^{na4.ú}$níg.bùr.bùr ba.ba.za.^{d}íd numun ^{ú}eme.ur.gi$_7$ ú dili ka.a.ab.ba
	MM	$^{na4.ú}$níg.sù.sù[1] bá.bá.za.^{d}íd numun ⌜^{ú}⌝[..........g]i$_7$ *kar-áš tam-tim*
	NN	[...........s]ù.sù bá.bá.za.^{d}íd [.......................u]r.gi$_7$ *kar-áš tam-tim*
15	E	*mi-sis tam-tim ka-ra-áš tam-tim*
	I	*mi-sis* a.ab.ba
	YY	*mì-sis tam-ti*
	MM	*mi-sis tam-tim*
	NN	[..............*-ti*]*m*
16	E	[^{ú}nu.lu]h.ha ^{ú}*úr-nu-u* ^{ú}har.har
	I	^{ú}nu.lu[h.ha ....] ^{ú}har.har
	YY	^{ú}har.har ^{ú}nu.luh *ti-iá-tú* ^{ú}*úr-nu-u*
	MM	^{ú}har.har ^{ú}nu.luh.ha ^{ú}*ti-iá-tú* ^{ú}*ur-nu-u*
	NN	[......ha]r ^{ú}nu.luh.ha [..........] ^{ú}*ur-nu-u*
17	E	[$^{........}$*-bu*]*r-rat* ^{ú}*ha-hi-in* ^{ú}geštin.ka$_5$.a
	I	^{ú}*šib-bur-ra*[*t* ....]
	YY	luh.mar.tú ^{ú}*ha*$^{!}$*-hi-in* ^{ú}geštin.ka$_5$.a
	MM	⌜^{ú}⌝*šib-bur-ra-tu*$_4$ ^{ú}*ha-hi-in* [^{ú}geš]tin.ka$_5$.a
	NN	^{ú}*šib-bur-ra-tú* [................] ^{ú}geštin.ka$_5$.a [........]
18	E	[..............] ⌜ú⌝ babbar ^{giš}sila$_{11}$.gá šika nunuz.ga.na^{mušen}
	I	^{ú}lag.a.šà šika nunuz ga.n[u$_{11}$ ....]
	YY	^{ú}kur.ra ú babbar ^{ú}lag.gán šika nunuz.ga.nu$_{11}$^{mušen}
	MM	^{ú}kur.r[a$^{!}$ ú babb]ar [^{ú}lag].gán šika nunuz.[..............]
	NN	[............] ^{ú}lag.gán [................................ ....]
19	E	[.......................^{giš}]ma.nu $^{ú.zì}$nu.luh.ha
	I	[..]
	YY	numun ^{giš}*b*[*i-n*]*i* numun ^{giš}ma.nu ^{ú}*an-nu-ha-ru*
	MM	[................*-n*]*i* numun ^{giš}[....] ⌜^{ú}⌝[......h]a.ra
	NN	n]umun ^{giš}*bi-ni* [................... ^{ú}a]n.nu.ha.ra

[1] This is the mineral *sāpinu*, a flattened stone for smoothing, but this may not be the same as ^{ú}níg.sù.sù.

12–13 juniper, mussel, *ianiba*, alum, and 'donkey-vulva'(-shell); *ata'išu*, *sāpinu*,
14–15 *pallišu*-plant/stone, white gypsum, seed of 'dog's tongue', (var. 'single'-plant, coral)[1] sea-*missis*, sea leek,
16 *nuhurtu*, *urnû*, *hašû*-plant,
17 rue, *hahin* (thorny plant), fox-vine,
18 field-clod-plant (var. *nīnû*), 'white'-plant, *dough*, ostrich-egg shell,
19 tamarisk seed, seed of *erû*-wood, *nuhurtu*-flour, *alluharu*(-mineral).

[1] probably an error in Ms. YY (BAM 161), reading *ú-aš* ka.a.ab.ba for var. *karaš tamti*.

20	E	[............................... ^{giš}]nu.úr.ma
21	E	[.... g]al gú.níg.àr
	I	gú.gal gú.níg.àr.ra
	YY	gú.gal gú.níg.àr.ra
	MM	gú.gal g[ú].n[íg...]
	NN	[......................r]a
22	E	[...] 36 ú.hi.a
	I	^{giš}h[ab ....] 36 ú.meš
	YY	^{giš}hab šika ^{giš}*nu-úr-ma-a* ^{ú}*nu-ṣa-ba* 36 ú.hi.a
	MM	^{giš}hab ši[ka .....-*ú*]*r-ma-a* ^{ú}*nu*-[............] 36 ⸢ú⸣.[meš]
	NN	^{giš}h[a]b [.................................*n*]*u-ṣa-b*[*u* ....]
23	E	[..................................*l*]*u ina* geštin nag
	I	*mu-ṣi šá* [...................... *i*]*na* geštin *lu ina* kaš n[ag ....]
	YY	šeš diš-*niš* gaz sim *lu ina* geštin *lu ina* [ka]š *lu ina* ga na[g-*ma* ti]
	MM	[*mu-ṣ*]*i šá* gar.meš mah.meš
	NN	[.......................... ma]h.meš

24	E	[....................................
25	Ex	[.................................

26	E	diš ki.min x [.......................................
27	E	x [..

20 [.........], pomegranate,
21 peas, pulses,
22 madder, pomegranate-rind, and *nuṣābu*, 36 plants (in all)
23 (var. for discharge, regarding the major characteristics), pound and sieve these together and he drinks them either in wine or in beer or in milk [and he will recover].

(rest broken).

No. 6 = BAM 115

F	=	VAT 8693 (BAM 115) (collated 30-8-02)
A	=	CBS 19801 (BAM 396) [text no. 1] = ll. 2′–9′.
B	=	K 2405 + (= AMT 31,1 + 59,1 + 61,1) [text no. 2] = ll. 10′–12′

2′	F	gi.du$_{10}$.ga šim.hi.⸢a⸣ [.......................................]
	A	gi.du$_{10}$.ga šim.hi.a *ka-li-šu-ma* hi.[hi] *ina ka-li*$^{!}$(text at)-*tu* bún-*ma i-na a-h*[*e-e*] igi *mùš-tin-ni-su* nu
3′	F	dab-*bat ru-ub-ṣa i-di-ka-a* [.......................]
	A	dab-*bat ru-ub-ṣu i-de-ek-ke-e-m*[*a*$^{?}$]
4′	F	*i-tab-ba-ka ul* tag-*su ni*$^{?}$ [.......................]
	A	gig nu zu *ú-ṭa-ab-šu* suhuš ^{ú}eme.ur.gi$_7$ gu$_7$-*ma i-ne-*[*eš*]

5′	F	^{na4}zálag ^{na4}kur.nu.dib ^{na4}*mu-ṣu* an.záh ^{na4}peš$_4$.anše [............
	A	^{na4}*za-la-qu* ^{na4}ka.gi.na *mu-ṣa-am* an.záh ^{na4}peš$_4$.anše ^{šim}šeš
6′	F	[......................] šika nunuz ga.nu$_{11}$^{mušen}an.záh níta *u* munus ^{ú}*a-a-*[.........
	A	šika ^{giš}nu.ur.ma šika nunuz ga.n[u$_{11}$^{mušen}] an.záh.ge$_6$ nita *u* munus ^{ú}kù.babbar numun ^{giš}šinig
7′	F	ka.a.ab.ba ^{na4}níg.bùr.bùr ^{giš}tara.muš ^{ú}gír-*h*[*a-*.........................]
	A	ka.a.ab.ba ^{ú}níg.bùr.bùr ^{ú}tara.muš ^{ú}gír-*uh-ha-a*[*h*] numun ^{ú}eme.ur.gi$_7$ ^{ú}eme.ur.gi$_7$
8′	F	numun ú dili téš.bi *ta-ša-*[*qa*]-*a*[*l*] *ta-sàk ina* ì.giš *ù* ì.giš bára.ga hi.hi
	A	numun ú dili *mal-ma-liš ta-šá-qàl* súd *ina* kaš.sag [........................]
9′	F	[.....................] *tuš-bat ina še-rim* nag *la i-sa-dir ina* a šeg$_6$ [....................................]
	A	*ana* igi mul.úz *tuš-bat ina še-ri* nag.na[g] *la i-*[*s*]*a-a-dar ù ina* a šeg$_6$ *ir-ta-na-haṣ-*[*m*]*a* [*i*]-⸢*ne-eš*⸣

10′	F	ì.giš bára.ga *ù* kaš.sag *ina* mud zabar *ana* [gìš-*šú* dub-*ak*]
	B	ì.giš bára.ga *u* kaš.sag *ina* m[ud..........................du]b-*ak*
11′	F	[i]llu ^{šim}buluh *ina* izi šeg$_6$-*šal ta-šá-hal ana* [.........]
	B	illu ^{šim}buluh *ina* izi šeg$_6$-*šal ta-šá-hal ana* gìš-*šú* dub
12′	F	[ú] babbar *ina* ì.bára.ga *u* kaš.sag ki.min ^{im}sahar.na$_4$.kur.r[a] x
	B	ú babbar *ina* ì.giš [bára.ga *u* kaš.šag] x ^{im}sahar.na$_4$.kur.ra *ina* ì.giš *u* kaš.sag ki.min

---

13′	F	[diš na] *ša* a.meš nag *u ma-gal* zi.meš egir-*šú* t[i]

14′	F	[diš.n]a *ina* ki.ná-*šú* kàš-*šú iš-*⸢*tin* šu⸣ ^{d}*be-let*-dingir.meš t[i]

15′	F	[dù.d]ù.bi giš.ná *šu-a-tú ta-za-qap ana* [x] ha šub-*di* x [..........]
16′	F	[...] x ^{šim}li gar-*an* kaš x x x [....................]

17′	F	[...........] x x [..] x *i-di* [......................]
18′	F	[..........................] x limmu [................]

TRANSLATION

1′ [If a man suffers from a calculus ...(?)][1]

2′ mix 'sweet' reed, all of the aromatics, blow them into the kidney; the opening of his urethra should not be grasped by (its) sides.

3′ He shall remove the flux [..

4′ he pours out, it should not affect him ... [.............] (var. and it will make him better in respect to the undiagnosed disease, he will eat root of 'dog-tongue'-plant and he will get better).

5′ You weigh out and crush together (var. equally, l. 8′) *zalāqu,* haematite, *muṣu*, frit, 'donkey-vulva'(-shell), myrrh,

6′ pomegranate-rind, shell of ostrich egg, 'male' and 'female' black frit, 'silver-rosette'-plant, tamarisk seed,

7′ coral, *pallišu*-plant/stone, *taramuš, uhhahu*-thorn, seed of 'dog's tongue', 'dog's tongue',

8′ seed of 'single'-plant. Mix them in oil and in pressed oil (var. premium beer),

9′ you leave them out overnight facing the Goat-star and he keeps drinking it in the morning; no time should elapse and he should keep bathing in hot water and he will get better.

10′ You pour pressed oil and premium beer in a bronze tube into [his penis],

11′ you boil over a fire and filter the *baluhhu*-resin, pour (it) into his penis,

12′ ditto (= you mix) 'white'-plant in pressed oil and premium beer, (alternatively): ditto alum in oil and premium beer.

13′ [If (the patient) is a man] who drinks water and repeatedly rises (to urinate),[2] eventually he will recover.

14′ [If a] man urinates when he lies down, it is the hand of (the goddess) Bēlet-ilī, he will recover.

15′ Its ritual: you set up that bed, you put ....[...].

16′ you set up [...] and juniper, [...........] beer ...[.............]

17′–18′ ....

---

[1] This line has been restored from the duplicate (text No. 1), although the restoration is not certain.

[2] or 'is constantly erect'.

rev.

1′ F (traces)
2′ F [........]eme.ur.gi$_7$ ^{šim}l[i ....]
3′ F [..........] x *lu ina* geštin *lu ina* [ka]š x [.................]

4′ F [diš.na *ina* k]i.ná-*šú* kàš.meš-*šú* ⌜*iš-tin*⌝-[*ma* ....
5′ F [.........] ú.meš *ina pi-šir-t*[*i* ....
6′ F [.........] ú babbar ^{ú}*šá-na-di* [.....................
7′ F [.............*ta*]*l-l*[*a*]*-li-ia* [....................

8′ F [...............]⌜^{ú}⌝ukuš-*ti-gil-la* [.................

9′ F [...............] ⌜^{ú}⌝níndu edin múd [....................

10′ F [...............] ki.ná *šá ana* ugu x [.................
11′ F [........... a].gar.gar *a-sur-re-e*[1] x [.......
12′ F [.............] x súd *ina* kaš nag.meš-*m*[*a* ....

13′ F [....... *a*]*n* ⌜*mu*⌝-*ur*![2]-*ru ta-d*[*i* ....
14′ F [.......] ⌜*a*⌝-*bu-ru-ṣa-na* x [..........................

15′ F [.......................] x a n[a$^?$ ....]

[1] see CAD A/2 351, 'damp course', but now suggested by A. George as a word for toilet or latrine. George's idea is supported by an expression in the Babylonian Talmud which uses the Dreckapotheke 'dust of the toilet' as materia medica, corresponding to the use of *eper asurrê* as a secret name for Dreckapotheke in Akkadian; see F. Köcher, *Uruk die Gräber*, ed. R. M. Boehmer et al. (Mainz, 1995), 204 f., and M. J. Geller, 'Akkadian Therapy in the Babylonian Talmud' (Max-Planck-Institut für Wissenschaftsgeschichte Preprint 259 [2004], fn. 126).

[2] The collated sign looks like /ama/, which makes little sense here, and hence Köcher's reading as copied is adopted.

rev.

1′ ....

2′ [........], 'dog's tongue'-[plant], juniper, [...............

3′ [he drinks ......] either in wine or beer ...[................

4′ [If a man] urinates when he lies down [and ....

5′ [.........] drugs in a solution [...........

6′ [.......] 'white'-plant and *šanadu*-plant(?)[1] [..........

7′ ....

8′ [........] cucumber [...............

9′ [..........] *illūru*-plant of the steppe, blood [of ...

10′ [..........] a couch, which is above [..........

11′ Crush [........] excrement of the latrine [...............

12′ and he keeps drinking it in beer and [he will get better].

13′ [.......] .. myrrh[?], ..[.................

14′ ......, *a.*-insect ....

15′ ....

(rest fragmentary)

---

[1] This is usually a disease name, although see, similarly, the plant name [ú]*samānu*, Text No. 4: 38.

No. 7 BAM 116

G	=	A 267 + VAT 13743 (BAM 116) (collated 27-08-02)
MM	=	K 9684 + (BAM 431 iv 42–46) (list of medicinal plants) [text no. 18] = 4–8
ZZ	=	A 234 (BAM 164: 18–21) (list of medicinal plants from Kiṣir-Assur) = rev. 6′–9′
B	=	K 2405 + (AMT 31,1 +) [text no. 2] = 10′–13′
YY	=	A 239 (BAM 161 v 3–6) = 1–3.

obv.

1	G	[..................] gig ^{šim}gúr.gúr ^{ú}kur.kur
	YY	diš na *mu-ṣa* gig ^{šim}gúr.gúr ^{ú}kur.kur
2	G	^{šim}šeš $^{\text{na4}}$*ga-bi-i* diš-*niš* súd
	YY	^{šim}šeš $^{\text{na4}}$*ga-bé-e* téš.bi súd
3	G	*ina* geštin.kala.ga *la pa-tan* nag.meš
	YY	*ina* geštin.meš kala.ga nu *pa-tan* nag
4	G	diš ki.min ^{ú}*zi-im*-kù.babbar ^{ú}numun *pu-qut-te*
	MM	(om.) ^{ú}z[*i*-......].babbar numun ^{ú}*pu-qu-tú*
5	G	^{ú}níg.bùr.bùr ^{ú}níg.[s]ù.sù illu ^{šim}buluh
	MM	$^{\text{na4.ú}}$[....... n]umun ^{ú}*a-zal-la* ^{šim}šeš [.......] ^{šim}buluh
6	G	$^{\text{na4}}$peš$_4$.[anše] šika nunuz gá.nu$_{11}$^{mušen}
	MM	$^{\text{na4}}$peš$_4$.[anše] šika nunuz gá.n[u$_{11}$^{muše}]^{n}
7	G	^{šim}šeš ka.ab.ba 9 ú.meš
	MM	ka.ab.ba 9 ú
8	G	*mu-ṣ*[*i l*]*at-ku-ti ina* geštin nag.meš
	MM	*mu-*⌜*ṣi*⌝ *lat-ku*
9	G	diš ki.min ^{ú}sikil *up-pat* ^{šim}gúr.gúr ^{giš}*š*[*u-nim*]
10	G	^{šim}hab ^{šim}šeš illu ^{šim}buluh
11	G	numun ^{giš}*šu-nim* numun ^{ú}*tara-muš*$_8$ ^{šim}gam.ma
12	G	⌜ì.⌝udu ^{giš}*šuq-di* 11 ú.meš *an-nu-ti*
13	G	[súd] *ina* ì.nun šeg$_6$-*šal šu-*⌜*hi-šú*⌝
14	G	[^{uzu}ú]r.kun-*šú* [..............]
15	G	(trace)

rev.

1′–2′	G	(traces)
3′	G	[....................] *ana* šà šub-*di ana* gìš-*šú* du[b]
4′	G	diš ki.min ^{ú}*úr-ni-i* min min min
5′	G	[diš k]i.[m]in ^{ú}geštin.ka$_5$.a súd min.min.min
6′	G	[g]ú.tur ^{šim}šeš naga.si
	ZZ	gú.tur ^{šim}šeš naga.si
7′	G	ka.a.ab.ba $^{\text{na4}}$*ga-bi-i* 5 ú.meš
	ZZ	ka.a.ab.ba $^{\text{na4}}$*ga-bi-i* 5 ú.meš
8′	G	diš na *ana* kàš.meš-*šú ma-gal* zi.zi-*bi*
	ZZ	diš na *ana* gìš.meš-*šú ma-gal* zi.zi-*bi*
9′	G	*lu ina* kaš *lu ina* geštin ⌜*lu*⌝ *ina* a.meš nag.meš
	ZZ	*lu ina* kaš *lu ina* geštin *lu ina* a.meš [........]

TRANSLATION

1 [If a man] suffers [from discharge], crush together *kukru*, *ata'išu*,
2 myrrh, and alum,
3 and he drinks it in strong wine on an empty stomach.

---

4 If ditto, 'silver-lustre'-plant, *puquttu* seed,
5 *pallišu*-plant/stone, *sāpinu*, (var. *azallû* seed), *baluhhu*-resin,
6 ['donkey]-vulva'(-shell), shell of ostrich-egg,
7 myrrh, coral; (total) 9 drugs
8 for discharge, checked, he keeps drinking it in wine.

---

9 If ditto, 'pure'-plant, 'mole-cricket', *kukru*, *šunû*,
10 madder, myrrh, *baluhhu*-resin,
11 *šunû* seed, *taramuš* seed, *ṣumlalu*,
12 fat, and almond(wood); [crush] together these 11 drugs
13 and boil them in ghee, his thighs
14 (and) his buttocks [...............
15 ....

rev.

1′–2′ ....
3′ put [............] into it and pour it into his penis.

4′ If ditto, *urnû*, ditto, ditto, ditto.

5′ [If di]tto, crush fox-vine, ditto, ditto, ditto.

6′ Pea, myrrh, and horned alkali,
7′ coral, alum; 5 drugs.
8′ If a man repeatedly rises[1] because of his urine,
9′ he keeps drinking (the drugs) either in beer or in wine or water.

---

[1] or has an erection.

10′	G	^{ú}igi-*lim* ^{šim}šeš šika nunuz gá.nu$_{11}$^{mušen}
	B	^{ú}igi-*lim* ^{šim}šeš šika nunuz ga.nu$_{11}$^{mušen}
11′	G	$^{\text{na4}}$an.zah.ge$_6$ diš-*niš* súd *ina* 3 *u*$_4$-*me* *ina* al.us.sa.k[u$_6$][1]
	B	an.záh.ge$_6$ 1-*niš* sú[d.....]
12′	G	2 *u*$_4$-*me* *ina* geštin.šur.ra 3 *u*$_4$-*me* *ina* a.meš
	B	3*u*$_4$-*mi* *ina* geštin.šur.ra 2 *u*$_4$-*mi* *ina* a
13′	G	$^{\text{[gi]š}}$*nu-ur-m*[*i*]-*i* nag.meš-*ma*
	B	^{giš}nu.úr.ma nag.meš ti
14′	G	[*ana hi-n*]*iq-tú* ⸢ud.zal$^?$.sa$_9$⸣
15′	G	[*ana mal-su-ti-š*]*ú za-mar* zi-[*ha*] = colophon[2]

---

1 CAD Š/3 100, sauce made of fish. A fish sauce also occurs in the Babylonian Talmud.

2 Cf. BAM 106 rev. 12.

10′ Crush together *imhur-lim*, myrrh, ostrich-egg shell,
11′ black frit, for 3 days in garum,
12′ for 2 (var. 3) days in drawn wine, and for 3 days in
13′ pomegranate-juice he keeps drinking it (var. he will recover).
14′ [For a] stricture of *midday.*

15′ Hurriedly excerpted for his [lecture] (colophon)

No. 8 AMT 66,7

H	=	S 261 (AMT 66,7) (Babyloniaca 14 65 ff., 107 ff.) (collated)
D	=	VAT 9870 + 10095 [text no. 4] (BAM 112: 9′–12′; 14′) = 1–4
F	=	VAT 8693 (BAM 115: 10′) [text no. 6] = l. 6
G	=	A 267 + VAT 13743 [text no. 7] (BAM 116) = l. 7
YY	=	A 239 (BAM 161 v 3–6) = l. 7
A	=	CBS 19801 (BAM 396 i 23′–31′) [text no. 1] = 18–21

1	H	^{na4}zálag ^{na4}an.zah ^{na4}a[n..]
	D	$^{[n]a4}$zálag ^{na4}an.zah ^{na4}an.zah.ge$_6$ ^{na4}níg.bùr.bùr ^{na4}[...^{n}]^{a4}*mi-si-sa*
2	H	[....................]munus ^{na4}gi.dub-*tam-tim* ^{n}[^{a4}..]
	D	^{na4}šuba níta *u* munus ^{na4}gi.dub-*tam-tim* ^{na4}x na$_4$.pa ^{ú}*a-ku-ṣi-ma-na* 37 ú.hi.a šeš
3	H	[.........................]-*liš tu-šam-ṣa šum-ma ina* geštin.šur *šum-ma ina* [..................................]
	D	diš-*niš* súd *mal-*[*ma-liš t*]*u-šam-ṣu šum$_4$-ma ina* geštin.šur.ra *šum$_4$-ma ina* kaš *u* ì.giš *hal-ṣú* gaz nag.me[š]
4–5	H	[............................]-*šú* gim *šur-šum-me* kaš ki.min kàš [................]
	B	[*šum$_4$-ma*] kàš.meš-*šú* gim *šur-šum-me* kaš na.bi *mu-ṣa* gi[g]
6	H	[......................................] mud zabar *ana* gìš-*šú* dub-*ak* [...............]
	F	ì.giš bára.ga *ù* kaš.sag *ina* mud zabar *ana* [....................................]
7	H	[...-*b*]*i-i* diš-*niš* súd *ina* geštin kala.ga nu *pa-tan* [...]
	G	[.............] gig ^{šim}gúr.gúr ^{ú}kur.kur ^{šim}šeš ^{na4}*ga-bi-i* diš-*niš* súd *ina* geštin.kala.ga *la pa-tan* nag.meš
	YY	diš na *mu-ṣa* gig ^{šim}gúr.gúr ^{ú}kur.kur ^{šim}šeš ^{na4}*ga-bé-e* téš.bi súd *ina* geštin.meš kala.ga nu *pa-tan* nag
8	H	[....................^{ú}kur].kur ú dili diš-*niš* súd *ina* kaš.sag nu pa-tan nag-[*ma* ti]
9	H	[...........................] x ú dù.a.bi sig[1] diš-*niš* súd *ina* geštin kala.ga nu *pa-tan* nag-*ma* ti
10	H	[.......................... *g*]*a-bi-i* diš-*niš* súd *ina* a zú.lum.ma nu *pa-tan* nag-*ma* ti
11	H	[.............................. geštin].ka$_5$.a diš-*niš ina* kaš nu *pa-tan* kal nag-*ma* ti
12	H	[.........................] x a diš-*niš* súd *ina ha-šu-ri ša-ah-li*[2] nu *pa-tan* nag-*ma* ti
13	H	[............ še$_{10}$ e]me.šid *iz-zi*[3] diš-*niš* súd *ina* geštin nag.meš *ina mar-ha-ṣi* ra-*su*
14	H	[...... ^{ú}nu.luh].ha ^{ú}har.har illu li.dur ki dida gu$_7$ zé gú.bí^{ku6} nag
15	H	[................did]a ^{buru5}úš.ku$_6$[4] ú babbar diš-*niš* súd *ina še-rim* nu *pa-tan* nag-*ma* ti

[1] This might be sig = *qatnu* or alternatively sig for sig$_7$.
[2] CAD Š/1 98 'strained'; hapax: 'in strained *hašurru* (oil)'.
[3] < *nezû*, see Text No. 16 ii 13′, še$_{10}$ eme.diri *iz-zi*, 'faeces excreted by a lizard'. An alternative reading is *igāru*, since a 'wall lizard' (eme.šid iz.zi) is attested in Hh. xiv 210, and it is difficult to tell which meaning may apply to a particular context. Cf. CAD Ṣ 255, citing KAR 196 r. i 16, (eme.šid *šá* IZ.ZI), as a variant from AMT 67,1 iv 9.
[4] See PSD B 216, known only lexically, see MSL 8/2 108.

TRANSLATION

1 Crush together *zalāqu*-stone, frit, black frit, *pallišu*-stone, [...]-stone, *misisu*,
2 male and female agate, 'stylus of the sea', ..., mussel, *akuṣīmānu*: crush these 37 drugs,
3 you use them in equal amounts, you pound them either in drawn wine or in beer and pressed oil, and he keeps drinking it.

4–5 [If] his urine is like beer dregs, that man suffers from 'discharge'. Urine [...........]

6 You pour pressed oil and premium beer in a bronze tube into his penis [........

7 If a man suffers from discharge, crush together *kukru*, *ata'išu*, myrrh, and alum, and he drinks (var. keeps drinking) it in strong wine on an empty stomach.

8 [Ditto.] Crush [........], *ata'išu* and 'single'-plant together and he drinks it in premium beer on an empty stomach [and he will recover].

9 [Ditto]. Crush together [.........].., all of the *fresh / fine* plants, and he drinks it in strong wine on a empty stomach and he will recover.

10 [Ditto.] Crush together [..... and] alum and he drinks it in date juice on an empty stomach and he will recover.

11 [Ditto.] <Crush> [... and fox]-wine together and he drinks it *all* in beer on an empty stomach and he will recover.

12 [Ditto.] Crush together ..[........] and he drinks it in strained *hašurru*-oil on an empty stomach and he will recover.

13 [Ditto.] Crush together [.....] lizard [dung]; he keeps drinking it in wine and you bathe him.

14 [Ditto.] He eats *nuhurtu* and *hašû* and *abukkatu*-resin with *billatu*-beer, and he drinks eel gall.

15 [Ditto.] Crush together *billatu*-[beer] and ...-locust and 'white'-plant, he drinks it in the morning on an empty stomach and he will recover.

16 H [...............] x *ur* ì.giš ka-*ka* diri *ana* kir$_4$ gìš-*šú* *tu-qar-ra-ar*

17 H [.............g]a ki ^{šim}gig ì.giš *ta-mah-haṣ ba-lu pa-tan* 3 *u$_4$-me* nag-*ma ina-eš*

---

18 H [..]-*šú* kàš-*šú* gim kàš anše babbar-*a* egir kàš-*šu* múd *ú-kal-lam* na.bi

A diš na ^{uzu}éllag-*su* gu$_7$-*šu* murub$_4$-*šú* tag.tag-*šú ù* kàš-*šú* gim kàš anše babbar egir kàš-*šu* múd *ú-kal-la-ma* na.bi

19 H [...] 2 gín illu ^{šim}buluh 1/2 sìla a.geštin.na *ina* ^{dug}kam *t*[*u*-............]

A *mu-ṣa-am* gig 2 gín ^{šim}šeš 2 gín illu *ba-lu-hi-im* 2 sìla a.geštin.na téš.bi *ina* ^{dug}kam *tu-šab-šal*

20 H [.. m]ud zabar *ana* gìš-šú dub-*ak*! ud.sa$_9$? kaš.sag šub-*di* [.........]

A šed$_7$ ì.giš bára.ga *ma-al-ma-liš* hi.hi *mi-iš-lam ina* mud zabar [*a-n*]*a mùš-tin-ni-su*! *ta-ša-pak* [*mi-i*]*š-lam ina* kaš.sag hi.hi

21 H [...$^{gi]š}$*šu-ši ina* ì.giš *hal-ṣi u* kaš nu *pa-tan* na[g-*ma* ....]

A [*ina* mul$_4$ *tu*]*š-bat ba-lum pa-tan* nag-*ma i-ne-eš*

22 H [... geštin. kal]a.ga hi.hi *e-nu-ma* tag-*šú* nu *pa-tan* [*ina-eš*]

16 [Ditto.....]..., fill your mouth with oil and you sprinkle the tip of his penis.

17 [..........]... with *kanaktu*, stir in oil, he drinks it for 3 days on an empty stomach and he will get better.

---

18 If a man has pain in his kidney, his groin hurts him, and his urine is white like donkey-urine, and later on his urine shows blood, that man

19 suffers from 'discharge'-disease. You boil together in a jug 2 shekels of myrrh, 2 shekels of *baluhhu*-resin, 2 *sila*-measures of vinegar;

20 cool it and mix it equally in pressed oil, and half of (the mixture) you pour into his urethra [in] a bronze tube, and the other half mix in premium beer,

21 [..], (var. you leave it [over night]), he drinks *šūšu* in pressed oil and beer on an empty stomach and he will get better.

22 [......................], mix strong [wine], when it affects him on an empty stomach, [he will get better].

Text No. 9 AMT 82,1 + duplicates = Tablet 3 diš na éllag-*su* gu$_{7}$-*šú* (plates 4–8)

I		K 4957 + 11742 + S 110 + 516 + 679 + 761 + 2058 (= AMT 82,1 + unpub. + unpub. + OECT 6 pl 16 + AMT 58,4 + AMT 61,5 + AMT 39,9); i 26–54, ii 24′–45′; iv 1′–28′.
J	=	K 2960 + 10268 + 14977 (AMT 58,3) + Rm. II, 315 (AMT 62,1); obv. and rev. are reversed, as in Ms. K below [text no. 10] = i 1–32; ii 3′–13; iii i′–13′; iv 20′–31′.
K	=	VAT 9024 = KAR 73 [text no. 10]; see Langdon, OECT 6, 56–57; obv. and rev. are reversed, as in Ms. J above; see new copy here. Edition: Ebeling ZDMG 74 (1920), 185 ff. and Landsberger, ibid. 443 f.; i, 46–ii 17.
E	=	VAT 13734 [text no. 5] (BAM 114) (collated 27-08-02) = ii 20–38
D	=	VAT 9870 + 10095 (BAM 112: 13′–16′) [text no. 4]; (collated 27-08-02) = ii 20′–23′.
YY	=	A 239 (BAM 161 iv 1′ ff.) = ii 28′–38′.
MM	=	K 9684 + (BAM 431 iv 27 ff.) [text no. 18] = ii 31′–38′.
NN	=	K 4164 + (BAM 430 iv 32′ ff.) [text no. 40] = ii 31′–38′. See also No. 40.
AAA	=	A 199 + VAT 9586 (BAM 171 44′–48′); (lines collated 27-08-02) = iv 10′–14′.
BBB	=	VAT 13789 (BAM 158 iv 26–33) = iv 10′–14′.
VV	=	YBC 7123 +, No. 9c + 9d: 9′; iv 31′ [text no. 48]

(**NB.**: ll. ii 39′–43′ appear similar to No. 11 6′–8′).

col. i

1	J	diš na da[b éllag-*su*		
	K	diš na dab éllag-*su* [..] x lá gig		
2	J	*lu* kàš [...		
3	J	2 gín [....................................	2 gín...........................	2 gín.............]
4	J	2 gín [....................................	2 gín..............................	2 gín.............]
5	J	2 gín [....................................	2 gín...........................	2 gín.............]
6	J	2 ⸢gín⸣ ^{ú}*kur-ka-n*[*u*	2 gín	2 gín ....]
7	J	2 gín ^{ú}*mir-gi-ra-nu*	2 g[ín	2 gín ....]
8	J	2 gín ^{ú}*sa-ma-num*	2 gí[n] x [.......	2 gín ....]
9	J	2 gín ^{ú}*pu-qut-tu*	2 gín ^{ú}*a-zal-l*[*e*	[2 gín ....]
10	J	2 gín ^{ú}geštin.ka$_{5}$.a	2 gín ^{ú}geštin.hád.du.a	[2 gín ....]
11	J	2 gín ^{ú}úkuš.ti.gil.kur.ra	2 gín ^{ú}úkuš.hab	[2 gín ....]
12	J	2 gín ^{ú}hab	2 gín ^{ú}*ak-tam*	[2 gín ....]
13	J	2 gín suhuš ^{ú}nam.tar níta	2 gín ^{ú}*lip* šáh[1]	[2 gín ....]
14	J	2 gín ^{šim}li	2 gín ^{šim}gam.ma	[2 gín ....]
15	J	2 gín illu li.dur	2 gín ^{šim}man.du	[2 gín ....]
16	J	2 gín $^{šim.d}$nin.urta níta	2 gín $^{šim.d}$maš mí	[2 gín ....]
17	J	2 gín ^{ú}nu.luh.ha	2 gín ^{ú}*úr-nu-u*	[2 gín ....]
18	J	2 gín ^{ú}hur.sag	2 gín ^{ú}*šu-mut-t*[*u*$_{4}$]	[2 gín ....]
19	J	2 gín ^{ú}kur.zi	2 gín ^{ú}zi-*a*[*h* zé][2]	[2 gín ....]
20	J	2 gín ^{na4}*nit-ku*	2 gín ^{na4}s[a......	2 gín ....]
21	J	2 gín gú.gal	2 gín g[ú.tur...........	2 gín ....]
22	J	2 gín ^{giš}hab 2 gín ^{giš}*nu-úr-ma*	2 [gín	2 gín ....]
23	J	2 gín numun ^{giš}ma.nu	[2 gín	2 gín ....]

[1] Presumably this is a 'pig-fat'-plant, like the 'fat of the gecko'-plant, see CAD L 204a.

[2] See DAB 235, 'plant to remove gall'.

TRANSLATION

1 If a man is affected, his kidney [....................] ... is ill,
2 or urine [..

---

3 2 shekels of [....., 2 shekels of ...., 2 shekels of .....
4 2 shekels of [....., 2 shekels of ...., 2 shekels of .....
5 2 shekels of [....., 2 shekels of ...., 2 shekels of .....
6 2 shekels of *kurkānû*, [2 shekels of ...., 2 shekels of ....
7 2 shekels of *mirgirānu*, 2 shekels [of ...., 2 shekels of ....
8 2 shekels of *samānu*, 2 shekels of [..., 2 shekels of ....
9 2 shekels of *puquttu*, 2 shekels of *azallû*, [2 shekels of ....
10 2 shekels of fox-vine, 2 shekels of raisins, [2 shekels of ....
11 2 shekels of cucumber, 2 shekels of gherkin, [2 shekels of .....
12 2 shekels of madder, 2 shekels of *aktam*, [2 shekels of ....
13 2 shekels of root of male mandrake, 2 shekels of 'pig-fat'-plant, [2 shekels of .....
14 2 shekels of *burāšu*-juniper, 2 shekels of *ṣumlalû*, [2 shekels of .....
15 2 shekels of *abukkatu*-resin, 2 shekels of *suādu*, [2 shekels of ....
16 2 shekels of male *nikiptu*, 2 shekels of female *nikiptu*, [2 shekels of ....
17 2 shekels of *nuhurtu*, 2 shekels of *urnû*, [2 shekels of ....
18 2 shekels of *azupīru*, 2 shekels of *šumuttu*, [2 shekels of .....
19 2 shekels of *samīdu*, 2 shekels of 'detox'-plant, [2 shekels of ....
20 2 shekels of *nitku*, 2 shekels of ...., [2 shekels of ....
21 2 shekels of peas, 2 shekels of lentils, [........, 2 shekels of ....
22 2 shekels of madder, 2 shekels of pomegranate, 2 [shekels of ...., 2 shekels of ....]
23 2 shekels of seed of *e'ru*-wood, [2 shekels of ...., 2 shekels of .....]

24	J	2 gin ^{ú}*šu-nu-'u*	[2 gín	2 gín ....]
25	J	2 gín ka.a.ab.b[a ...	2 gín peš$_4$] ⌜a⌝.ab.ba⌜	2⌝ [gín ....]
26	I	2 [gín ....]		
	J	2 gín gi.dub [*tam-ti*	2 gín ^{na4}pe]š$_4$.anše	2 gí[n ....]
27	I	2 g[ín...]		
	J	2 ⌜gín⌝ [............	2 gín ^{n}]^{a4}*mu-ṣa*	2 gín x [..............]
28	I	2 gí[n ....]	[2 gín ka$^?$.]a.ab.ba	⌜2⌝ [gín ^{n}]^{a4}an.zah.g[e$_6$]
	J	[....................	2 gín ^{n}]^{a4}an.zah	2 gín ^{n}[^{a4}an.zah.ge$_6$]
29	J	[2 gín ^{ši}]^{m}gam.⌜ma⌝	2 gín [^{na4}·]^{ú}níg.bùr.bùr	2 gín $^{na4.⌜ú⌝}$[níg.sì.s]ì
	I	2 gín [...........]	[2 gin...........bù]r	⌜2 gín⌝ $^{na4.ú}$níg.sì.sì
30	I	2 gín x [........................]	[2 gín .... ku]r.ra	2 gín ^{im}sahar.na$_4$.kur.ra
	J	[2 gín ^{im}sahar].⌜bábbar.kur.ra⌝	2 gín ^{im}sahar.ge$_6$.kur.ra	2 gín ^{im}saha[r.na$_4$.kur.r]a
31	I	2 gín x [..]	[2 gín ^{giš}níg].na$_4$	2 gín šika nunuz.ga.nu$_{11}$^{mušen}
	J	[...........^{n}]^{a4}*a-bat-te*	2 gín kak.[.................]	2 gín šika nunu[z.ga.nu$_{11}$^{muš}]^{en}
32	I	2 gín m[un ...]	[2 gín] ⌜*a*⌝*-ma-nim*	2 gín mun *buh-ri*
	J	[...............k]ù.pad$^?$	⌜2⌝ [gín] x [.............]	[2 gí]n mun *b*[*uh-ri*]
33	I	*šá-niš* 1/2 gí[n ....]	mun.meš	

34 I šu.nigin 90 [ú.hi.a *šá*] *hi-níq-ti* gal-*ú*[1]
35 I ú.hi.a *ina* x [.............] x *ina* ^{na4}na.zà.hi.li àr-*en*
36 I diš-*niš* hi.hi *ina* g[a ....] *ina* ge$_6$ *ana* igi mul.ud$_5$ gar-*an*
37 I níg.na ^{šim}l[i .... gar-*an* sisk]ur bal-*qí* ^{dug}a.da.gur$_5$ gub-*an*
38 I én [.....................-*t*]*u$_4$* 3-*šú* šid-*nu*

---

39 I én ⌜^{d}⌝[gu.la................] ⌜x *at-ti-ma*⌝ dingir.mah *at-ti-ma mu-bal-li-ṭa-at* a[d$_6$]
40 I *ú-* x [........................ -*š*]*ú-nu* igi.bar-*ma* nag-*šu lib-*⌜*luṭ*⌝
41 I [...................... na]m.dingir-*ti-ki* gal-*tu$_4$ lid-lul* tu$_6$ é[n]

---

42 I [........................] x *ina* kaš *lu ina* kaš.sag lú.tin.[na]
43 I ⌜*lu ina* geštin$^?$⌝ [n]ag.meš-*ma* ^{na4} ⌜*i la*⌝ x x [......................] x ti

---

44 I én ^{d}gu-la nin an-ta gal [an-ú]r-ta n[am-t]a-[è]
^{d}min gašan ⌜gal-*tu$_4$ is*⌝-[*tu i-šid* AN]-*e ina a-ṣi-*⌜*i-ki*⌝

---

45 I dingir-re-e-ne-k[e$_4$ ad-gi$_4$-gi$_4$ an-ú]r-ta nam-ta-è *ma-li-kát* [*ilī i-šid* AN-*e*] *ina a-ṣi-i-ki*

---

46 I ⌜mah-di⌝ [.......................................an-ú]r-ta nam-ta-è
K [...............] ⌜réme x x x ⌝ [...]
I *ti-*[*iz-qa-ar-tu šá* ....] *ú-dam-ma-qu* min
K [.......................] *ana* lú *re-e-ma* tuk-⌜*ú ú-dam*⌝-*m*[*a-*..] ki.min

---

47 I ud-g[im zálag .... an-ú]r-ta nam-ta-è
K [.................] an-zíb še-ga an-úr-ta nam-ta-è
I *te-*[*li-tu* ....-*t*]*i ma-gir-tu* min
K [x] *tu* [x] gim *u$_4$-me šu-pa-ta ma-gir*$^!$*-tu* ⌜ki.min⌝

---

1 *rubbû*, 'soak'.

24 2 shekels of *šunû*, [2 shekels of ......, 2 shekels of ....]
25 2 shekels of coral, 2 shekels of] sea-pebble, 2 [shekels of ....],
26 2 shekels *sea-stylus*(-insect), 2 shekels of] 'donkey-vulva'-shell, 2 shekels of [................],
27 2 shekels [of ....], 2 shekels of *muṣu*-stone, 2 shekels of [............],
28 2 shekels [of ...., 2 shekels] of frit, 2 shekels of black frit,
29 [2 shekels of] *ṣumlalû*, 2 shekels [of] *pallišu*-stone, 2 shekels of *sāpinu*-stone,
30 2 shekels of] *alluharu*, 2 shekels of *qitmu*, 2 shekels of alum,
31 2 shekels of *pumice*, 2 shekels of ... [........], 2 shekels of ostrich-egg shell,
32 2 shekels of block salt, 2 [shekels] of red salt, 2 shekels of steamed salt,
33 alternatively, half of shekel [.........] of salts.

---

34 Total, 90 [drugs] soaked [for] stricture.
35 ... the drugs in [.........], you grind up in a mortar,
36 mix (it) together, in milk? [...............] and place it at night before the Goat-star.
37 [You place] a censer (with) juniper [before Šamaš(?)], you perform a sacrifice, you set up an *adagurru*-vessel,
38 you recite the incantation [......] 3 times.

---

39 Incantation. [Gula ....] you indeed are the Bēlet-ilī, you indeed resurrect the dead,
40 she [.............], she noticed their [...], and may the one who drinks it be healthy.
41 Let him praise [..............] your (fem.) great divinity. Incantation spell.

---

42 He keeps drinking [.................] in beer or in premium tavern-beer
43 or in *wine* and....... -mineral [..............], he will recover.

---

44 Incantation. Gula, great lady from heaven, when you come up from the horizon,

---

45 O counsellor [of] the gods, when you come up from the [horizon],

---

46 highly [regarded one who], having mercy for the patient, makes (things) better when you come up from the horizon,

---

47 capable, brilliant like daylight, welcome one, when you come up from the horizon,

---

48	I	n[in é-šu-me-ša$_4$ ....]-gi-a ^{d}en-líl-lá ki-ág-gá ^{d}utu-u$_{18}$-lu
	K	[...] x [... siki]l mah-ke$_4$ é-gi$_{16}$-a ^{d}en-líl-lá ke$_4$-ág-gá ^{d}utu-u$_{18}$-lu-ke$_4$
	I	[........................ ....]-*tu kal-lat* ^{d}*en-líl* ⸢*na*⸣-*ram-ti* ^{d}*Ninurta*(maš)
	K	[GAŠA]N$^?$ ⸢*é-šu*⸣-*me-š*[*a*$_4$ si]kil[1]-*tú ṣir-tú kal-lat* ^{d}BE *na-ram-tu* ^{d}*Nin-urta*
49	I	g[á-e .... šà-an-s]ù-ud-da gù mu-ra-an-dé
	K	gá-e ìr ^{d}[gu-la ....]-sù-da gù-mur an-da
	I	*ana-k*[*u arad* ^{d}*gu-la ina qe-reb*] an-*e ru-qu-ti al-si-ki*
	K	*a-na-k*[*u* .... *qé*]-*reb* an-*e ru-qu-ti al-si-ki*
50	I	dili-m[u ....] du$_{11}$-ga gá-e geš-tuk-ma-ab
	K	di[li] gub-[................]-da-gar giš-tuku-a ugu-na
	I	⸢*e*⸣-[................ -*a*]*z-ki a-qab-bi ši-man-ni ia-a-ti*
	K	⸢*e-diš*⸣-[*ši-ia*] *a-za-az-ki a-qab-bi ši-man-ni a-a-ši*
51	I	mu ud x [..........-e]n igi-zu-šè a-ì gub-bu-da-a-mu
	K	mu gig-ga me-en ⸢igi⸣-zi-šè a-a gub-ba ad-mu
	I	*á*[*š*-...............................*m*]*a-har-ki az-ziz a-hu-lap-ia*
	K	*áš-šú mar-ṣa-ku-ma ma-*⸢*hir*⸣-*ki a-zi-iz a-hu-la-a-pí-ia*
52	I	g[al ......] gig-ga gá-e dili-mu a-mu
	K	gal ì-zu gig-ga gá-e dili-⸢mu⸣ a-a ad-mu
	I	[............................*m*]*ur-ṣi e-diš-ši-ia a-hu-lap-ia*
	K	⸢*ra-bi-tu*$_4$ *mu*⸣-*da-at mur-ṣi e-diš-*[*š*]*i-ia a-hu-la-a-pí-ia*
53	I	[...................... na]m-ti-la-ke$_4$ za-e-me-en
	K	igi mah ⸢zi⸣[2]-ba nam-⸢ti⸣-la-ke$_4$ za-e me-en
	I	[.............................. *na*]-*piš-ti ba-la-*[*ṭi*] *at-ti-ma*
	K	*ru-ba-tú ṣir-tú qa-i-šat na-piš-ti ba-la-ṭí at-*⸢*ti-ma*⸣
54	I	[..................................].gá tuku-ma-ra-ab
	K	[gaš]an-mu mu-⸢hun⸣-a hun-gá arhuš tuku-ma-ra-áb
	I	[.............................] *re-e-ma ri-ši-i*
	K	⸢*be-el-tu*⸣ *nu-hi-ma re-e-mu ri-še-e*
55	K	[...........n]u$^?$ gig nu ì$^!$-zu š[u]-mu mu-ni-in-dab
	K	[*mu*]-*še-zi-bat na-*⸢ *piš-ti*⸣ *mur-ṣi* ⸢*la*⸣ *i-du-ú qa-ti ṣab-ti*
56	K	en ud-da ti-la me-en ud gul (?) mu-un-ni-gá-gá
	K	*a-di u*$_4$*-mu ba-laṭ-ku*[3] *lud-lul*$^?$[4]*-ki*
57	K	⸢lú⸣-igi-du$_8$-a nam-dingir-zú [h]é-è
	K	[*a-mi*]-*ri li-ta-'-id* ⸢dingir⸣-*ut-ka*
58	K	[en na]m-ti-la me-en nam-mah-zú-⸢a⸣ du$_{11}$-ga
	K	[*a-di*] ⸢*bal-ṭa*⸣-*ku-ma nàr-bi-ki lu-uq-bi*
59	K	[gá-e lú-m]u$_7$-mu$_7$ ir$_{11}$-zú ka-tar-zú hé-me-s[i]l
	K	[*a-na-ku a-ši*]-*pu a-rad-ki da-lil-li*$^!$(text kal)-*ki lud-lul*

[1] For restoration, see CAD K 82a.
[2] or nam? Note that igi in this line is phonetic for egi.
[3] presumably for *balṭāku*.
[4] sign looks like lugal(!)

48 pure exalted Lady of Ešumeša, daughter-in-law of Enlil, beloved (wife) of Ninurta,

49 I, [Gula's] servant, have called on you in the midst of the remote heavens.

50 Alone I stand before you, I am speaking, listen to me!

51 Because I am ill, I stood before you, woe is me!

52 Great one who knows illness, I am alone, woe is me!

53 You are the august queen who grants good life and good health.

54 My lady, be calmed and have pity.

55 O she who saves lives -- help me (lit. take my hand, Sum. took my hand) with this unknown sickness,

56 (and) to as long as I am alive let me praise you.

57 May the onlooker praise your divinity,

58 (and) as long as I am alive let me praise you.

59 [I], your servant [the] incantation-priest, will praise you.

gap

col. ii

1′	K	⸢én⸣ *a-ta-mar* [*pa*]-⸢*né-e*⸣-*k*[*i* ^{d}gu-la *a-s*]*u-gal-la-tú ṣir-tú*
2′	K	x x [..................]-*šum at-ti-ma šu-luh-tú šu-pu-tú*
3′	J	⸢*a*⸣-*t*[*a-mar* ....]
	K	*e*[*b*]-*bé-ta a-t*[*a-mar ša*]*m-mu an-na-a šá-a ina* igi-*ki* íl-*ku*
4′	K	*ina u*$_4$*-me an-né-*⸢*e*⸣ [*lu p*]*àr-dan-nu lu šá-hi-hu*
	J	*ina u*$_4$*-mi* ⸢*an-né-e lu*⸣ [....................................]
5′	J	*lu mu-ṣu lu* dúr.gig ⸢*lu* murub$_4$ gig⸣ [..
	K	*lu mu-ṣu* / *lu hi-niq-tu l*[*u* dúr.gi]g *lu ta-ti-ka-te šá* kàš.meš tuku-*ši lu* gim *sin-niš-ti* g[iš.tu]kul sìg-*iṣ lu mim-ma mur-ṣu šá mar-ṣa-ku-ma*
6′	J	*at-ti* zu-*ú ana-ku* nu zu nag-*ti* [.............................]
	K	*at-ti ti-de-e a-na-ku la i-du-ú* / *šam-mu an-na-a* nag
7′	J	*ina šam-mi an-né-e lu-úb-luṭ ina šam-mi an-n*[*é-e* ....
	K	ú.meš *an-né-e lu-úb-luṭ lu-uš-lim lu*-si.sá
8′	J	⸢lál *ì*⸣-*lí* dingir-*ti-ki* gal-*tu*$_4$ *lud-lul* [tu$_6$.én]
	K	*da-lil* dingir-*ti-ki* gal-*ti lud-lul*[1]

9′	J	[én *a*]-*na* ^{d}*gu-la lik-tar-ra-ba ka-liš* [.......]
	K	*a-na* ^{d}*gu-la li*[*k-r*]*u-bu ka*$_{15}$(kak)-*liš* ub.meš
10′	J	[.... *tu*]-*du-qa-a ù bul-lu-ṭa š*[*u-*.........]
	K	*ša* tu$_6$.du$_{11}$.ga-⸢*šu*⸣ *bul-lu-ṭu šu-tu-rat*
11′	J	[......] *a-sa-ta mu-bal-li-ṭa-at* [....................]
	K	gal-*at a-su-tú mu-bal-li-ṭa-at* ^{d}*gu-la pa-líh-a*
12′	K	*ina qí-bit* ^{d}*ba-ba*$_6$ *ú-šar-bi* mu-*šá ana* dù.un.meš *a-zak-kar*
	J	[.........................] ⸢*ú-šar-bi*⸣ mu.ne *ana* dun.dun.meš [........]
13′	K	*ina* igi-*šá ki-i al-*⸢*li*⸣-*ka* 3-*šú tu-šad-bab-šú* ki.za.za
	J	[.............................b]i? ⸢x *kín* mu *ú*⸣-[......................]
14′	K	⸢*šá*⸣-*mu an-na-a* ⸢nag⸣-*ma* ki.za.za ur$_5$.gim du$_{11}$.ga
15′	K	[*šam-m*]*u ba-lá-ṭi šá* gašan-*ia* ⸢*al*⸣-*ta-ti a-na-ku*
16′	K	[.....-*a*]*l*?-*tú u ab-ta-luṭ* 3-⸢*šú*⸣ du$_{11}$.ga-*ma uš-ka-na*
17′	K	[.............]-⸢*ku šam*⸣-*mu an-na-*⸢*a* nag.meš-*ma*⸣ ti-⸢*uṭ*⸣

gap

20′	E	[.................................. gi]m kàš anše n[a.bi ....]
	D	[*šum*$_4$*-ma*] kàš.meš-*šú* gim kàš anše na.bi *mu-ṣa* gig
21′	E	[... -*šu*]*m-me* kaš na.bi *m*[*u-*.......]
	D	[*šum*$_4$*-ma*] kàš.meš-*šú* gim *šur-šum-me* kaš na.bi *mu-ṣa* gi[g]
22′	E	[..] *šur-šum-me* geštin [min]
	D	[*šum*$_4$*-ma*] kàš.meš-*šú* gim *šur-šum-me* geštin na.bi *mu-ṣa* gi[g]
23′	E	[.................................. g]im še.gín *he-li-ti* [min]
	D	[*šum*$_4$*-ma*] kàš.meš-*šú* gim še.gín *he-li-ti* [min]
24′	I[2]	él[lag ....
25′	I	kà[š ....
26′	I	*šum*$_4$*-*⸢*ma* kàš-*šú* gim a.m[eš ....
	E	[......................] gim a.meš gazi^{sar} na.bi ud.da k[ur-*id*]

---

[1] There is no ruling in KAR 73.

[2] This is the first preserved line of col. ii.

col. ii

1′ Incantation. I beheld your face, [O Gula], august healer,
2′ [..........], you are supreme and pre-eminent (var. the pure one),
3′ I beheld this drug which I hold up before you.
4′ On this very day, (the patient) has either *pardannu* or *šahhihu*-diseases,
5′ either discharge (var. or stricture) or rectal disease or loin disease, or dribbling of urine, or one is struck by a weapon like a (menstruating) woman, or whatever illness with which I am sick,
6′ and you know what I do not know: am I to drink this drug?
7′ With these drugs let me be healthy, let me be well, let me be happy,
8′ so that I may praise your great divinity! [Incantation spell].

9′ Incantation. In every corner let them bless Gula,
10′ who is supreme in spells and healing,
11′ great is her medicine, Gula heals those who revere her.
12′ By the command of Baba I will praise and call her name to everyone,
13′ when I go before her. Three times you will have him recite it (the incantation) and he will bow down,
14′ he will drink this drug and bow down, and recite thusly:
15′ 'I drank this healing drug of my goddess,
16′ [..] and I was cured'. He says this three times and bows down.
17′ [........] he keeps drinking this drug and he will recover.
18′–19′ (fragmentary)

Ms. A col. ii with duplicates

20′ [If] his urine is like an ass' urine, that man suffers from discharge.
21′ [If] his urine is like beer dregs, that man suffers from discharge.
22′ [If] his urine is like wine dregs, that man suffers from discharge.
23′ [If] his urine is like clear paint / glue, that man suffers from discharge.
24′ kidney [......................................
25′ urine [.......................................
26′ If his urine is like *kasû*-juice, that man is overcome by sun-fever.

27′	I	*šum$_4$-ma* kàš-*šú* s[ig$_7$ ....]
	E	[m]in sig$_7$ *hi-niq-ti* murub$_4$ [gig]
28′	I	*šum$_4$-ma* kàš-*šú* babbar-*ma e-ba-a* [
	E	min babbar-*ma e-ba-a* na.bi na$_4$ *šá-hi-h*[*u* gig][1]
	YY	[...] gig
29′	I	*šum$_4$-ma* kàš-*šú* gim $^{na4!}$duh.ši.a [............]
	E	min gim ^{na4}duh.ši.e na.bi na$_4$ [gig]
	YY	*šum$_4$-ma* kàš-*š*[*ú* ....] duh.ši.a na.bi na$_4$ g[ig]
30′	I	*šum$_4$-ma* kàš-*šú* gim *šá gi-na-a* murub$_4$^{2}-*šú u* [..........
	E	min gim *šá gi-na-a* murub$_4$.meš-šú *u* sag šà-*š*[*ú* x x] na.bi *hi-niq-ti* dúr gig
	YY	*šum$_4$-ma* kàš-*šú* gim *šá gi*-[...] murub$_4$.meš-šú *u* sag šà-*šú* gu$_7$-[*šú*] na.bi *hi-niq-ti* éllag gig

---

31′	I	*ana* ti-*šú* ^{ú}*tara-muš* ^{ú}igi-*lim* ^{ú}ig[i-*ešra* ....
	E	*ana* [....] ^{ú}*tara-muš* ^{ú}igi-*lim* ^{ú}igi-*ešra* ka.a.ab.ba ^{š}[^{im} ...]
	YY	*ana* ti-*šú* ^{ú}*tara-muš* ^{ú}igi-*lim* ^{ú}igi-*ešra* ka.a.ab.ba
	MM	om. ^{ú}*tara-muš* ^{ú}igi-*lim* ^{ú}igi-*ešra* ka.a.ab.ba
	NN	^{ú}*tara-muš* ^{ú}igi-*lim* ^{ú}igi-*ešra* [.... a]b.ba
32′	I	^{na4}*ga-bi-i* na$_4$.pa ^{na4}n[i.bu ....
	E	^{šim}li na$_4$.pa ^{na4}ni.bu ^{na4}*ga-*[*bi-i*] ^{na4}peš$_4$.anše ^{ú}kur.kur ^{ú}níg.sù.s[ù]
	YY	^{šim}gúr.gúr ^{giš}li ^{na4}*ga-bi-e* na$_4$.pa ^{na4}*iá-ni-ba* ^{na4}peš$_4$.anše ^{ú}kur.kur ^{ú}níg.sù.sù
	MM	^{šim}gúr.gúr ^{šim}li ^{na4}*ga-be-e* na$_4$.pa ^{na4}ni.bu ^{na4}peš$_4$.anše ^{ú}kur.kur $^{na4.ú}$níg.bùr.bùr
	NN	^{šim}gúr.gúr [...l]i ^{na4}*ga-be-e* na$_4$.pa [....].bu ^{na4}peš$_4$.anše [......k]ur ^{ú}níg.bùr.bùr
33′	I	^{na4ú}níg.bùr.bùr ba.ba.za.^{d}í[d ....]
	E	^{ú}níg.bùr.bùr ba.ba.za.^{d}íd numun ^{ú}eme.ur.g[i$_7$]
	YY	$^{na4.ú}$níg.bùr.bùr ba.ba.za.^{d}íd numun ^{ú}eme.ur.gi$_7$ ú dili ka.a.ab.ba
	MM	$^{na4.ú}$níg.sù.sù bá.bá.za.^{d}íd numun ⸢^{ú}⸣[..........g]i$_7$ *kar-áš tam-tim*
	NN	[..........s]ù.sù bá.bá.za.^{d}íd [........................u]r.gi$_7$ *kar-áš tam-tim*
34′	I	*mi-sis* a.ab.ba ^{ú}nu.lu[h.ha ....
	E	⸢*mi*⸣-*sis tam-tim ka-ra-áš tam-tim* [^{ú}nu.lu]h.ha ^{ú}*úr-nu-u*
	YY	*mì-sis tam-ti* ^{ú}nu.luh *ti-iá-tú* ^{ú}*úr-nu-u*
	MM	*mi-sis tam-tim* ^{ú}nu.luh.ha ^{ú}*ti-iá-tú* ^{ú}*ur-nu-u*
	NN	[.............-*ti*]*m* ^{ú}nu.luh.ha [..........] ^{ú}*ur-nu-u*
35′	I	^{ú}har.har ^{ú}*šib-bur-ra*[*t* ....
	E	^{ú}har.har [........*bu*]*r-rat* ^{ú}*ha-hi-in* ^{ú}geštin.ka$_5$.a [..............
	YY	^{ú}har.har luh.mar.tú ^{ú}u$_4$$^{!}$.hi.in ^{ú}geštin.ka$_5$.a ^{ú}kur.ra
	MM	^{ú}har.har ⸢^{ú}⸣*šib-bur-ra-tu$_4$* ^{ú}*ha-hi-in* [^{ú}geš]tin.ka$_5$.a ^{ú}kur.r[a$^{!}$]
	NN	[......ha]r ^{ú}*šib-bur-ra-tú* [................] ^{ú}geštin.ka$_5$.a [........]
36′	I	^{ú}lag.a.šà šika nunuz ga.n[u$_{11}$ ....
	E	⸢ú⸣ babbar ^{giš}sila$_{11}$.gá šika nunuz.gá.na^{mušen}[.........................^{giš}]ma.nu $^{ú.zì}$nu.luh.ha [.......................^{ú}]nu.úr.ma [.....................]
	YY	ú babbar ^{ú}lag.gán šika nunuz.ga.nu$_{11}$^{mušen}numun ^{giš}*b*[*i-n*]*i* numun ^{giš}ma.nu ^{ú}*an-nu-ha-ru*
	MM	[ú babb]ar [^{ú}lag].gán šika nunuz.[................................-*n*]*i* numun ^{giš}[....] ⸢^{ú}⸣[......h]a.ra
	NN	[............] ^{ú}lag.gán [................................. n]umun ^{giš}*bi-ni* [....................] [^{ú}a]n.nu.ha.ra

---

1 see YBC 7123 + 22′ (text No. 48), na$_4$ *šah-hi-hu* gig

27′ If his urine is yellow, that man [suffers] from stricture of the groin.
28′ If his urine is white and thick, that man [suffers] from a dissolving calculus.
29′ If his urine is like *dušû*-stone, that man [suffers] from a calculus.
30′ If his urine is as normal, his groin and epigastrium hurt [him]; that man suffers from stricture of the kidney (var. rectum).

31′ To cure him: *taramuš*, *imhur-lim*, *imhur-ešra*, coral,
32′ alum, mussel(-shell), *janibu*-stone, and 'donkey-vulva'-shell; *ata'išu*, *sāpinu*,
33′ *pallišu*-plant/stone, white gypsum, seed of the 'dog's tongue', 'single'-plant, coral,
34′ sea-*missis*, *nuhurtu*, sea leek (var. *tiātu*), *urnû*,
35′ *hašû*, rue, *hahin* (thorny plant), fox-vine, *nīnû*,
36′ field-clod plant (var. 'white' plant), ostrich-egg shell, tamarisk seed, *e'ru*-wood seed, *annuharu*,

37′	I	gú.gal gú.níg.àr.ra ^{giš}x.[..
	E	[...g]al gú.níg.àr [...
	YY	gú.gal gú.níg.àr.ra ^{giš}hab šika ^{giš}*nu-úr-ma-a* ^{ú}*nu-ṣa-ba*
	MM	gú.gal g[ú].n[íg...] ^{giš}hab ši[ka .....-*ú*]*r-ma-a* ^{ú}*nu*-[....]
	NN	[.........................r]a ^{giš}h[a]b [..........................*n*]*u-ṣa-b*[*u*]
38′	I	36 ú.meš *mu-ṣi šá* gar.m[eš................ *i*]*na* geštin *lu ina* kaš n[ag ....]
	E	36 ú.hi.a [............................*l*]*u ina* geštin nag
	YY	36 ú.hi.a šeš diš-*niš* gaz sim *lu ina* geštin *lu ina* [ka]š *lu ina* ga na[g-*ma* ti]
	MM	36 ⸢ú⸣.[meš *mu-ṣ*]*i šá* gar.meš mah.meš
	NN	[.. ma]h.meš
39′	I	diš na *lu* na$_{4}$ *mu-ṣa* gig [....................................
40′	I	*lu* si tùm[1] ....[...
41′	I	^{ú}*zi-im* kù.babbar ^{ú}níg.⸢bùr.bùr⸣ [...................]
42′	I	^{na4}peš$_{4}$.anše šika.nunuz.ga.nu$_{11}$^{mušen} ka.a.[a.ba]
43′	I	diš-*niš* ⸢súd *lu*⸣ *ina* kaš.sag *lu ina* geštin na[g-*ma ina-eš*][2]
44′	I	⸢dub 3⸣.[kám] diš na éllag-*su* [gu$_{7}$-*šú*][3]
	C	diš ki.min x [..................................]
45′	I	[........... š]à$^{?}$ gìš-*šú ip-pu-uš* ^{šim}šeš x [..................

(bottom of tablet)

rev. col. iii

1′	J	(traces)
2′	J	*ina* a gazi^{sar} luh [.........................
3′	J	diš ki.min ^{giš}geštin.ka$_{5}$.a *tur-ár* súd šà gìš-*šú* diri [.......[4]
4′	J	diš ki.min numun ^{ú}*tu-lál tur-ár* súd šà gìš-*šú* diri [.......[5]
5′	J	diš ki.min ^{na4}peš$_{4}$.anše *tur-ár* súd šà gìš-*šú* diri [.......[6]
6′	J	diš ki.min ^{na4}áš.har *ina* ì.nun sú[d ....
7′	J	diš ki.min ^{na4}áš.har ^{na4}an.zah *ina* ì.nun súd [..........
8′	J	diš ki.min numun ^{giš}esi gaz sim *ina* a gazi^{sar} *u* ga *tara-ba*[*k* ....[7]
9′	J	diš na šà gìš-*šú* gig-ma kàš-*šú* bi.iz.bi.iz gazi^{sar} *tur*-[*ár* ....
10′	J	*ana* igi gìš-*šú* mar *ina* a gazi^{sar} kúm.meš-*ti* luh-*šú* a x [........[8]
11′	J	[diš k]i.min ^{giš}geštin.ka$_{5}$.a súd šà gìš-*šú* diri gim ùb$^{?}$ *pi-lu-ú ina* a gazi$^{s[ar}$ ...][9]
12′	J	[................ s]úd šà gìš-*šú* diri gim ⸢ùb$^{?}$ x x⸣ [................
13′	J	[.............................] ⸢šà gìš-*šú* diri gim⸣ [..................

1 See Sm 467 = AMT 58,5 : 3 (text No. 2, B$_{4}$), sa tùm, although both contexts are obscure.
2 Lines 39′–43′ here are similar to Text No. 11 below, ll. 6′–8′, but are not duplicates.
3 See Rm II, 375 : 6′ (text No. 13), and YBC 7123 + No. 9c: 8′ (text No. 48).
4 Probably a simplicium.
5 Probably a simplicium.
6 Probably a simplicium.
7 Simplicium.
8 Possibly a simplicium.
9 Possibly a simplicium.

37′ peas, pulses, madder, pomegranate-rind, *nuṣābu*,

38′ 36 plants for the principal symptoms of 'discharge' [...] (var.: pound and sift), he drinks them in wine or beer (var. or milk) [and he will recover].

39′ If a man either suffers from stone / discharge, [...................

40′ or ... [...

41′ 'silver-lustre'-plant, bore-stone, [.....................

42′ 'donkey-vulva'(-shell), ostrich-egg shell, coral,

43′ crush together, he drinks it either in premium beer or in wine, [and he will get better].

44′ Tablet 3 of: 'If a man's kidney [hurts him]'.

45′ [....................], the *shaft* of his penis has expanded, myrrh, ... [..........................

rev. col. iii

2′ Wash him in *kasû*-juice [............].

3′ If ditto, dry out and crush fox-vine and soften the *shaft* of his penis [......].

4′ If ditto, dry out and crush seed of *tullal*[1], soften the *shaft* of his penis [......].

5′ If ditto, dry out and crush 'donkey-vulva'(-shell), soften the *shaft* of his penis [......].

6′ If ditto, crush *ashar* in ghee [.......................]

7′ If ditto, crush *ashar* and frit in ghee [......].

8′ If ditto, pound and sift the seed of *ušû*(-wood), you stir it in *kasû*-juice and milk, [........

9′ If a man is 'ill' in the *shaft* of his penis, constantly dribbling urine, you dry out *kasû*, [.....

10′ daub it on the opening of his penis, cleanse it in hot *kasû*-juice and juice of [.......].

11′ If ditto, crush fox-vine, soften the *shaft* of his penis like *a drum* in *kasû*-juice [....].

12′ [If ditto,] crush [...], soften the *shaft* of his penis like *a drum* [.........................]

13′ [If ditto ......] soften the *shaft* of his penis like [a drum? ....].

[1] lit., 'you purify'-plant.

col. iv

1′	I	⸢a.meš x⸣ [...............................]
2′	I	^{ú}hur.[sag[1] ....]
3′	I	*sah-lé-e* [..................................]
4′	I	gazi^{sar} im [...............................]
5′	I	*a-na na-šá-hi* [...........................][2]
6′	I	*ana* im *ka-li-t*[*e ka-le-e* ....]
7′	I	^{ú}*la-ha-ga* ⸢*u*⸣ [...][3]
8′	I	$^{[n]a4}$lagab.munu$_4$ *ta-šar-*[*rap*.............................]
9′	I	[*ina*] ^{urudu}šen.tur *tara-*[*bak ina* ^{kuš}edin sur-*re* lá-*ma* ...]
10′	I	[*ana š*]*i-me-er-te ka-li-te š*[*u-* ....]
	AAA	*ana ši-me-er-te ka-liš-ma šu-*⸢*ṣe*⸣*-e* lú ti.la ^{šim}gúr.gúr
	BBB	*ana ši-me-er-te ka-li-šu šu-ṣe-e* lú ti ^{šim}gúr.gúr
11′	I	[.................. nu]mun ^{ú}*tara-muš*$_8$! [...........................]
	AAA	^{šim}li ^{ú}har.har numun *tara-muš*$_8$ ⸢^{ú}⸣[.........] ^{ú}*ba-ri-ra-t*[*ú*]
	BBB	^{šim}li ^{ú}har.har numun *tara-muš*$_8$ ^{ú}*ka-man-tú* ^{ú}*ba-ri-ra-tú*
12′	I	[.......... *an-nu*]*-ti te-ṭe*$_4$*-*[*en*..............]
	AAA	6 ú.meš *te-ṭe*$_4$*-en* [....] zà.li!.a^{sar}
	BBB	6 ú.hi.a šeš àr-*en* sim *sah-lé-e*
13′	I	[....................... téš].bi hi.h[i ....]
	AAA	*i-na* dida [..................] *ina* šen.tur *ta-*⸢*rab*⸣*-*[*bak*]
	BBB	ki dída sig$_5$.ga [téš].bi hi.hi *ina* šen.tur *tara-bak*
14′	I	[........................] x [...............]
	AAA	*ina* ^{kuš}edin *te-ṭá-*[*ri* ....]
	BBB	[*ina* ^{k}]^{uš}edin.a šur.re lá-*su-ma* ti
15′	I	[..................] x x [................] ud [.....]
16′	I	[..........] *ana* ugu *tu-*x x [.....................]
17′	I	[.........] x ^{šim}li súd [................^{ú}igi-*lim*]
18′	I	[^{ú}]igi-*ešra ina* ì.giš hi.h[i ....]
19′	I	[diš n]a šir-*šú mun-ga* dab *ta-tak-kip-ma mun-g*[*u* ....
20′	I	diš na šir-*šú* lugud *ú-kal ta-mah-haṣ-ma nab-ra-a* [.............
	J[4]	[............................] ⸢*ú-kal ta-mah-haṣ*⸣*-*[.........................
21′	I	diš na *mi-qit ir-ri* tuku eme.šid.edin.na há[d.a ......]
	J	[...........*-q*]*it ir-ri* tuku eme.šid.edin.na hád.a gaz s[im]
22′	I	eme.šid.edin.na sum^{sar}.šir.dili [.............]
	J	[....ši]d.edin.na sum^{sar}.šir.dili šeg$_6$-*šal* g[u$_7$]
23′	I	gír.tab ti.la ud.3.kam *ana* ì.giš šub [...]
	J	[........] ti.la ud.3.kam *ana* ì.giš šub ki.ta-*šú* šéš

[1] or ú.har.[har.

[2] CAD N/2 s. v. hapax: 'to have diarrhoea'

[3] see BAM 171 39′.

[4] This was given by Thompson (AMT 62,1) as col. i.

col. iv

1′–5′ (fragmentary)
6′ In order to [restrain] 'flatulence' of the kidneys, [............
7′ *lahagu*-plant, ...[..
8′ you burn lumps of malt [................
9′ you decoct (everything) into a small vessel [spread it on a leather strip and tie it on....]

10′ To rid a healthy man (var. entirely) of *šimertu*-disease of the kidneys: *kukru*,
11′ juniper, *hašû*, seed of *taramuš*, *kamantu*, *barīrātu*,
12′–13′ you grind up and sift these 6 plants; mix *sahlû* together with *frothy*[1] *billatu*-beer and decoct (it) into a small vessel,
14′ you spread it on a leather-strip and bind it on him and he will recover.

15′ ....
16′ ....
17′ crush [........], juniper, mix [...................*imhur-lim*]
18′ and *imhur-ešra* in oil [...and he will recover].

19′ [If a] man's testicle is affected by stiffness, you prick (it) and the stiffness [......]

20′ If a man's testicle contains pus, you stir (the *materia medica*) and *a vessel* [.........]

21′ If a man has shown symptoms of 'collapse of the intestines', you dry out, pound and sieve a desert-lizard [......],
22′ you boil a desert lizard and a single-clove garlic and he eats (it).
23′ Put a live scorpion in oil for 3 days, anoint his lower parts.

---

[1] sig_5 = *našpu*, with the meaning inferred from *našāpu*, 'to blow'.

24′	I	diš ki.min eme.šid.zi.da šeg$_6$-*šal* gu$_7$ ^{š}[^{im}..]
	J	[.....................š]id.zi.da šeg$_6$-*šal* gu$_7$ ^{šim}im.man.du illu ^{šim}bulug ^{šim}⸢li⸣ [...]
25′	I	^{šim}gúr.gúr ^{šim}šeš ^{ú}*b*[*a*-..]
	J	[............ ^{š}]^{im}šeš![1] ^{ú}*ba-ri-ra-ta ina* dè ^{giš}kiši$_{16}$ *tu*-[*qat*]-*tar*
26′	I	diš lú.tur *šá* mí n[u].z[u ....]
	J	[.......................n]u.zu *mi-qit ir-ri* tuku *up-pat tim-bu*-[*ut-t*]*a*
27′	I	hád.a súd [..]
	J	[................................ *in*]*a* kaš nag *ina* ì [šé]š
28′	I	*šum*$_4$-⸢*ma*⸣ x [..]
	J	*šum*$_4$*-ma* x [..................-*t*]*i nap-šal-ti* nu.⸢dug$_8$⸣?
29′	J	*šum*$_4$*-ma* šir 1[5 ....*ina*] maš.sìla 150-*šú* kúm [gar]-*an*
30′	J	*šum*$_4$*-ma* šir 15[0 .... *ina*] maš.sìla 15-*šú* k[úm gar]-*an*
31′	J	(catchline): diš na *ina la si-ma-ni-šú* murub$_4$.[meš-*šú* gu$_7$.meš-*šú* du$_{10}$.gam?.me]š?-⸢*šú*?⸣[2] x ga x [..........] x
	VV	DUB 3 KÁM diš na *ina la si*-[..] x na
	J	colophon = BAK No. 329, same as No. 24 below

[1] erasure.
[2] see AMT 43,1 (text No. 22) and YBC 7123+ 11′ (text No. 48).

24′ If ditto, you boil an *anduhallatu*-lizard and have him eat it, (aromatics:) you fumigate *suādu*, *baluhhu*-resin, juniper,
25′ *kukru*, myrrh, and *barīrātu* on *ašagu*-thorn coals.
26′ If a virgin boy has 'collapse of the intestines', dry out and crush *mole cricket*
27′ [....................] he drinks it in beer and rub him in oil.

28′ If [his ....]., a salve not ....
29′ If [his] right testicle [...], heat and place [........ on] his left shoulder,
30′ If [his] left testicle [...], heat and place [......... on] his right shoulder.

31′ If a man [has pain in his] groin prematurely. (Catchline)
Tablet 3 of éllag.gig and catchline of Tablet 1 of *ina lā simānišu*.

No. 10 KAR 73 (plates 9–10)
Ms. K = VAT 9024 (= KAR 73) rev. 1–14

1 [*e-nu-m*]*a* diš na *lu-u pàr-dan-nu lu-u š*[*a*]*ḫ-ḫi-ḫ*[*u*]
2 [*mu*]*-ṣu lu-u ḫi-niq-tú* ⸢*lu-u*⸣ dúr gi[g]
3 [*ta*]*-ti-ka-te šá* kàš.meš tuku-*ši*[1]
4 *lu-u ki-ma sin-niš-ti kak-ku* sìg-*i*[*ṣ*]
5 *lu-u mim-ma mur-ṣu šá-niš-ma la-a* zu-*ú*
6 dù.dù.bi *ina* igi ^{d}*gu-la ina* ùr ki kéš
7 a.meš ^{šim}li kù.meš sù gi.guḫšu(sig$_4$+sig$_4$.šú) ⸢tur$^?$ gar⸣-*an*
8 zú.lum.ma *tas-qé-e* dub-*aq* ninda.ì.dé.a ⸢làl ì.nun.na⸣ gar-*an*
9 ^{dug}a.da.gur$_5$ gub-*an lu* siskur kù *l*[*u ik-ri-b*]*u*(?) dù-*uš*
10 uzu.zag.lu uzu.me.ḫé uzu.ka.izi gar-*an*
11 ^{ú}ḫar.ḫar ^{ú}kur.kur ú *mat-qu* ú dili $^{⸢ú⸣}$sumun.dar *saḫ-lé-e*
12 diš-⸢*niš*⸣ súd *ina* kaš.sag šub-*di a-na* igi ^{d}*gu-la* gub-*an*
13 ⸢lú.gig⸣ dùg.gam$^!$-*su-ma* šu-*ka ina muḫ*-⸢*ḫi-šú*⸣ *tu*-[*qa*]*t*-⸢*tar*⸣(?)
14 *te-re-qam-*[*m*]*a*[2] kaš.sag *ša* gub-*nu* gig.bi *ina* šu-[*šú* í]l-*ma* ur$_5$.gim du$_{11}$.ga

---

[1] See text No. 9 ii 5′.
[2] Cf. CAD R 267, passim in rituals.

TRANSLATION

1 When (it is the case): if a man (suffers from) either *pardannu* or *šahhihu*-disease,
2 discharge or stricture or a rectal disease,
3 he constantly has dripping urine,
4 or (as if) being struck by a weapon like a (menstruating) woman,
5 or whatever other illness which is not recognised,
6 its remedy (lit. ritual): in front of Gula, on a roof, the place of ritual preparation,
7 you sprinkle pure juices of juniper, you set up a *small* alter,
8 (on which) you sprinkle dates and *sasqû*-flour, you place *mirsu*-cakes of honey and butter,
9 you set up an *adagurru*-vessel (and) you either make a pure offering or a *prayer.*
10 You set (on the alter) the shoulder, the fatty meat and the roast-meat,
11 crush together *hašû*, *ata'išu*, sweet-plant, 'single'-plant, *šumuttu*, *sahlû*,
12 place (them) in premium beer, place it before Gula.
13 Have the patient kneel and you *fumigate* your hand over him,
14 you withdraw and that patient raises up in [his] hand the premium beer which you set out and recite thus: (incantation follows, see above, text No. 9 col. ii 1′ – 17′).

No. 11 Ms.L = K 6493 + 6811 + Bu 91-5-9, 52 (+) K 10676 (unpubl.) (plates 11–12)

The non-physical join is not based upon textual parallels but on the distinctive similarities in appearance of the tablets.

1′ (trace)
2′ [..g]a$^{?}$ ^{giš}nu.ú[r.ma ....]
3′ [..] x ^{giš}nu.úr.m[a ....]
4′ [..] x *lu ina* kaš *lu ina* [geštin]
5′ [..] nu *pa-tan* nag [ti]

6′ [...] ⸢^{ú}⸣níg.bùr.bùr peš$_4$.anše ka *tam-t*[*i*]
7′ [...] x šika nunuz.ga.nu$_{11}$^{mušen} numun ^{giš}kiš[i$_{16}$]
8′ [...] *lu ina* kaš *lu ina* geštin na[g][1]

9′ [1 gín ....] ⸢gín⸣ [.............................. 1 g]ín ^{ú}*tara-muš* 2 gín ^{ú}x
10′ ⸢1⸣ [gín] ^{ú}igi-*li*[*m* ....] ⸢1⸣ gín ú dili 1 gín numun ^{ú}[..]
11′ 2 gín *úr-n*[*é-e* ....] ⸢2⸣ gín ^{ú}gur$_4$.hab[2] 2 gín ^{ú}tur.[ra^{3}]
12′ 2 gín ^{ú}ku[r.kur ....*nu-ṣa*]-⸢*bu*⸣ 2 gín ^{ú}*a-ra-r*[*i-a-nu*]
13′ 2 ⸢gín ^{ú}⸣.[...] ⸢^{ú}*sa*⸣-*ma-nu* 2 gín ^{ú}[.......]
14′ 2 gín ⸢^{ú}⸣gír [...] x x 2 gín ^{ú}ú[kuš..hab]
15′ 1 gín ⸢ú⸣ babbar 2 g[ín ....] x 2 gín na$_4$.[......]
16′ 1 gín ⸢^{ú}⸣úkuš.ti.g[i.la ....] ⸢gín⸣ [............]
17′ 1 gín ⸢^{ú}⸣hab 2 g[ín ....]
18′ 1 [gí]n ⸢$^{ú.giš}$⸣*šu*-⸢*šum*⸣ 2 ⸢gín x⸣ [...]
19′ [..................] x a 2 ⸢gín ^{ú}x⸣ [...]
20′ 1 [gín ....] ⸢*pa-har*⸣ [...]
21′ 2 g[ín ...]-*tu$_4$* ⸢2 gín ^{ú}⸣[...]
22′ 2 gí[n ....] ⸢2⸣ gín ^{šim}gam.m[a] ⸢2 gín x⸣ [..................................]
23′ 1 g[ín ....] 2 gín šika nunuz.ga.⸢nu$_{11}$^{mušen}⸣ [.........................]
24′ [x gín .... ^{ú}k]ur.ra 2 gín x x [..]
25′ [x gín ....] ka *tam-*[*ti* ....]
26′ [x gín ....] gu x x [...]
27′ (traces)

rev.
28′ 2 ⸢gín⸣ ^{na4}*mu-ṣa* 2 gí[n ....] ⸢2 gín ^{na4}an.zah⸣ [....]
29′ 2 gín ^{na4}*si-mi* 2 gín níg.na$_4$[4] ⸢2⸣ gín <gín>*a-bat-ti* 2 ⸢gín⸣ [.........]
30′ 2 gín ⸢^{na4}⸣peš$_4$.anše 2 gín ^{na4}peš$_4$.a.ab.ba 2 gín ^{na4}x [...............]
31′ 2 ⸢gín⸣ $^{na4.ú}$níg.sù.sù 2 gín na$_4$.zálag 2 gín gú.[ga]l$^{?}$ 2 g[ín gú.tur]
32′ 2 gín gú.níg.àr.ra 2 gín ^{ú}hab-*a-nu*[5] 2 gín naga.si 2 gín [.......]
33′ 2 gín ^{šim}gig 2 gín illu li.tar 2 gín ^{ú}*zi-bu-u* 1/2 g[ín ....]
34′ 1/2 gín mun.ku.pad[6] 1/2 gín mun *a-ma-nim* 1/2 gín mun [*buh-ri*][7]

---

[1] Ll. 6′–8′ are similar to No. 9 ii 39′–43′.
[2] A variant for ^{ú}gír.hab = *dadānu*? The reading kiši$_{16}$ for ú.gír follows the giš-determinative.
[3] See DAD 203 (= *haltappānu*, although not in AHw).
[4] See text No. 4 : 21, in which gi$_6$.na$_4$ is a variant for gi$_6$.pàr.
[5] = *bušānu*?
[6] for kù.pad (*šibirti ṭabti*)
[7] Cf. No. 9: 32 above.

TRANSLATION

2′ [..], ... pomegranate, [.............
3′ [..],.. pomegranate, [..............
4′ [..].. either in beer or in [wine],
5′ [..................................], he drinks it on a empty stomach [and he will recover].

6′ [..], *pallišu*-stone, 'donkey-vulva'(-shell), coral,
7′ [...].. ostrich-egg shell, acacia seed,
8′ [.......................................] he drinks it either in beer or in wine.

9′ [1 shekel of ...., x] shekels of [................, 1] shekel of *taramuš*, 2 shekels of ...
10′ 1 [shekel] of *imhur-līm*, [1 shekel of ...] 1 shekel of 'single'-plant, 1 shekel of seed of [...]
11′ 2 shekels of *urnû*, [x shekels of .. ..] 2 shekels of *dadānu*$^{?}$, 2 shekels of *hašû*,
12′ 2 shekels of *ata'išu*, [............... 2 shekels of] *nuṣābu*$^{?}$, 2 shekels of *arariānu*,
13′ 2 shekels of ..[........, 2 shekels of ...., 2 shekels of] *samānu*-plant, 2 shekels of [...]
14′ 2 shekels of *ṣadānu*, [x shekels of ....., 2 shekels of] ..., 2 shekels of cucumber,
15′ 1 shekel of 'white'-plant, 2 shekels [of ....], 2 shekels of [....]-stone,
16′ 1 shekel of gourd, [2 shekels of ....]...
17′ 1 shekel of madder, 2 shekels [of ....
18′ 1 shekel of *šūšu*-tree$^{?}$, 2 shekels of ..[...
19′ [x shekels of ....] ... 2 shekels of ... [..................................
20′ 1 [shekel of ....] .... [..
21′ 2 shekels [of .....]..., 2 shekels of ...[....................................
22′ 2 shekels [of ....], 2 shekels of *ṣumlalû*, 2 shekels of [...........
23′ 1 shekel of [...............], 2 shekels of ostrich-egg shell, [.................
24′ [x shekels ...., x shekels of] *nīnû*, 2 shekels of ... [..............
25′ [x shekels of ...., x shekels of] coral, [.......................
26′ [x shekels of ....] .....[...................................
27′ ....

rev.

28′ 2 shekels of *muṣu*-stone, 2 shekels [of ....], 2 shekels of frit, [...]
29′ 2 shekels of *simu*-stone, 2 shekels of *lipāru*$^{?}$, 2$^{?}$ shekels of pumice, 2 shekels of [.....]
30′ 2 shekels of 'donkey-vulva'(-shell), 2 shekels of seashore-pebble, 2 shekels of [...]-stone,
31′ 2 shekels of *sāpinu*-stone, 2 shekels of bright-stone, 2 shekels peas, 2 shekels of [lentils]
32′ 2 shekels of pulses, 2 shekels of *bušānu*, 2 shekels of horned alkali, 2 shekels of [....],
33′ 2 shekels of *kanaktu*, 2 shekels of *abukkatu*-resin, 2 shekels of black cumin, half shekel [of ...]
34′ half shekel of block-salt, half shekel of red salt, half shekel of steaming salt.

35′ pap 93 ú.hi.a *hi-níq-ti* gal-*ú* gaz sim *ina* ud sù.s[ù ....][1]
36′ kéš.kéš *lu* siskur bal-*qí* uzu.zag uzu.me.hé uzu ka.[izi ....]
37′ ú.hi.a *ina* múl.ug$_5$ gar-*an* én ^{d}⸢*gu*⸣-*la* n[in an-ta-gal]
38′ én *a-ta-mar* <*pa-né-e-*>*ki lu-úb-luṭ* én.meš *an-na-ti ana* ugu [...........][2]

39′ én [^{d}g]*u*-[*l*]*a* nin an-⸢ta⸣-gal an-ú[r-ta nam-ta-è][3]

40′ [................................] ⸢^{na4}gig⸣ *lu* ^{na4}*mu-ṣa lu* [.............
41′ [..gi]g *lu ti-ti* [................
42′ [..] *lu mim-ma* [...........

43′ [... g]azi^{sa}[^{r} ....

Ms. L$_2$ = K 10676 probably belongs to K 6493+ (plate 12)

1′ [...........] x x [..............
2′ [................^{šim}m]ug ^{šim}šal [..............
3′ [..............^{šim}ma]n.du ^{ú}nu.luh.h[a..............
4′ [....................naga].si ú nam.ti.la *mar-haṣ šá* [.........

5′ [...................]x nu ^{giš}šur.mìn ^{šim}gír ^{ši}[^{m}............
6′ [................] ⸢^{ú}⸣har.har ^{ú}*ši-mur-tú*[4] ⸢^{ú}⸣[...........
7′ [................^{š}]^{im}šeš lagab.munu$_4$ x [...............
8′ [................] ⸢^{ú}⸣*ár-kan-nu* ⸢^{ú}⸣[..........
9′ [.....................] x igi [................

10′ [...................] x ⸢igi⸣ [........

---

[1] Cf. No. 9 : 34 above, and note gal = *rubbû*, 'soak'.
[2] Cf. No. 9 ii 1 above.
[3] Cf. No. 9 44 above.
[4] The word *šimurtu* appears in Thompson, DAB 323, but not in CAD or AHw.

35′ Total, pound and sift 93 drugs for soaking a stricture, in the day sprinkle [......]
36′ bind on or make a sacrifice – shoulder meat, abdominal fat, roast meat, [...].
37′ Set out the drugs under Corvus. The incantation, 'Gula, [great] lady',
38′ (and) the incantation 'I beheld your (face)... let me be healthy', – these incantations [recite] over [him].

39′ Incantation. Gula, great lady, [when you exit] from the horizon.

40′ [....................], ..., or *muṣu*-stone or [................
41′ [.......................]... or *figs* [...
42′ [...].. or whatever [.......................

43′ [.....................................] *kasû* [....................................

TRANSLATION (K 10676)

2′ [........], *ballukku*, *šimeššalû*, ...[..............
3′ [...............], *suādu*, *nuhurtu*, [............
4′ [...............] horned alkali, 'health'-plant, a lotion which [.......

5′ [...................].., *šurmēnu*, *ṣadānu*, ..[.............
6′ [...................] *hašû*, *šimurtu*, ..[..........
7′ [..................] myrrh, a lump of malt, ..[.............
8′ [.................], *arkannu* ..[.................
(rest broken)

additional texts

No. 12
Ms. M = K 11829 (plate 11)

1′ traces
2′ [...] ⸢tu$_6$ én⸣

3′ [....................................]-ra dingir-bi
[..............................] x du$_8$-a tu$_6$ én

5′ [..............................] én 3-*šú* šid-*nu*

6′ [................k]a ^{šim}man.du ^{šim}gám-ma
7′ [..................] *šur-šum-ma* kaš
8′ [...............................] *u* te-*su* lá

9′ [................................n]u tuh.še.giš.ì súd
10′ [................................ ^{kuš}edin su]r-*re* lá-*ma* ti

---

11′ [diš na ....]-*ra ik-ṣu-ra*
12′ [................................] ⸢*ina* kaš⸣ hi.hi *ina* geštin.šur.[ra]
13′ [.................................] x ⸢še⸣ gud$^?$ gešt[in...]
14′ (trace)

TRANSLATION

2′ [..] incantation-spell.
3′–4′ (too broken for translation, but also ends with ‘incantation-spell’).

5′ [..........................], recite the incantation 3 times.

6′ [.......................] ... *suādu*, *ṣumlalû*,
7′ [........................] beer dregs,
8′ [.....................] and bandage his cheek.

9′ [...], crush sesame residue,
10′ spread it [on a leather-strip ...], tie it on and he will improve.

11′ [If a man’s ....].. have been compacted,
12′ mix [......................] in beer, in drawn wine
13′ [.....................................] sesame[?], wine,
14′ (broken)

No. 13 AMT 39,6

Ms. N = Rm II, 375 (AMT 39,6), see Thompson, AfO 11, 337

1′ traces
2′ [............................] en ki x x x [....................
3′ [................................*t*]*al-ha-am-ma*[1] *in*[*a-eš*]

4′ [..........................] ^{ú}*áp-pár-ha-nu*(?) ^{ú}[..........
5′ [..........................] $^{na4.ú}$*bu-ka-nu*[2] ^{ú}[...................

6′ [dub.x.kam] diš na éllag-*su* [gu$_7$-*su*][3]

7′ [diš na *i-te-ni*]*k-ki-ik* na.bi na$_4$ *šá-hi-ih-ta*[4] [gig ....
8′ [...................... *in*]*a* kaš.sag šub-*di* nag-*ma* [*ina-eš*]

9′ [................ ^{n}]^{a4}an.zah.ge$_6$ šika nunuz ga.nu$_{11}$^{mušen} ^{šim}li diš-*niš* [súd ...
10′ [...............] geštin.šur.ra nag-*ma* [*ina-eš*]

---

1 see CAD L 38, rarely attested.
2 pestle, cf. CAD B 308 (citing our passage as uncertain), since the word is not attested in other medical texts.
3 See the catalogue of incipits, text No. 48: 8′ and 10′.
4 See YBC 7146: 21′ (text No. 48), [na$_4$] *šah-hi-hu* gig.

TRANSLATION

1–2′ broken

3′ [...................... and] you will brew beer(?) and he will get [better].

4′ ....

5′ ....

6′ [Tablet x:] 'if a man's kidney [hurts him]'.

7′ [If a man] constantly scratches (his penis?), that man [suffers from] a dissolved calculus.

8′ Put [.......................] in premium beer, he drinks it and [he will get better].

9′ [Crush ....] black frit, ostrich-egg shell, and juniper, [....

10′ [.......................], he drinks it in drawn wine and [he will get better].

No. 14 AMT 89,4 + AMT 53,8 (plate 13)
Ms. O = K13405 + S 804 + 926 (all AMT 89,4) + 2160 (AMT 53,8)

1′ (trace)
2′ lá sag [...
3′ *ina* kaš [...

4′ diš na *hi-níq-ti* m[urub$_4$ ....
5′ [k]a.a.a.ab.ba x [...............................

6′ [diš n]a [n]a$_4$ gig x [................
7′ *ina* ˹kaš? *ina*˺ g[a ....

8′ diš na na$_4$ *š[a]h-hi-hu* x [..................
9′ ^{na4}šà.˹gissu˺ ^{giš}*si-h[u?* ....

10′ ^{ú}*nu-ṣa-bu* ^{ú}*ka-n[a-ak-tu*................
11′ ^{šim}šeš *mi-ṣi* ú.3.m[eš ....
12′ ^{ú}níg.bùr.bùr ga![1] nunuz g[a.nu$_{11}$^{mušen} .....
13′ 9 ú.hi.a *hi-níq-ti* x x [..........................

14′ numun eme.ur.gi$_7$ ^{ú}nu.luh.ha ˹^{ú}x˺ [....
15′ ^{šim}šeš numun ^{giš}gír.hab numun gazi^{sar}
16′ numun ^{giš}šinig 7 ú.meš *hi-níq-ti*

17′ ^{ú}igi-*lim* ^{ú}*nu-ṣa-bu* ^{ú}*pu-qut-ti*
18′ ^{ú}x x [e]me.ur.gi$_7$ ^{šim}šeš
19′ [*lu ina* kaš *lu*] *ina* ga súd! 7 ú.hi.a! hád
(bottom)

rev.

20′ [........................... ^{ú}k]ur.ra 1 gín naga.si
21′ ˹2˺ g[ín ....] x 2 gín ^{ú}nu.luh.ha
22′ di x x x [.. g]ín ^{ú}*tara-muš*
23′ 5 ú.meš *a[n-nu-t]i* $^{<ú>}$kur ^{giš}ásal![2]
24′ gaz sim *ina* x [..........] x ga súd
25′ gur!-*ma* hád.a g[u$_7$ *ina* k]aš ˹lú˺.kaš.tin.na
26′ nag

27′ 5 gín ˹^{na4}*ga-bu*˺-*u* 5 [gín ....
28′ 5 gín [......... k]a.a.ab.[ba ....
29′ 5 gín ^{ú}[nu.luh].ha x [..............
30′ 5 ú.hi.a [*an-nu*]-*ti* nu [*pa-tan* nag ....
31′ *lu ina* kaš *ina me-[e*...................

---

[1] error for šika.
[2] text: a.áš.ṭúb

TRANSLATION

1′–2′ ....
3′ in beer [..

4′ If a man [suffers from] stricture of the groin [......................
5′ coral, [..

6′ [If a] man suffers from a calculus ...[.....................
7′ in either beer or milk [........................

8′ If a man, (in order) for the stone to dissolve, .. [...................
9′ ...., *sību* [...............

10′ *nuṣābu* and *kan*[*aktu* ....
11′ myrrh, *a little bit*, 3 days [.......
12′ *pallišu*-stone, shell of [ostrich-egg .....
13′ 9 drugs for stricture of [................

14′ Seed of 'dog's tongue', *nuhurtu*, ...
15′ myrrh, *dadānu* seed, *kasû* seed,
16′ tamarisk seed, 7 drugs for stricture.

17′ *imhur-lim*, *nuṣābu*, *puquttu*,
18′ ...., 'dog's tongue'-plant, myrrh
19′ crush [in either beer or] in milk, dry out the 7 drugs.

rev.

20′ [.................x shekels of] *nīnû*, 1 shekel of horned alkali,
21′ 2 shekels of ....., 2 shekels of *nuhurtu*,
22′ .... [x] shekels of *taramuš*,
23′ these 5 drugs; *nīnû* and *ṣarbatu* (?)
24′ pound and sieve, crush (them) in [beer$^{?}$ or] milk,
25′–26′ dry it a second time, he *eats* [it], he drinks it [in] brewer's beer.

27′ 5 shekels of alum, 5 [shekels of ....]
28′ 5 shekels of [.......5 shekels of] coral,
29′ 5 shekels of *nuhurtu*, ...
30′ [he drinks] these 5 drugs [on an] empty [stomach ....],
31′ either in beer or in water [..]

No. 15 AMT 2,7

Ms. P = K 1847 (AMT 2,7)

This text is cited because of the stone in l. 3′; it is not a kidney-disease text *per se.*

1 (traces)

2′ [.................]-*nu* ^{šim}li ^{ú}x [.................

3′ [diš na .... gi]g-*a* na$_4$ gig-*ma*[1] ⸢*la ṣa-a*⸣-[*du* ....

4′ [........ *ip*]-*pu-uš ina* šu lú.a.zu gur-*ti*[2] [gig tuk-*ši*][3]

5′ [..........] ⸢^{ú}⸣*tara-muš* numun ^{giš}še.ná.a diš-*niš* gaz si[m ......

6′ [*ina* ^{kuš}edi]n.sur-*re šu-hi-šú ra-pal-ti-šú* lál x [......

7′ [.................] x *ina* geštin.du$_{10}$.ga nag.meš-*ma* ^{ú}*su-pa-lu* súd *ina* ì.g[iš .....

8′ [diš na ....] x šub-*a* gi.gíd hur.meš-*šú ú-na-qar-šú*[4] [............

9′ [....................] x ⸢su⸣-*šú* tar-*is* na.bi hur.meš-*š*[*ú* gig .....

10′ [.......................... ^{ši}]^{m}gam.m[a ....

---

[1] For this incipit, see text No. 1 ii 25.

[2] Read *tūrti.*

[3] dupl. AMT 101 3, 15, cited CAD A/2 345, 'he has a relapse in spite of the ministrations of the physician'. See also text No. 38 below, in which the same phrase occurs.

[4] CAD N/1 332 (hapax in a medical context).

TRANSLATION

2′ [.........], juniper, ... [..............

3′ [If a man's ...] are ill and (he) suffers from a calculus, and (it) is not moving [.................]
4′ [the shaft of his penis(?) has] expanded (i. e., it is tumescent), [he has a relapse] while in the care of the 'physician',
5′ [...................], pound and sift together *taramuš* (and) seed of *šunû*-shrub,
6′ spread it [on a leather]-strip, bind (it) on his buttocks (and) haunches, ... [...............
7′ he keeps drinking [..........] in sweet wine and crush *supālu*-juniper, in oil, [.........

8′ [If a man's ...] produces ..[...], his windpipe 'erodes' him, [..........
9′ [..................], his body is stopped, that man [is sick in] his lungs [.....
10′ [...................................] *ṣumlalû*, [.......................................

No. 16 AMT 66,11 + (plate 14)

Q	=	K 11230 + 11280 + 16437 (AMT 66,11 +) + S 126
A	=	CBS 19801 (BAM 396 ii 5′–12′; 22′) [text no. 1] = ll. 18–22
C	=	VAT 9871 + 10397 (BAM 111) [text no. 3] = ll. 18–22

col. i

1′	Q	[..] *ša*[*p-l*]*i*
2′	Q	[..] *tara-muk*
3′	Q	[..] nag
4′	Q	[................ mud za]bar *ana* gìš-*šú* mú
5′	Q	[....................... u]d.3.kam *i-šah-hu-úh*
6′	Q	[diš na..............] x *ù* kàš-*šú it-ta-na-aṣ-ba-ta*
7′	Q	[...................] šeg$_6$-*šal bi-rit pi-ni-te-šú*[1]
8′	Q	[...................] na$_4$ *i-šah-hu-uh*
9′	Q	[diš ki.min .... u]d.3.kam šub-*di ina* mul$_4$ [*tu*]*š-bat* nag
10′	Q	[................] ⸢^{ú}⸣*tara-muš a*-⸢*ár*⸣-kù.babbar
11′	Q	[........numun ^{ú}eme.]ur.gi$_7$ numun ^{ú}dili num[un ^{ú}nu.lu]h.ha$^{!}$(ha over ni)
12′	Q	[.........gi].dub *tam-ti mi-si*[*s* a.a]b.ba
13′	Q	[...... a.a]b.ba ^{na4}la-[.............r]u
14′	Q	[............] ^{na4}min babbar ^{na4}min ge$_6$ x [....... me]š
15′	Q	[....... gešti]n.ka$_5$.a ^{šim}šeš [^{šim}] x
16′	Q	[.....] x *ina* kaš.lú.tin.na nag.n[ag-*ma*] *ina-eš*
17′	Q	[diš.na ... g]ig numun ^{ú}eme.ur.gi$_7$ hád.a gaz ti-*ut*
18′	Q	[diš na ... g]ig *ana* ti-*šú* ^{šim}šeš ^{šim}buluh
	A	^{šim}šeš $^{na4.ú}$níg.bùr.bùr ^{ú}*a-ar*-kù.babbar
19′	Q	[........n]umun ^{ú}eme.ur.gir$_7$ numun ^{ú}gír.hab
	A	numun ^{ú}eme.ur.gi$_7$ numun ^{ú}gír-*uh-ha-*[*ah*]
	C	[n]umun ^{ú}eme.ur.gi$_7$ [.............................]
20′	Q	[........... šika nun]uz ⸢ga.nu$_{11}$⸣^{mušen} téš.bi gaz sim
	A	^{na4}peš$_4$.anše šika nunuz ga.nu$_{11}$$^{m[ušen]}$ ú.hi.a *an-nu-ti* téš.bi *ta-sàk*
	C	[.. p]eš$_4$.anše šika nunuz gá.nu$_{11}$^{mušen}
21′	Q	[........................] x x *ina* mud zabar *ana* gìš-*šú* mú
	A	*ina* kaš.sag *ba-lu pa-tan* nag-*šu ina* mud zabar *ana*(šè) *mùš-tin-ni-su* mú-[*ah*]
	C	[...] kaš nu *pa-tan* nag-*ma* [...........................] *ana* gìš-*šú* mú-*ah*
22′	Q	[.............. sah]ar munu$_4$ *ki-šú-ma* ti
	C	[.....................] x e$_{11}$-*šú* sahar munu$_4$ [.......................................] *ina-eš*
23′	Q	[..........-š]*ú* ⸢*ed*$^?$-*de*⸣-*eh u ha*⸣- x [..]

[1] see AHw 854 *birit pēmi/pēni.*

TRANSLATION

1′ [..] below.

2′ You bathe [the patient ....
3′ He drinks [...
4′ Blow [.......] into his penis [through] a bronze [tube ......
5′ [................] and on the 3rd day (the stone) will dissolve.

6′ [If a man suffers from ....] and his urine has been constantly 'seized',
7′ boil [..................], his crotch
8′ [......................], the stone will dissolve.

9′ [Ditto], place [....] on the 3rd day and set it under the stars and he drinks it,
10′ [...............], *taramuš*, 'silver-rosette'(-plant),
11′ [seed of] 'dog's [tongue]'-plant, seed of 'single-plant', *nuhurtu* seed
12′ [..........] 'sea-stylus', sea-*misis*,
13′ [.... of the] sea, ...
14′ [......] white and black (ditto)-stone, ...
15′ [...] fox-vine, myrrh, ...
16′ he drink keeps drinking [....] in brewer's beer [and] he will get better.

17′ [If a man] suffers from [.....], dry out and pound seed of 'dog's tongue'-plant, and he will recover.[1]

18′ [If a man] suffers [from ....] in order to cure him, crush and sieve together myrrh, *baluhhu*,
19′ [..........], seed of 'dog's tongue', *dadānu* seed,[2]
20′ 'donkey-vulva'(-shell), ostrich-egg shell, pound together all of these drugs,
21′ and he drinks it in premium beer on an empty stomach, blow it into his urethra through a bronze tube.
22′ Remove [..................] and take ...... malt-powder [.........] and he will [get better].

23′ [If a man's ....] *is covered* and ...[..]

[1] Simplicium.
[2] Ms. A differs.

col. ii

1′ Q 1. [šu ....
2′ Q 1.šu ^{ú}[.............
3′ Q 1.šu dù.me[š ....
4′ Q 1.šu ^{ú}igi.[*lim* ....
5′ Q 1.šu ^{ú}sumun.da[r ....
6′ Q 1.šu ^{ú}níg.b[ùr.bùr...........
7′ Q 1.šu ^{ú}a [..................
8′ Q 1.šu ^{ú}a [..........
9′ Q 1.šu ⸢ú⸣ [................
10′ Q 1.šu ^{ú}*šá-ga-⸢bi-gal-zu* 1⸣.[šu ....
11′ Q 1.šu ^{ú}ugu-*kul-la* 1.šu [........
12′ Q 1.šu ^{ú}*pad-da-nu* 1.šu [..........
13′ Q 1.šu še$_{10}$ eme.diri *iz-zi* 1.šu [..........
14′ Q 1.šu numun ^{giš}li 1.šu numun ^{giš}al-[..........
15′ Q 1.šu numun ^{giš}esi 1.šu numun ^{ú}x[.........
16′ Q téš.bi gaz sim *šum$_4$-ma in*[*a* ....[1]
17′ Q ⸢*š*⸣*á-ram-ma tu-sa-m*[*ah*[2] ....

18′ Q (traces)

---

[1] Cf. text No. 4: 12, *šum$_4$-ma ina* geštin.šur.ra *šum$_4$-ma ina* kaš *u* ì.giš *hal-ṣú*.
[2] For *summuhu*, see Goltz, *Heilkunde* 42.

col. ii

1′ 1 [handful of ....

2′ 1 handful of [.............................

3′ 1 handful of ....

4′ 1 handful of *imhur-lim*, [................

5′ 1 handful of *šumuttu*, [................

6′ 1 handful of *pallišu*-plant, [...............

7′ 1 handful of ....

8′ 1 handful of ....

9′ 1 handful of ....

10′ 1 handful of *šagabigalzu*, 1 [handful of ......

11′ 1 handful of *elkulla*, 1 handful of [.........

12′ 1 handful of *paddānu*, 1 handful of [.............

13′ 1 handful 'wall-lizard' excrement, 1 handful of ....

14′ 1 handful of juniper seed, 1 handful of seed of ...[...

15′ 1 handful of seed of *ušû*, 1 handful of seed of ....

16′ pound and sift together, whether in ....

17′ you mix *the grains*[1] [.....................

---

[1] See AHw 1325 s. v. *tarammu* (var. *šarammu*), usually referring to a pile of grain.

No. 17 BAM 113

Ms. R = VAT 10818 (BAM 113)

1′ [................................] ^{šim}šeš ⸢ú⸣[............................

2′ [................. ú *a*]*n-ni-*⸢*ti*⸣ téš.bi súd š[im ....

3′ [diš na ......] x *-dir-šú* ⸢bar uzu⸣.meš-*šú ši-ši-t*[*u ma-li*]

4′ [.........] u_4-*mi u* ge_6 *la i-*[*ṣal*]*-lal* na.bi [*hi-niq-ti* bún][1]

5′ [gig] *ana* ti-*šú* ^{ú}igi-*lim* súd *ina* ì ^{giš}buluh[2] *i-*[.....

6′ [diš na ....] *ú-ta-na-har* na.bi *hi-niq-*[*ti* bún ....

7′ [..........] ⸢ú⸣hab k[aš.sa]g nu *pa-tan* n[ag ....

8′ [........ì.g]iš *hal-ṣi* hi.hi *ina* [mud zabar ....]

9′ [........ *hi-niq-t*]*i* bún-*šú* [..................

10′ [........... ì].giš *hal-ṣi* hi.hi *ina* mud za[bar ....

11′ [........... ì.gi]š *hal-ṣi* hi.hi šeg_6-*šal* du[b-*ak* ....

12′ [.............] illu šim [.......................

13′ (trace)

---

[1] See text No. 2: 5.

[2] For ^{giš}buluh, see BAM 167: 7.

TRANSLATION

1′ [..............................], myrrh, ..[........................

2′ pound these [...] plants together ...[...........

3′ [If a man's....] .... him, the skin of his flesh is [covered with] a membrane,

4′ [.....] day and night he cannot sleep, that man [suffers from stricture of the bladder].

5′ In order to cure him, pound *imhur-līm*, [......] it in oil of *baluhhu*-wood.

6′ [If a man's .....] is dried up, that man [suffers from] stricture [of the bladder].

7′ [......... he] drinks madder (and) premium beer on an empty stomach [.....

8′ Mix [........and] pressed oil in a bronze tube [and insert it ....

9′ [......], stricture[?] of his bladder [......................

10′ Mix [.... and] pressed oil in a bronze tube [and insert it ....

11′ Mix [..... and] pressed oil, heat it up (and) pour [it ....

12′ ....] resin of ..... [.......................................

Kidney-desease drugs

No. 18 BAM 431, see also below, text No. 39.

MM	=	K 9684 + 9999 + S 341 + Rm 328 (BAM 431 v 11′–32′;)
NN	=	K 4164 + (BAM 430 v 15′–37′) [text no. 40]
S$_1$	=	VAT 9467 + 10300 + 10414 (BAM 165) ii 15′ ff.
YY	=	A 239 (BAM 161) vi 7–19
ZZ	=	A 234 (BAM 164 5–9) (listing of medicinal plants from Kiṣir-Assur)
S$_2$	=	VAT 13913 (BAM 163) 1′–4′
S$_3$	=	VAT 11819 (BAM 162) 2′–4′
X	=	K 6545 + 8355 + 9030 (AMT 40,5) [text no. 23] = ll. 11–14

11′	MM	$^{\text{⸢ú}}$*tara-muš*$_8$ $^{\text{ú⸣}}$igi-*lim* ^{ú}igi-*ešra*
	S$_1$	^{ú}*tara-muš*$_8$ ^{ú}igi-*lim* ^{ú}igi-*ešra*
	YY	^{ú}*tara-muš*$_8$ ^{ú}igi-*lim* ^{ú}igi-*ešra*
	NN	[.*ta*]*ra-muš*$_8$ ^{ú}igi-*lim* ^{ú}igi-*ešra*
	X	^{ú}*tara-muš* ^{ú}igi-*lim* ^{ú}[..............]
12′	MM	[...........] ^{ú}hab
	S$_1$	^{ú}*ak-tam* ^{ú}hab
	YY	^{ú}*ak-tam* ^{ú}hab
	NN	$^{\text{⸢ú⸣}}$[*a*]*k-tam* ^{ú}hab
	X	[..............] ^{ú}hab
13′	MM	[............... ^{ú}]úkuš.<*ti*>-*gi-la*
	S$_1$	^{ú}úkuš.hab ^{ú}úkuš-*ti-gi-la*
	YY	numun ^{ú}úkuš.hab ^{ú}úkuš-*ti-gi-la-a*
	NN	$^{\text{⸢ú⸣}}$[............... ha]b ^{ú}úkuš-*ti-gi-la*
	X	úkuš.hab úkuš-*ti-gi-li*
14′	MM	[...............] bún *a-bat-t*[*i*]
	S$_1$	bún *a-bat-te* ^{ú}níg.bùr.bùr[1]
	YY	bún *a-bat-ti* $^{\text{na4.ú}}$níg.bùr.bùr
	NN	numun [.... bú]n *a-bat-ti*
	X	bún *a-bat-ti* ^{ú}níg.bùr.bùr
15′	MM	[...................] x nu [.........]
	S$_1$	[numu]n eme.ur.gi$_{15}$ numun ^{giš}šinig
	YY	numun ^{ú}eme.ur.gi$_{15}$ numun ^{giš}*bi-nu*
	NN	numun [.............] numun ^{giš}[........^{ú}]níg.bùr.bùr
16′	MM	(traces)
	S$_1$	[numun] ^{giš}ma.nu
	YY	numun ^{giš}ma.nu
	NN	[num]un ^{giš}ma.ni
17′	MM	$^{\text{⸢šim}}$li ^{ú}*nu*⸣-*ṣa-b*[*u*]
	S$_1$	^{ú}*nu-ṣa-bu* [x ^{ši}]^{m}li
	YY	^{ú}*nu-ṣa-bu*
	NN	[num]un x [......... *ṣ*]*a-bu*
18′	MM	$^{\text{⸢ú⸣d}}$maš ka.a.ab.ba
	S$_1$	*ni-kip-tu*$_4$ [*im-bu tam-ti*]*m*
	YY	numun ^{giš}li *ni-kip-tú* ka.a.ab.ba

[1] Good example of a drug which appears in kidney but not in anus texts.

19′	MM	[*qan-ṭ*]*up-pi*[1] *tam-tim* gi.šeš *tam-tim*
	S_1	gi.dub.ba *tam-tim* [................]
	YY	*mi-sis tam-ti*[2] gi.dub *tam-ti*
20′	MM	[..*m*]*u-ṣa* ^{na4}an.zah ^{na4}an.zah.ge$_6$
	YY	^{na4}*mu-ṣa* ^{a4}an.zah ^{na4}an.zah.ge$_6$ ^{na4}babbar
21′	MM	[^{n}]$^{a4.šim}$šeš
	S_1	[........] x mu kil
	YY	^{šim}šeš
22′	MM	[..] ^{giš}*nu-úr-ma-a* gazi^{sar}
	YY	pa ^{giš}nu.úr.ma
23′	MM	[šika nu]nuz gá.nu$_{11}^{mušen}$ numun ^{ú}in$_6$.úš
	YY	šika nunuz gá.nu$_{11}^{mušen}$ gazi^{sar} numun ^{ú}dili
24′	MM	[^{n}]^{a4}peš$_4$.anše ^{na4}peš$_4$ a.ab.ba sa$_5$
	YY	peš$_4$.anše peš$_4$ *tam-tim*
	NN	[^{n}]^{a4}peš$_4$.anš[e ....]
25′	MM	[..] ⸢ú⸣ éllag.meš
	YY	31 ú éllag gig *ina* kaš.lú.tin.na nag
	NN	30 ú [....................................]
26′	MM	[^{ú}h]ar.har ^{ú}*úr-nu-u*
	ZZ	^{ú}har.har ^{ú}*úr-nu-u*
	S_3	^{ú}har.har [..........]
	NN	^{ú}har.ha[r ....]
27′	MM	[.........] ^{ú}kur.kur
	ZZ	^{ú}kur.kur
	NN	ú babbar ⸢ú⸣ [.....]
28′	MM	[........] x *sah-lé-e*
	ZZ	^{ú}*ti-ia-tú sah-lé-e*
	S_2	[.........] *sah-lé-i* x
	NN	*sah-lé-e* [..........]
29′	MM	[......] x ^{ú}eme.ur.gi$_{15}$
	ZZ	numun ^{ú}si.sá ^{ú}*zi-bu-u*
	S_2	[..................] ^{ú}*zi-bu-u* x
	S_3	numun ^{ú}x [..................]
	NN	^{ú}eme.u[r.gi$_{15}$ ....]
30′	MM	[.....^{n}]$^{a4.im}$sahar.na$_4$.kur.ra
	ZZ	gazi^{sar} $^{na4.im}$sahar.na$_4$.kur.ra
	NN	^{im}sahar.na$_4$.[......................]
31′	MM	[..... *š*]*u-un-hu*
	ZZ	^{ú}x x
	S_2	^{ú}*šu-un-hu-'u* im.s[ahar.na$_4$.kur.ra]
32′	MM	[...] éllag^{2}.meš
	ZZ	11 ú.meš éllag *ina* geštin nag.meš
	S_2	11 ú.meš éllag *ina* kaš x ⌊.......]
	S_3	11 ú.hi.a éllag [............
	NN	11 ú.[................................]

[1] not in CAD Q 81 (*qanduppu*).
[2] Note the variant gi.šeš *tamti* in Ms. MM.

No. 19 Ms. T = VAT 8903 (Köcher, KADP No. 36) vi 14–26

Inventory, mentioning a bandage for kidneys, etc.; cf E. Ritter, *Studies Landsberger* (Assyriological Studies 16, 1965), 313 f., E. Reiner, *Bibliotheca Orientalia* 15 (1958), 102, Goltz, *Heilkunde* 57, H. Limet, *Oikumene* 5 (1986), 82 f. (ref. court. M. Stol), and W. Farber, Iraq 39 (1977), 223 ff. [ref. court. R. Biggs].

14	^{ú}*qúl-qúl-la-nu*	(plant)
15	*maš-qi-a-te*	potions
16	*qutārī*(kù.gi.meš)	fumigations
17	*te-qi-a-te*	ointments
18	*nap-šal-a-te*	salves
19	*alla-nu*.meš	suppositories
20	*mar-haṣ*.meš	lotions
21	zì.da.meš	flours
22	*kup-pa*$^{!}$*-tin*$^{!}$	pill[1]
23	⌜*x x*⌝*-šal-tú*	......
24	*naṣmadi*([lá]^{di}) *ša* éllag	bandage for the kidney
25	lá-*di ša* sag.ki	bandage for the head
26	lá-*di ša* umbin	bandage for the nails

[1] See Goltz, *Heilkunde* 328, for a justification of reading this line as *ap-is-lat*, as derived from the disease name *apišalû*, although a disease name is hardly likely in the present context.

Anus disease texts

No. 20 HS 1883 rev. 15–18 (BAM 393) Old Babylonian

see M. Haussperger, 'Medizinisches Kompendium aus altbabylonischer Zeit', *Würzburger medizinhistorische Mitteilungen* 16 (1997), 131–148.

15 *šumma*$_x$(àš.šár) *a-wi-lum šu-bu-ra-am ma-ru-uṣ ši-ir na-ap-ša-tim*
16 *tu-ra-ar-ma i-na e-li-im tu-uš-te-te-ma tu-ka-ṣa-a-ma i-né-a-aš*
17 *šumma*$_x$(àš.šár) *iš-tu ur*[1]*-šu ú-za-qá-at-sú ši-im-ṭam ši-im-tam ú-pí-tam ta-ša-dul*$^{?}$*-ma i-né-a-aš*

15 If a man is ill in the anus: dry out raw meat
16 and you mix (it) in sesame oil and you *heat* it[2] and cool (it) and he will get better.
17 If after an abscess stings him, you *extend* plucked wool[3] (var. a baked branding-iron)[4] and he will get better.

---

[1] Note that the *ep*-sign in this tablet usually has several verticals in the middle of the sign, whereas this sign does not.

[2] *etēmu / šutētumu* 'mix'(?), cf. CAD E 383, but we are assuming a root *emēmu*, 'to be hot',

[3] as a bandage

[4] *šimṭam* and *šimtam* are alternative readings. See obv. l. 17, *ši-im-ta-am e-mi-ta-am ta-ša-k*[*a-an-m*]*a*, 'place a hot branding-iron' on the patient, which may be a reference to scarification. The word *upītu* here is taken as derived from *epû*, 'to bake', and the expression is parallel to *ši-im-ta-am e-mi-ta-am* in obv. 17, cited above.

No. 21 BAM 95 forerunner to diš na *ina lā simānišu*[1]

V	=	VAT 13752 + (BAM 95)
AC	=	K 3550 (AMT 22,2) [text no. 50]; ll. 1–4.
AD	=	VAT 10170 (BAM 152 iii 1–7; ii 8–11) = ll. 1–4; 36–37.
HH	=	VAT 9138 (BAM 168: 78–81) [text no. 34] = ll. 8–9, 16–18.
AE	=	STT 197 iii = ll. 10–15; 37.
dd	=	S 1283 + 1947 (AMT 40, 4 + 57,5 and duplicates) [text no. 30] = ll. 21–22
II	=	VAT 13726 (BAM 99: 25–26) [text no. 35] = ll. 27–28.
CC	=	VAT 10092 (BAM 104: 34) [text no. 28] = l. 37.
AA	=	HE 331 + VAT 8694 + 14118 (BAM 96 ii 16–17) [text no. 26] = l. 38
AF	=	VAT 8027 (BAM 54 18–19 text mostly *suālu*) = ll. 8–9
PP	=	Ass. 13955/k* (BAM 101: 4–11) [text no. 42] = ll. 34–35
W	=	S 36 + (and duplicates) (AMT 43,1 +) [text no. 22] = ll. 16–18.
AG	=	A 250 (BAM 108: 15–18) = ll. 1–2; 16–18

1	V	[...............] ^{ú}har.har ^{ú}x x x ^{ú}kur.r[a ....
	AC	[.................. ^{ú}a.zal].lá ^{ú}kur.kur ^{ú}kur.ra
	AD	[..............] ^{ú}har.]..
2	V	[...].⸢du mun⸣ na[ga..] ⸢*sah-le-e*⸣ [............] x x [..]
	AC	^{ú}⸢*úr-né*⸣-*e* ^{ú}nu.luh.ha [........................^{ši}]^{m}man.du ⸢mun x ì$^{?}$.giš$^{?}$⸣ udu *lu-u* máš.gal
	AD	^{ú}*úr-nu-u* ^{ú}nu.luh.ha ^{ú}[............................] ^{šim}man.du mun naga.si *sah-le-e* ^{giš}x ^{ú}tál.[tál]
3	V	[..]ì udu x [......................l]um.ma ì [.............. ....] gaz.ga[z]
	AC	[.......................................] x meš lú [.............] x x *qí-lip* zú.lum.ma x x [...........]
	AD	^{ú}*a-ši-i* pa úkuš.hab 15 ú.hi.a šeš diš-*niš* gaz sim *ina* ì.udu *u qí-lip* zú.lum.ma hi.hi gur-*ma ina* ^{giš}nàga ga[z]
4	V	[.....] tag.[tag ....] gar im [.......................-*ṭ*]*u lat-ku*
	AC	ì.giš [..................] x [........] x x ⸢*ú*$^{?}$⸣-*na-šar*$^{?}$ [.....................]-*lum* è.a x x x x a
	AD	ì.giš tag.tag *alla-nu* dù-*uš* ì.nun sù *ana* dúr-*šú* gar-*ma* im *eṣ-lu* è.a *bul-ṭu lat-ku*
5	V	[^{ši}]^{m}gúr.gúr x x ^{šim}[.........] x igi [....................................] 7 ú.meš š[eš.meš]
6	V	[diš-*niš* s]úd *ina qí*-[*li*]*p* zú.lum.ma hi.hi gur-*ma ina* ^{giš}nàga gaz ì.gi[š ....] x
7	V	[*ina* dú]r-*šú* gar-*an* im *eṣ-lu*$_4$ è [*bu*]*l-ṭu lat-k*[*u*]
8	V	[z]ú.lum.ma dilmun^{ki} naga.si ì.udu éllag udu.níta ^{šim}gúr.gúr ^{giš}l[i ....] illu li.t[ar .....]
	HH	zú.lum.ma dilmun^{ki} naga.si *tur-ár* ì.udu éllag udu.ní[ta] ^{šim}gúr.gúr ^{giš}li ^{šim}gam.ma illu ^{šim}buluh illu li.tar 8 ú.meš
	AF	[.............] dilmun^{ki} naga.si ì.udu éllag udu.níta ^{šim}gúr.gúr [.................................]
9	V	[*all*]*a-nu lat-ku šá* im kud-*si* [.....] gar-[*an*]
	AF	[.................]-*ku šá* i[m ....]
	HH	*alla-nu* im kud-[*si*] *ana* dúr-*šú* gar-*an bul-ṭu lat*-[*ku*]

[1] See F. Köcher's comments on this tablet in BAM I xxii, 'Rezepte gegen innere Erkrankungen, die später z.T. in die Tafelserie diš na *ina la simānišu* eingearbeitet worden sind.' Although one cannot prove that this tablet is a 'forerunner', it is the only tablet in the corpus written in a landscape format, and the text repeats the formula labelling passages as ***bulṭu latku***, 'a proven recipe', which is not a common feature of these texts.

TRANSLATION

1 [..................] *hašû*, *azallû*, *ata'išu*, *nīnû*,

2 *urnû*, *nuhurtu*, ..., *suādu*, horned alkali salt, *sahlû*, *urânu* (var. sheep or goat fat),

3 *ašû*, leaf of cucumber – these 15 drugs you pound and sieve together, mix them in fat and date-rind, repeat and pound them in a mortar.

4 You smear oil and make a suppository, sprinkle ghee (on it) and put it into his anus, so that pent-up flatulence comes out. A proven remedy.

---

5 *Kukru*, ... [.........] ... [..................................], crush these 7 drugs

6 [together], mix (them) in date peel, repeat and grind it in a mortar, [.................] oil

7 and put (it) [in] his anus, (so that) pent-up flatulence comes out. A proven remedy.

---

8 You dry out Dilmun dates, horned alkali, fat of the kidney of a male sheep, *kukru*, juniper, *ṣumlalû*, *baluhhu*-resin, *abukkatu*-resin,

9 (var. 8 drugs), put a proven suppository into his anus which is to stop 'wind' (flatulence). (Var. adds: a proven remedy).

10	V	diš na *ur-šu dan-nu* ká.mud-*šú* dab-*ma* ká.mud úš-*hi*[1] numun ^{giš}g[i.zú.lum.ma] *šá* ugu nindu [..]
	AE	diš na *ur-šu dan-nu* [....................]-*ma* [..................] x ugu ni[ndu$^?$]
11	V	naga.si ^{ú}kur.ra diš-*niš* súd *ina* ì.udu éllag udu.níta hi.hi *al*[*la-nu* dù-*uš*] *ana* dúr-*šú* g[ar-*an*]
	AE	[......] ^{ú}kur.ra diš-*niš ta-sàk* ì.udu éllag udu.nít[a ....] *alla-nu* dù-*uš ana* dúr-*šú* [...]
12	V	*a-na ur-še* gaz *um-ṣa-a-ti qut-tu-pi* ká.mud-*šú mu-*⸢*uṣ*⸣-[*ṣi* ....] úkuš.hab ge$_6$ [.....
	AE	*a-na ur-še* gaz.meš-*e um-ṣa-a-ti qut-tup-pi* ká-mu[d-.........-*ṣ*]*i-i* še.sa.⸢a⸣
13	V	^{ú}kur.ra *sah-lu-u* ú babbar u$_5$.gar.ib^{mušen} mun.kù.pad diš-*niš* gaz s[im ....] *ana* dúr-*šú* gar-*a*[*n*]
	AE	^{ú}kur.ra x x x naga.si *sah-*[..]-*e* ^{ú}[..]-*e* ú babbar u$_5$.gar.ib^{mušen} mun.kù.pad 8 ú.hi.a šeš téš.bi gaz sim *ina* ì.udu hi.[hi u dù-*u*]*š ana* dúr-*š*[*ú*] gar-*ma bul-ṭu* igi.bar
14	V	diš na dúr-*šú ha-niq-ma* dúr-*šú ur-še u um-ṣa-a-ti* diri *ana* ti-*šú* ^{ú}kur.[r]a ^{šim}li ^{šim}gig ^{ú}na[m.t]i.la
	AE	diš na dúr-*šú ha-niq-ma* dúr.gig *um-ṣ*[*a-t*]*e* diri *ana ti-šú*
15	V	*mal-m*[*a-*.........súd] *ina* ì.udu u illu ^{šim}buluh hi.hi *u* dù-*uš ana* dúr-*šú* gar-*an-ma* ti
	AE	*mal-ma-liš* diš-*niš* súd *ina* ì.udu u illu ^{šim}buluh h[i...] dù-*uš ana* dúr-*šú* gar-*ma* ti
16	V	diš na *ina* [.....-*m*]*a-ni-šú* murub$_4$.meš-*šú* gu$_7$.meš-*šú* gìri^2.meš-*šú i-ta-á*[*r-raṣ*] *kim-ṣa-a-šú i-ka-ṣa-a-šú* na.bi *ina meṣ-hi-*⸢*ru-ti*⸣
	W	diš na *ina la si-ma-ni-šú* ⸢murub$_4$-*šú*⸣ gu$_7$.meš-*šú kim-ṣa-a-š*[*ú i-za-qata-š*]*ú bur-ka-šu i-kaṣ-ṣa-ṣa-šú* na.bi *ina meṣ-hi-ru-ti-šú*
	HH	diš na *ina la si-ma-ni-šú* murub$_4$.meš-*šú* gu$_7$.meš-*šú kim-ṣa-a-šú i-za-qata-šú* úr.meš-*šú i-tan-na-ah bur-ka-šu i-kaṣ-ṣa-a-šú* diš na *ina meṣ-hi-ru-ti-šú*
	AG	[......] *ina la si-ma-ni-šú* murub$_4$.meš-*šú* gu$_7$.meš-*šú* [........]-*a-šú i-za-qata-šú* úr.meš-*šu* [.........]-*ah bur-ka-šú i-kaṣ-ṣa-ṣa-šú* [....] *meṣ-hi-ru-te-šú*
17	V	dúr.gi[g] *ana* t[i-*šú*] ^{ú}kur.ra ^{šim}li ^{šim}gúr.gúr ^{šim}gig ú nam.ti.la *mal-ma-liš* súd
	W	[....g]ig *ana* ti-*šú* ^{ú}kur.ra ^{šim}li ^{šim}gig ^{šim}gúr.gúr ú nam.ti.la *mal-ma-liš* súd
	HH	dúr.gig *ana* ti-*šú* ^{ú}gamun.ge$_6$ ^{ú}kur.ra ^{šim}gig ú nam.ti gazi^{sar}*mal-ma-liš* súd
	AG	dúr.gig gig
18	V	*ina* ⸢ì⸣[u]du [.... nag]ar-*nu* dù-*uš* ì.giš šur.min sù *ana* dúr-*šú* gar-*an-ma* ti
	W	*ina* ì.udu hi.hi al.la.na dù-*uš* ì.giš šur.min sù *ana* dúr-*šú* gar-*an-ma ina-eš*
	HH	*ina* ì.udu hi.hi *alla-nu* dù-*áš* ì.giš ^{giš}šur.mìn sù *ana* dúr-*šú* gar-*an-ma* ti
19	V	diš na *kim-ṣa-*⸢*a*⸣-[*šú*] zi *e-sil ši-hat* uzu tuk-*ši* múd dub.meš na.bi dúr.gig šu ^{d}nam.érim
20	V	*ana* ti-*šú* ^{ú}[kur.r]a *sah-lu-u* naga.si diš-*niš* súd *ina* ì.udu hi.hi *alla-nu* [dù-*uš*]-*ma ana* dúr-*šú* gar-*an-ma* [ti]
21	V	[diš na d]úr.gig-*ma* dúr-*šú e-sil* u$_5$.gar.ib^{mušen} suhuš ^{giš}[........................*all*]*a-nu* dù-[*uš*]
	dd	diš na dúr gig-*ma* dúr-*šú e-sil* gar.ib.u$_5$^{mušen} [s]uhuš ^{giš}nam.tar níta súd hi.hi diš-*niš tu-kap-pat*
22	V	[*an*]*a* dúr-*šú* gar-*an-ma* [ti]
	dd	*ana* dúr-*šú* gar

[1] see CAD Š/3 192, citing similar contexts where this incipit occurs.

10 If a man's anal opening is affected by a tough *uršu*-blister and his anal-opening is blocked, crush together *kūru*-seed which is over the oven [...].
11 Crush together horned alkali and *nīnû*, mix (them) in fat of the kidney of a male sheep, make a suppository, and insert it into his anus.

---

12 In order to smash the *uršu*-abscess, to cut off the haemorrhoids[1], (and) to spread his anal-opening, pound and sieve together (l. 13) roasted-barley, black cucumber,
13 *nīnû*, *sahlû*, 'white'-plant, bat guano, and block-salt (var.: these 8 drugs),[2] mix in fat, make a suppository and insert it into his anus, and he will experience good health.

---

14 If a man's anus is constricted and his anus is full of *uršu*-blisters and haemorrhoids, to cure him, crush together in equal measure *nīnû*, juniper, *kanaktu*, 'health'-plant,
15 mix (them) in fat and *baluhhu*-resin, make a suppository and put it into his anus and he will improve.

---

16 If a man's groin hurts him at an inappropriate time, he stretches out his feet, his shins gnaw at him with pain, that man suffers from rectal disease (already) during his youth –
17 to cure him, crush in equal amounts *nīnû*, juniper, *kanaktu*, *kukru*, 'health'-plant,
18 mix them in fat and make a suppository, sprinkle (on it) cypress oil, put it into his anus and he will get better. (NB. for variants, cf. text No. 22 1–4).

---

19 If a man pulsates in his shins, is constipated, and he is wasting away, his blood drains away, that man is ill in the anus, (it is) Hand of the Oath –
20 to cure him, crush together *nīnû*, *sahlû*, and horned alkali, mix (them) in fat, [make] a suppository and put it into his anus [and he will improve].

---

21 If a man has rectal disease and is constipated in his anus, pound bat guano and the root of male mandrake, mix and roll them together into a pill (var. make a suppository),
22 insert (them) into his anus and [he will improve].

---

[1] The reference to 'plucking' (*qatāpu*) or 'cutting off' this type of lesion may point to haemorrhoids or piles rather than abscess.

[2] Ms. AE has 2 additional plants listed which do not appear in Ms. V, and hence the discrepancy with listing 8 drugs.

rev.

23	V	[diš na] *n*[*ik*]<*-kim*>*-ti*[1] dúr gig šà$^{!}$.meš-*šú* mú.meš-*hu* na$_4$ [........] 2 gín ésir 1/2 gín il[lu...]
24	V	[lá-*i*]*t* ì.giš ^{giš}*dap-ra-ni* mes$^{\text{he-pí}}$ *šum$_4$-ma* gig *t*[*u-*...........] x *alla-nu* gar-*an* *šum$_4$-ma* gig x [...]
25	V	$^{\text{min}6}$*ru-ku-us*[2] *sah-lé-e* gazi^{sar} hi.hi kéš en x [......] [t]ùn-*šú* *ina* a kúm luh-*si* ^{síg}àka [ì.giš sù][3]
26	V	*ana* dúr-*šú* gar-*an* *ṭúr-ri-iš* gazi^{sar}lá [*h*]*i-ṭa* x [........ *b*]*ul-ṭu lat-ku šá ina* šu *ka-a-a-ma-a*[*n-ti*]
27	V	diš na dúr.gig gig múd *i-te-ez-zi qé-reb* dúr-*šú i-ha-*[.................... $^{\text{ši}]\text{m}}$buluh ^{šim}gig bar zú.lum.ma *ina* ì.udu hi.hi
	II	diš na dúr.gig gig múd *i-te-ez-zi qé-reb* dúr-*šú i-ha-áš ana* [ti-*šú*] ^{šim}buluh ^{šim}gig bar zú.lum.ma *ina* ì.udu hi.hi
28	V	u dù-*uš* [.....]-*šú* gar-*an*
	II	*ana* dúr-*šú* gar-*an-ma* t[i]
29	V	diš na múd *ina* dúr-*šú ú-tab-ba-ka* na.bi *qer-bé-ni* dúr gig *ana* [t]i-*šú* ^{šim}gúr.gúr ^{giš}li naga.si ^{ú}kur.kur ^{ú}kur.ra[4]
30	V	*sah-lé-e* illu ^{šim}buluh 7 ú.meš *an-nu-ti* diš-*niš* súd *ina* ì.udu éllag udu níta hi.hi *alla-nu* dù-*uš ana* dúr-*šú* gar-*an-ma* ti
31	V	^{ú}kur.ra ú babbar *sah-lu-u* naga.si gibil.meš $^{\text{na}4}$*ga-bi-i* ^{ú}nu.luh.ha ^{šim}gúr.gúr ^{šim}li
32	V	^{šim}gam.m[a] illu ^{šim}buluh ^{šim}šeš ^{šim}hab mun 1[3] ú.meš šeš diš-*niš* gaz sim *ina* ì.[ud]u ⸢éllag udu⸣.níta
33	V	[g]aba.làl illu ^{šim}buluh hi.hi *ina* izi šeg$_6$-*šal alla-nu* [d]ù-*uš ana* dúr-*šú* gar-*an-ma* ti nagar [*lat-ku*(?)]
34	V	[ì].udu éllag gud ì.udu éllag udu.níta ì.nun gaba.làl [ì] az du.du ì *hal-ṣa* úš ^{giš}e[ren]
	PP	ì.udu éllag gud níta : ⸢ì⸣.[udu ....] ì.nun.na gaba.[làl] ì a[z] ⸢du.du x⸣ [..] ì *hal-ṣu* úš ^{giš}ere[n]
35	V	[$^{\text{ši}]\text{m}}$šeš ^{šim}hab ^{šim}buluh illu ^{šim}buluh illu li.tar ú babbar diš-*niš* súd dúr-*šú* eš.meš *nap-šal-t*[*i* ....]
	PP	^{šim}šeš ^{šim}hab ^{ši}[^{m}......] [i]llu [...........................] ú [..] *nap-šal-t*[*i* dú]r.g[ig]
36	V	diš na dúr gig ^{šim}gúr.gúr ^{šim}li ^{šim}še.li babbar diš-*niš* súd *ina* ì.nun hi.hi dúr-*šú te-te-ni-qí-ma* ti
	AD	diš na dúr gig ^{šim}gúr.gúr ^{šim}li ^{šim}še.li [..] gaz *ina* ì.nun súd *ina* dúr-*šú* mar.meš-*ma* t[i]

1 see BAM I xxiii for emendation.

2 The TAB sign at the beginning of l. 25 appears to be a marginal notation, perhaps referring to '2', hence the reading min$_6$. It is not clear to what it refers.

3 Restored BAM 104 61.

4 This incipit also occurs as the first incipit in text No. 35: 1 (BAM 99).

23 [If a man] suffers from bloating of the anus (and) his bowels are swollen, bind [...]-stone, 2 shekels of bitumen, one half shekel of resin of [....],

24 oil of *daprānu*, ... If he is (still) ill, you [......], insert a suppository; if he is (still) ill, .. [.....]

25 tie ditto, mix *sahlû* and *kasû*, bind (them), until ..[....], wash his *belly* in hot water, [moisten] a wad of wool [in oil]

26 and put (it) into his anus. Bind *kasû* into a binding(?), ... [...]. A tested recipe from a trustworthy hand.

---

27 If a man suffers from a diseased anus, defecates blood and the middle of his rectum 'hastens'[1], to [heal him], mix *baluhhu, kanaktu,* date-rind in fat,

28 make a suppository put it into his anus (var. and he will improve).

---

29 If a man passes blood from his anus, that man is suffering internally in the rectum, to cure him, *kukru*, juniper, horned alkali, *ata'išu*, *nīnû*,

30 *sahlû*, *baluhhu*-resin: crush 7 drugs together, mix (them) in fat of a kidney of a male sheep, make a suppository, put it into his anus and he will get better.

---

31 Fresh *nīnû*, 'white' plant, *sahlû*, and horned alkali, alum, *nuhurtu*, *kukru*, juniper,

32 *ṣumlalû*, *baluhhu*-resin, myrrh, *ṭurû* and salt; pound and sieve together these 13 drugs, mix them in fat of the kidney of a male sheep,

33 (with) wax and *baluhhu*-resin, boil them over a fire, make a suppository, insert it into his anus and he improve. A [proven(?)] suppository.

---

34 Crush together fat of ox kidney, fat of the kidney of a male sheep, ghee, wax, oil of creeping myrtle, pressed oil, cedar 'blood',

35 myrrh, *ṭūru*, *baluhhu*, *baluhhu*-resin, *akukkatu*-resin, and 'white' plant, keep smearing his anus – a salve for rectal disease.

---

36 If a man (suffers from) a diseased rectum: crush (var. pound) together *kukru*, juniper, and white *kikkirânu*, mix (them) in ghee, and keep daubing (the patient's) rectum (with it) and he will improve.

---

[1] 'has diarrhoea', < *hâšu* (lit. 'hasten')?

37 V $^{⌜ú⌝}$kur.ra [naga].si še$_{10}$ gud sa$_{5}$ *ina* gissu hád.a gaz sim *ṭà-pu šá* dúr.gig *te-ṭe-ni-pi-ma* dúr.gig zi-*hi*

AD ^{ú}kur.ra naga.si še$_{10}$ gud sa$_{5}$ *ina* gissu hád.a g[az] *ṭi-pu*[1] *šá* dúr.gig *te-ṭ[e-n]i-pi-ma* dúr.gig [...]

AE [..........nag]a.si še$_{10}$ gud diri *ina* gissu hád.a [g]az sim [....................] *te-ṭe-ni-pi-ma* dúr.gig zi-*hi* ti$^{?}$

CC [.........nag]a.si še$_{10}$ gud [.......] gissu hád.a gaz sim *ṭi-pu šá* dúr.gig *te-ṭe-ni-*[................]

---

38 V [^{š}]^{im}gúr.gúr ^{giš}li ^{ú}kur.kur ^{ú}*šib-bur-ra-tú* a.gar<.gar> maš.dà ^{šim}gig illu ^{šim}buluh illu li.tar *ina* dè ^{giš}kiši$_{16}$ dúr-*šú tu-qat-tar*

AA ^{šim}gúr.gúr ^{giš}li ^{ú}*šib-[bur-r]a-tú* ú [.........] a.gar.gar maš.dà pap x [še]š *ta-[sàk* ....]

---

colophon = Hunger, BAK No. 196

[1] AHw 1392, 'bandage' or perhaps 'addition'.

37 Dry out in the shade *nīnû*, horned alkali, and dung of a red ox, pound and sieve, keep adding a bandage for the diseased rectum and diseases of the rectum are removed (var. and he will improve).

38 You fumigate his anus (with) *kukru*, juniper, *ata'išu*, rue, gazelle-dung, *kanaktu*, *baluhhu*-resin, and *abukkatu*-resin over acacia-reed coals.

(colophon)

No. 22 AMT 43,1 + AMT 57,6. (plates 15–18)
Text: diš na *ina lā simānišu*.

W	=	S 36 + 215 + 449 + 1245 + 1372 + 1452 + 1628 + 1646 (all = AMT 43,1) + K 7925 (AMT 43,2) + K 9091 (AMT 57,6) (+) K 3453 (AMT 53,9) (+) K 5955 (AMT 84,7) + 14453 (AMT 56,3), cf. RA 26 60 ff.
HH	=	VAT 9138 (BAM 168 = KAR 157, rev. 70–77) [text no. 34] = ll. 1–6
V	=	VAT 13752 + (BAM 95) [text no. 21] : 16–18 = ll. 1–4
II	=	VAT 13726 (BAM 99: 35–54) [text no. 35] = ll. iii 14–19; iv 1–2
VV	=	YBC 7126: 12′ (catchline Tablet 3) [text no. 48]
AG	=	A 250 (BAM 108: 15–18) = ll. 1–2
AA	=	EHE 331 + VAT 8694 + 14118 (BAM 96 ii 5–8) [text no. 26] = ll. 11–13

col. i

1	W	diš na *ina la si-ma-ni-šú* ⸢murub$_4$-*šú*⸣ gu$_7$.meš-*šú kim-ṣa-a-š*[*ú ....-qat*]*a*-[*š*]*ú*[1]
	HH	diš na *ina la si-ma-ni-šú* murub$_4$.meš-*šú* gu$_7$.meš-*šú kim-ṣa-a-šú i-za-qata-šú*
	V	diš na *ina* [.....-*m*]*a-ni-šú* murub$_4$.meš-*šú* gu$_7$.meš-*šú* gìri^2.meš-*šú i-ta-á*[*r-raṣ*]
	AG	[......] *ina la si-ma-ni-šú* murub$_4$.meš-*šú* gu$_7$.meš-*šú* [........]-*a-šú i-za-qata-šú*
2	W	*bur-ka-šu i-kaṣ-ṣa-ṣa-šú* na.bi *ina meṣ-hi-ru-ti-*⸢*šú*⸣ [.. g]ig
	HH	úr.meš-*šú i-tan-na-ah bur-ka-šu i-kaṣ-ṣa-a-šú* diš na *ina meṣ-hi-ru-ti-šú* dúr.gig
	V	*kim-ṣa-a-šú i-ka-ṣa-a-*[*š*]*ú* na.bi *ina meṣ-hi-*⸢*ru-ti*⸣ dúr.gi[g]
	AG	úr.meš-*šu* [.........]-*ah bur-ka-šú i-kaṣ-ṣa-ṣa-šú* [....] *meṣ-hi-ru-te-šú* dúr.gig gig
3	W	*ana* ti-*šú* ^{ú}kur.ra ^{šim}li ^{šim}gig ^{šim}gúr.gúr ú nam.⸢ti⸣.la
	HH	*ana* ti-*šú* ^{ú}gamun.ge$_6$ ^{ú}kur.ra ^{šim}gig ú nam.ti gazi^{sar}
	V	*ana* t[i-.] ^{ú}kur.ra ^{šim}li ^{šim}gúr.gúr ^{šim}gig ú nam.ti.la
4	W	*mal-ma-liš* súd *ina* ì.udu hi.hi *al-la-na* dù-*uš* ì.giš šur.min sù *ana* dúr-*šú* gar-*an-ma ina-eš*
	HH	*mal-ma-liš* súd *ina* ì.udu hi.hi *alla-nu* dù-*áš* ì.giš ^{giš}šur.mìn sù *ana* dúr-*šú* gar-*an-ma* ti
	V	*mal-ma-liš* súd *ina* ⸢ì⸣.[u]du [.... nag]ar-*nu* dù-*uš* ì.giš šur.min sù *ana* dúr-*šú* gar-*an-ma* ti
5	W	[diš ki.mi]n ⸢u$_5$⸣.gar.ib^{mušen} ^{ú}kur.ra illu ^{šim}buluh zú.lum.ma dilmun^{ki}
	HH	diš ki.min u$_5$.gar.ib^{mušen} ^{ú}kur.ra illu ^{šim}buluh ú babbar zú.lum.ma ^{mun}*eme-sal-lim*
6	W	[an.dah.šu]m mun 6 ú.hi.a *an-nu-tim alla-nu šam-ru*[2]
	HH	ì.udu gud 7 ú.meš *alla-nu* [....]
7	W	[diš ki.min ^{ú}]kur.ra ^{ú}kur.kur *sah-lé-e* $^{ú⸢}$*šar-ga-la*⸣-*te* ú babbar
8	W	^{ú}nu.luh.ha $^{na4⸢}$*ga-bi-i* ^{šim}gúr.gúr $^{šim⸣}$[..] ^{šim}šeš ⸢illu⸣ *a-bu-ka-tim*
9	W	mun 12 ú.hi.a *an-nu-ti a-he-en-*⸢*na-a* gaz⸣ x [..] x *ina* ⸢ì⸣.udu gaba.làl
10	W	⸢*u*? illu $^{šim⸣}$buluh šeg$_6$-*šal* hi.hi *al-la-an* dù-*uš i*[*na* dúr-*š*]*ú* gar-*an-ma ina-eš*

---

[1] This incipit is known from the Assur catalogue, probably as the opening of the first tablet of anus-disease texts; see below, No. 48: 11′: diš na *ina la si*[*-ma-ni-šú* murub$_4$.meš-*šú* gu$_7$.meš-*šú*].

[2] Thompson, RA 26 60 translates 'powerful,' which can also be found in CAD Š/1 332 (at end) describing drugs, although this passage is not cited.

TRANSLATION

1 If a man's groin hurts him at an inappropriate time, and his shins cause him a stinging pain (var. he stretches out his feet),

2 (var. he is weak in his thighs and) his knees (var. shins) gnaw at him with pain (var. are cold for him), that man suffers in the anus (already) during his youth,

3 to cure him, crush in equal amounts *nīnû* (var.black *kamūnu*), juniper, *kanaktu*, *kukru*, 'health'-plant (var. adds *kasû*),

4 mix them in fat and make a suppository, sprinkle cypress oil (on it) , put it into his anus and he will improve.

---

5 If ditto, bat guano, *nīnû*, *baluhhu*-resin, Dilmun dates (var. 'white'-plant, dates, gourmet-salt),

6 *andahšu*?, salt (var. ox fat), these 6 (var. 7) drugs (for a) *powerful* suppository.

---

7 [If ditto] *nīnû*, *ata'išu*, *sahlû*, *šargalatu*?, 'white'-plant,

8 *nuhurtu*, alum, *kukru*, ..., myrrh, *abukkatu*-resin,

9 and salt, pound these 12 drugs separately, boil and mix .... in fat and wax

10 and *baluhhu*-resin, make a suppository and put it into his [anus] and he will get better.

---

11 W diš ki.min ⸢ì⸣.[udu gud ì.ud]u éllag udu.níta ì.nun ⸢ì⸣ [*a-si*] du.du-*ki*[1]
AA ì.udu éllag gud ì.udu éllag udu.níta ì.udu ur.mah ì.nun ⸢ì⸣ [..........]
12 W ì mušen ì.giš ^{š}[^{im} ....] x ^{šim}šeš ^{šim}b[uluh i]llu li.tar
AA ì.giš mušen ì.giš $^{\text{⸢šim⸣}}$gír ì.giš ⸢x⸣-na ^{šim}šeš ^{giš}ere[n......] illu ^{šim}buluh illu li.dur
13 W ú babbar súd ⸢diš⸣-*niš* h[i.hi ...š]éš.meš [*nap-šal-ti* dú]r gig
AA ú babbar ^{ú}hab ^{šim}hab ì šé[š...] ì.udu úkuš.hab gazi^{sar} *ina* ^{síg}àka *ta-lap-pap ana* dúr-*šú* gar-[*an*]

---

14 W diš ki.min ^{šim}gúr.gúr ^{šim}li ^{š}[^{im}...] ^{ú}*pi-š*[*a-* ....*-n*]*i*
15 W ^{šim}šeš illu li.dur g[i.du$_{10}$.ga ì.giš ^{giš}g]ír *tu-qa-*[*at-tar*(?) ....]

---

16 W diš ki.min naga.si *qa-la-ti* [.........*n*]*u*? [....................................
17 W 5 ú.hi.a *an-nu-ti* ⸢*mal-ma-liš* súd⸣ [..
18 W zú.lum.ma dilmun^{ki} hi.hi *al-la-na* d[ù-*uš ina* dúr-*šú* gar-*an ina-eš*]

---

19 W diš na *ina meṣ-hi-r*[*u-t*]*i-šú* dúr gig na.bi z[i?.............
20 W ^{giš}*šu-ni*[*m* ..*-t*]*i* gazi^{sar} ^{ú}*a*[*k-tam* ....
21 W illu ^{šim}buluh [^{ši}]^{m}gúr.gúr gi.du$_{10}$.g[a ....
22 W diš-*niš ta-sàk ina* dè ^{giš}k[iš]i$_{16}$.⸢hab⸣ [*tu-qat-tar* ..

---

23 W diš na *ina meṣ-hi-ru-ti-šú* [dúr gig ....
24 W *il-bir-ma ina lam* x [................
25 W ^{giš}geštin.meš ^{giš}x̣ [...........
26 W [....] igi.d[u ....

col. ii

1 W *ina* a gazi^{sar} *tara-bak ina* ^{kuš}edin sur-*r*[*e* lá-*su-ma*]
2 W ^{ú}har.har *pa-ṣa-a-ti ina* ì.giš hi.[hi............

---

3 W diš ki.min šu.si-*ka mu-šá-ṭi* nigin làl sù
4 W ^{ú}naga.si ^{ú}*zi-ba-a* téš.bi *t*[*a-sàk* ....
5 W en múd è-*ni ta-kar*[2] *ki-ma* [.................
6 W *ina* ì.udu hi.hi *al-la-na* dù-*uš* [...................
7 W ^{ú}an.ki.an.di ^{šim}gúr.gúr ^{šim}[....................
8 W pa ^{ú}*ur-zi-ni* pa ^{giš}ása[l....................
9 W *ina* a ^{šim}gúr.gúr a zú.lum.ma ì.giš *u* [............
10 W *ina* ^{kuš}edin sur-*re* lál-*su-ma* [................
11 W *ina* dílim.a.bár ki làl hi.hi [...........

---

12 W diš na tùn gu$_7$-*šú* ⸢*ana* ti-*šú*⸣ [..............[3]
13 W k[uš ....] x x [....................................

gap
14′ W (traces)
15′ W [.......................................] x ⸢zì⸣.g[ig?] ⸢zì.gú⸣ zì.gú.gal
16′ W [.......................................*-i*]*š ra-bi-ki tara-bak ina* ^{kuš}edin sur
17′ W [.......................................m]eš *da-riš* nag.meš-*ma ina-eš*

---

1 See az du.du, No. 21: 34 and No. 42: 6, as well as No. 38: 3, ⸢ì⸣ *a-si mut-tal-li-ki*.
2 See Goltz, *Heilkunde* 36, described as 'sehr selten'.
3 see Cadelli, *Recherche* p. 299 f. for discussion, and 300 n. 76 and 78.

11 If ditto, crush and mix together fat of an ox kidney (and) of the kidney of a male sheep, (var. lion fat), ghee, oil of creeping [myrtle],
12 bird oil, myrtle oil, myrrh, *baluhhu*, *abukkatu*-resin, (var. adds cedar, *baluhhu*-resin),
13 (and) 'white'-plant, (var. madder, *ṭūru*), keep smearing (the anus) with oil, [a salve for] rectal disease. (Var. roll up fat, cucumber and *kasû* into wad of wool and insert it into his anus).

---

14 If ditto, *kukru*, juniper, [............
15 you *fumigate* myrrh, resin of *abukkatu*, [sweet] reed, and myrtle [oil, ...

---

16 If ditto, roasted horned alkali [..................
17 crush these five drugs in equal measure, mix [...................
18 (and) Dilmun dates, make a suppository [and insert it into his anus and he will get better].

---

19 If a man suffers from the anus during his youth, that man ..[........................
20 you crush together *šūnu*, ... *kasû*, *aktam*, [...................................
21 *baluhhu*-resin, *kukru*, sweet reed, [................
22 [fumigate] them on coals of *dadānu*-carob and [..................

---

23 If a man [suffers] from the anus during his youth, [...........
24 it has endured and .... [.............
25–26 vines, [...............................]..[................................

col. ii

1 You soak (the ingredients) in *kasû*-juice, spread it on a leather-strip, [bind it on him and]
2 mix crushed *hašû* in oil, [...

---

3 If ditto, wrap your finger with hair combings, sprinkle honey,
4 you [crush] together horned alkali and black cumin, [............,
5 you rub him until blood comes out like [..................],
6 you mix (the ingredients) in fat and you make a suppository, [........
7 *ankinute*, *kukru*, [...
8 leaf of *urzinu*, leaf of *ṣarbatu*, [.......................................
9 in *kukru*-juice, date-juice, oil and [.................................
10 spread on a leather-strip, bind it on him and [.................
11 Mix (it) in a salve with honey [.......................................

---

12 If a man's stomach hurts him, to cure [him ....
13 ....

gap

14′ ....
15′ [.................................]........, pea-flour,
16′ [...], you soak the concoction and spread (it) on a leather-strip,
17′ [...], ... he keeps drinking it and he will get better.

18′ W [..........t]uk.tuk-*ši* múd *ú-tab-ba-ka*
19′ W [..........] x šu ^{ú}kur.ra *sah-lé-e* ^{ú}naga
20′ W [..........*al-la-*]*na* dù-*uš ana* dúr-*šú* gar-*ma ina-eš*

21′ W [..........š]ed$_7$ dúr-*šú tu-qat-tar*

22′ W [..........]x *ter-ru* nigin[1] igi-*šú* ge$_6$
23′ W [..........] kúm šub-*ma* ^{giš}geštin.ka$_5$.a ^{ú}igi-*ešra*
24′ W [..........] a naga.si illu ^{šim}buluh
25′ W [..........] *ana* dúr-*šú* gar.gar-*an-ma ina-eš*

26′ W [..........] ⸢*mu-ṭa*⸣-*at*

---

rev. col. iii

1′ W [..........] x *ana* gig [zi]
2′ W [..........n]ag.meš-*ma* ti

3′ W [..........] x na$_4$ zú.lum.ma
4′ W [..........àr-*e*]*n alla-nu* múd tar-*si*

5′ W [..........] ⸢ú⸣in$_6$.úš
6′ W [..........]-⸢*e*?⸣ nag.meš
7′ W [..........].⸢meš⸣

gap

8′ W [..........m]eš

9′ W [.......... na]g

10′ W [..........^{ši}]^{m}li súd x x ⸢nag⸣

11′ W [..........] x ^{šim}hab nag

12′ W [.......... ^{ú}in.n]u.uš súd *ina* kaš nag

13′ W [.......... ^{im}sahar].na$_4$.kur.ra x x [.........-*m*]*a* nag *ina* a *ir-ta-na-haṣ*

14′ W [diš n]a [m]úd *ina* dúr-*šú* gim munus *ša na-a*[*h-šá-tú* šub.šub-*a t*]*a-hi-is-su-ma* dúr.gig.ga.kam
II diš na *ina* dúr-*šú* gim munus *ša na-ah-šá-te* šub.šub-*a ta-hi-su-ma* dúr.gig.ga.kám
15′ W [.. tu]k *ter-di-it*[2] *ir-ri* g[ig ....^{ú}nu.l]uh.ha súd *ina* kaš nag
II nu tuk *ter-di-it ir-ri* gig ^{im}kal.la ^{im}sahar.na$_4$.kur.ra nu.luh.ha súd *ina* kaš nag
16′ W [..K]U ^{na4}ka.gi.na dib.ba *ina* s[íg ....ere]n sù *ana* dúr-*šú* gar-*an*
II KU.KU[3] ^{na4}kur-*nu* dib.ba *ina* ^{síg}hé.me.da nigin-*mi* ì.giš ^{giš}eren sù *ana* dúr-*šú* gar-*an*
17′ W [.....-*n*]*é-e ina* kaš nag.meš *ina* a.meš [.......... ^{g}]^{iš}gi$_6$.pàr pa ^{giš}*šu-ši*
II *ur-né-e ina* kaš nag illu ^{šim}buluh *ina* a šed$_7$ *ir-ta-na-haṣ* pa ^{giš}gi$_6$.pàr pa ^{giš}*šu-še*

---

1 *sihir*, see CAD S 239, citing this passage.
2 AHw 1348 Darmgeschwür.
3 see CAD Q 208.

18′ [If a man's *anus*[?]] constantly has [........... (and)] it pours out blood,
19′ [...]..., *nīnû*, *sahlû*, horned alkali-plant,
20′ [....................................], make a suppository and insert it into his anus and he will get better.

21′ [.................................], cool (it and) you fumigate his anus.

22′ [.......................]..., the edge of his face/eye is black,
23′ put in hot [....................] and fox-vine, *imhur-ešra*,
24′ [............................] liquid of horned alkali, *baluhhu*-resin,
25′ [....................], keep inserting (them) into his anus and he will get better.

26′ ....

col. iii

1′ [...................................] to [remove] the illness,
2′ he keeps drinking [....................................] and he will recover.

3′ [.....................................] date stone,
4′ [grind] up [..................], a suppository to staunch blood.

5′ [...], *maštakal*,
6′ he keeps drinking .. [...].

7′ .....

gap

8′–12′ (broken, except for fragmentary phrases): he drinks...., pound juniper...., he drinks [..........] and *ṭūru*, crush [.....] and *maštakal* and he drinks it in beer.
13′ [......], alum, ..., and and he drinks it. He should continually immerse himself in water.

14′ If a man [passes] blood from his anus like a woman undergoing a haemorrhage, and he has no symptoms of ... and of a sore anus,
15′ he is suffering from diarrhoea. Crush yellow ochre, alum, and *nuhurtu*, he drinks it in beer.
16′ Wrap powder of magnetite in red wool and sprinkle cedar oil and insert it into his anus.
17′ He keeps drinking (var. drinks) *urnû* in beer. He should keep immersing *baluhhu* resin in cold water. Pound *lipāru*-leaf, *šūšu*-leaf,

18′ W [.....] eme.ur.gir$_7$ pa ^{giš}kiši$_{16}$-*h*[*a*-.... ..] ^{ú}<gìr.>naga.ga^{mušen} pa ^{giš}ma<.nu>
II pa ^{giš}eme.ur.gir$_7$ pa ^{giš}kiši$_{16}$-*ha-ah* pa ^{ú}gìr.naga.ga^{mušen} pa ^{giš}ma.nu
19′ W [... ú]r.tál.tál gaz *ina* kaš [...............] ⸢è⸣ gaz *ina* ì.udu hi.hi *ina* kuš *te-ṭer-re* lá
II pa ^{giš}úr.tál.tál gaz *ina* kaš *ta-la-aš* gur-*ma* è ga[z] *ina* ì.udu hi.hi *ina* kuš *te-ṭer-re* [..]

col. iv

1 W diš na mur[ub$_4$-*šú* gig$^?$-*s*]*u*[1] : 1/3 sìla a *u* ì.giš [................
II diš n[a ....

---

2 W 1 sìla zì.gig sim ^{dug}bur.zi a diri [............
II ⸢1 sìla zì.gig⸣ sim ^{dug}bur.zi a diri *ana* šà du[b ....

---

3 W diš na ninda gu$_7$-⸢*ma*⸣ *i-par-ru* kaš nag-*ma* [.................
4 W na.bi dúr.gi[g] *ana* ti-*šú* suhuš ^{gi}[^{š}.......
5 W *ina šèr-ti ba-l*[*u*] *pa-tan* nag-*šu* x [............
6 W x zì.kum hi.hi ur.gi$_7$ *šah-h*[*a-a*....
7 W [...] x x [......] illu ^{šim}buluh [..............

---

8 W traces

gap

9′ W [..........]-*te-šú tu-* x [.......................
10′ W [..........] igi diš-*niš* súd *i*[*na* ....

11′ W [........] x ri zi *pe-ṣi-t*[*i*....................
12′ W [......sú]d *ina* ì.udu hi.hi [........................

13′ W [..........] bar suhuš ^{ú}nu.luh.ha [...................
14′ W [..........] hi.hi *ana* dúr-*š*[*ú* gar-*an* ....

15′ W [...........] ^{giš}*šu-ši* im.gú.gar.rin.na[2] [..........

16′ W [...........] ^{giš}nam.tar níta úkuš.hab ú babbar diš-*niš* x [.......

17′ W [....... im.g]ú.gar.rin.na súd *ina* ì.udu hi.hi 2 [............
18′ W [...... g]i-*šú* gar.gar-*na* ú babbar ug[u nindu ....

19′ W [diš na *l*]*i-kis* dúr.gig šà.meš [........................... (catchline)
VV diš na *li*-[.. (catchline tablet 3)
20′ V [dub x kam] diš na *ina la si-ma-ni-šú* mur[ub$_4$.meš-*šú* gu$_7$.meš-*šú kim-ṣa-a-šú*]
colophon = Hunger, BAK No. 329

---

[1] See the similar incipit in text No. 4 (BAM 112) ii 15′, diš na murub$_4$^{2}-*šú* gig-*m*[*a* ... (kidney disease).
[2] a type of slime or mud, cf. CAD Q 53b, although the reading of the logogram is uncertain.

18′ 'dog's tongue'-leaf, and leaf of 'thorny plant', leaf of ...., *êru*-tree leaf,
19′ leaf of ***uzun lalî***, you knead it in beer and again take it out and pound it, mix it in fat and spread it on a leather strip and bind it on.

col. iv
1 If a man's hip[?] [hurts] him: one third *sila* of water or oil [..............

2 Sieve one *sila* of wheat-flour, fill a stone-jar with water, pour (the flour) into it [..............

3 If a man eats bread and vomits, drinks beer and [....................................
4 that man [suffers] from rectal disease. To cure him, [...........................
5 he drinks the root of [..........................] in the morning on an empty stomach ..[......
6 Mix .. of fine flour, a ... dog, [.......
7 ...., *baluhhu*-resin [...........]

8 ....

gap
9′ you ... [..
10′ you crush together in [............................

11′ white[?] ....[.....................................
12′ crush [..............], mix in fat, [...................

13′ [.........] peeling of root of ***nuhurtu*** [...............
14′ mix [........... and insert it] into his anus.

15′ [..................] *šūšu*, ...-mud, [..................

16′ [Crush] together [........], male mandrake, cucumber, and 'white'-plant [........]

17′ Crush [....] and ...-mud, mix them in fat, 2 [.......................
18′ keep putting [.....] on his [.....] 'white'-plant over [an oven[?] ....

19′–20′ (colophon)

No. 23 AMT 40,5, diš na *ina lā simānišu* Tablet 3[1] (plates 19–20)
rev. only preserved

X	=	K 6545 + 8355 + 9030 (AMT 40,5), cf. RA 26, 62 f.
ff	=	K 8248 (AMT 56,1) [text no. 32]
MM	=	K 9684 + (BAM 431 v 13′ ff.) [text no. 18] = ll. 16–17 (NB. lines cited here are composites of all manuscripts from Text No. 18 above)

NB: Cf. the opening lines of Ms. BB (text no. 27), which can be restored on the basis of this text.

rev. col. iii

0′	X	[.. a uzu]
1′	X	[udu.ní]ta *kab-ru-*⌜*ti*⌝ n[ag ....
2′	X	*la iš-šu-ma la iš-q*[*í-*..
3′	X	*ina* ud.5.kam *lu ina* ud.6.kam *lu ina* u[d.7.kam ....
4′	X	*ina* ud.14.kam *lu ina* ud.21.kam *lu ina* ud.23.ka[m ....
5′	X	*ina* ud.meš *an-na-ti* šéš-*su um-ṣa-te uq-ta-t*[*a-pa* ....
6′	X	*up-tar-ra-ru* KU.KU zú am.si KU.KU ^{giš}*e-lam-ma-ku* KU.KU ^{gi}[^{š}..........
7′	X	diš-*niš* ti-*qí* ^{giš}⌜kin⌝$^{?}$ gi.du$_{10}$.ga ^{šim}im.du ^{šim}gúr.gúr ^{šim}l[i ....
8′	X	dè[2] ^{giš}kiši$_{16}$ *ta-tab-bak* ká.bar.re[3]-*šú* ì.giš šéš gig *ina* ugu [..............
9′	X	diš na šà.meš-*šú* mú.mú ninda *u* kaš *muṭṭû*(lá) {*it*} *it-te-né-es-sil* na.bi *hi-ni*[*q-ti* dúr .....
10′	X	ì.udu úkuš.hab ki ì.udu ^{šim}hab illu ^{šim}buluh hi.hi *ana* dúr-*šú* gar-*a*[*n* ....
11′	X	*ta-tab-bal*[4] numun ^{giš}*šu-nim* a.gar.gar maš.dà ^{zì}kum ^{im}gú.gar.r[in.na .....
12′	X	*ina* a gazi^{sar} gim *ra-bi-ki tara-bak* kúm-*su ina* ^{kuš}[edin sur là]
13′	X	diš ki.min ú *zik-na* súd *ina* ì.udu hi.hi *al-l*[*a-na* dù ....
14′	X	diš na *mi-na-tu-šú* dub.dub gaba-*su u* sa.sal.meš-*šú* gu$_{7}$.meš-⌜*šú* á^{2}-*šú*⌝ *k*[*im-ṣa-a-šú u bir-ka-šú*][5]
	ff	[....................................... ga]ba-*su u šá-šal-la-*[*šú*] gu$_{7}$.meš-[*šú*.............................]
15′	X	gu$_{7}$.meš-*šú* éllag *bir-ki-šú lu šá* 15 *lu šá* 150 sìg-*su-ma ina mùš-tin-n*[*i-*..]
	ff	gu$_{7}$.meš-*šú* éllag *bir-ki-šú lu* šá 15 *lu šá* [15]0 [.......................................]-*šú*
16′	X	[.................................] na.bi *hi-niq-ti* dúr gig gig *ana* ti-*šú* ^{ú}*tara-muš* ^{ú}igi-*lim* ^{ú}[igi-*ešra* ...
	ff	múd *ú-kal-lam* na.bi *hi-níq-ti* dúr gig [...]
	MM	^{ú}*tara-muš*$_{8}$ ^{ú}igi-*lim* ^{ú}igi-*ešra* ^{ú}*ak-tam*
17′	X	^{ú}hab úkuš.hab úkuš-*ti-gi-li* bún *a-bat-ti* ^{ú}níg.bùr.bùr x [..............................
	MM	^{ú}hab ^{ú}úkuš.hab ^{ú}úkuš-*ti-gi-la* bún *a-bat-ti* $^{\text{na4.ú}}$níg.bùr.bùr numun ^{ú}eme.ur.gi$_{15}$
18′	X	^{ú}*nu-ṣa-bu* numun ^{šim}li $^{\text{na4}}$ka.a.ab.ba gi.dub.ba *tam-t*[*im* ....
19′	X	$^{\text{na4}}$an.zah bábbar $^{\text{na4}}$zálag gazi^{sar} numun ú dili 22 ú.hi.a *an-nu-ti* ga[z sim ....

1 Thompson, RA 26 64 points out that AMT 47,1 (K 2433) follows this tablet in sequence (see No. 24).

2 *pēntu*, CAD A/2 409.

3 See PSD B 104, 106, citing Kagal I 27 (MSL 13, 229), [*b*]*a-a*[*b ka-mu-u*], CAD K 126 f., although we interpret the meaning here as a metaphor for the anus, which is how Thompson attempted to understand the text with his translation (RA 26, 63): 'thou shall anoint the "gate" of his sore with oil'.

4 See Herrero, *Thérapeutique*, 49, citing AMT 2 2: 5 (now BAM 480), *du-muq-ši-na ta-tab-bal*, 'tu enlèveras leurs meilleures parties (des plantes médicinales)'.

5 Cf. text No. 2: 1.

TRANSLATION

0′ [..............................], he drinks thick [broth of the flesh of]
1′ male [sheep ....]
2′ (that) he did not *vomit*, he did not ....[........................
3′ On the 5th, 6th, or 7th day [..
4′ (or) on the 14th, 21st, or 23rd day [...............................
5′ on these days you should put salve on him, the haemorrhoids will be plucked off [and the ...
6′ dissolved. You take together powder of elephant tusk, powder of 'Elamite'-wood, powder of [....
7′ you pour out ..., sweet reed, *suādu*, *kukru*, juniper [......
8′ coals of *ašāgu*-(acacia), smear his 'outer-gate' with oil, the illness above ... [.......

9′ If a man's innards are inflamed and his (intake of) food and drink is diminished, he is always constipated, that man [suffers from] stricture of [the anus ...].
10′ Mix cucumber fat with fat of *ṭūru* (and) *baluḫḫu*-resin, insert it into his anus,
11′ you remove the [...], you decoct *šūnu*-seed, 'gazelle-excrement', *isqūqu*-meal (and) ...-mud
12′ in *kasû*-juice, like a concoction, when it is hot [you spread it] on a leather-strip [and bind it (on him)].

13′ If ditto, pound *bearded plant*[1], mix (it) in fat, [make a] suppository [and insert it into his anus].

14′ If his limbs are limp and his chest and back hurt him, his arms, shins, and knees
15′ hurt him, his right or left testicle aches him, and he shows blood in his urethra,
16′ that man suffers from stricture of a diseased rectum. To cure him: pound [and sieve] these 22 drugs – *taramuš*, *imḫur-līm*, [*imḫur-ešra*],
17′ madder, cucumber, gourd, ... pumice, *pallišu*-plant/stone, ... [...........
18′ *nuṣābu*, juniper-seed, coral, 'stylus'-insect (of the sea), [.........
19′ white frit, *zalāqu*-stone, *kasû*, (and) seed of 'single'-plant [.....

---

[1] Alternatively, one could read *šik-na*, but this plant does not appear in CAD Š/2, although *šiknu* can refer either generally to 'planting' (in OB usage) or to sediment in canals, etc., neither meaning of which is attested as a plant name.

20′ X ⌈^{ú}⌉*tara-muš* ^{ú}igi-*lim* ^{ú}igi-*ešra* ^{na4}*iá-artu*(pa)^{na4}*iá-ni-ba* ^{na4}*i*[*á-*...................
21′ X [........] x -⌈*ba*⌉ ^{ú}níg.sì.sì[1] ^{ú}níg.bùr.bùr ^{ú}níg.kud$^{?}$.da *kar-áš* [*tam-tim* ......
22′ X [...................................] x ⌈numun ^{giš}ma.nu ^{šim}⌉gúr.gúr ^{šim}[.........................
23′ X (traces)
24′–26′ (broken)
27′ X [.........^{gi}]^{š}geštin 21 ⌈ú⌉.[hi.a ....

28′ X ⌈pa⌉ ^{giš}pèš pa ^{giš}geštin [..
29′ X ^{ú}*ṣa-ṣu-um-*[*tu* ....
30′ X ^{ú}in$_{6}$.úš ^{giš}⌈eren⌉$^{?}$ [..
31′ X gazi^{sar}20 [ú.hi.a ....

32′–38′ (broken)
39′ X ⌈ka⌉ [...
40′ X ^{šim}gam.m[a ....

41′ X ka.a.ab.ba x [.......................................

42′ X ^{šim}gig ^{šim}gúr.g[úr ....

43′ X ^{šim}li suhuš ^{ú}x [....................................
44′ X naga.si ^{im}sahar.n[a$_{4}$.kur.ra ....

45′ X *he-pí eš-šú* ^{ú}*ṣa-*⌈*ṣu*⌉-[*um-tu*

46′ X *he-pí eš-šú* ^{šim}⌈li⌉ [...............................

47′ X [*he-pí eš*]-*šú* ^{šim}buluh [.......................................
48′ X [....... ^{ši}]^{m}g[ig ....
49′ X (traces)

rev. col. iv

1′–12′ (only ends of signs preserved)
13′–20′ (broken)
21′ X [................*i*]*t-qa ši-qit ad-*⌈*di*⌉ x x[...................
22′ X [..................] x -*ni-in-ni* gig *up-ta-a*[*s*]-*s*[*a-as*]
23′ X [................] x ⌈*ki ri*⌉ *ma ta-*⌈*par-ru*$^{?}$⌉ ú babbar *šá* illu[2] ^{giš}ásal *šum-šu*
24′ X [............] x ku$^{?}$ *šum-šú* ⌈^{šim}gig naga$^{?}$.si$^{?}$ *šum*⌉-*šú* ^{ú}*pi-zir* 1 *ma-na-at*
25′ X [............] NE gig *šá ub-búr*$^{?}$ ú x x *šum-*⌈*šu*⌉ ú.hi.a
26′ X [..........] x ì.udu si ⌈dara$_{4}$.maš hi.hi *it-qur*⌉-*ta*[*m*] ú$^{?}$ sa$^{?}$ x [.......
27′ X [.........] x *ka* nu.nu *tak-*⌈*ta-ad*⌉-*di* ì.udu *ina ap-pi* gar-*an*
28′ X [........... ì.ud]u šah ì.udu dara$_{4}$.maš *lu ka-*⌈*ia*⌉-*ma-an-ma*

29′ X [diš na ki.ná-*ma šit*]-⌈*ta-šú*⌉ ugu-*šú* du$_{10}$.ga zi-*ma i-ka-*⌈*šu-uš*⌉
30′ X [diš na *ina la si-m*]*a-ni-šú* murub$_{4}^{2}$-*šú* gu$_{7}$.meš-*šú*
(colophon, see Hunger BAK No. 318)

---

1 usually ^{ú}níg.sù.sù. This may not be the same as the flattening stone *sāpinu*, which presumably has a na$_{4}$ determinative. Can this be a *sāpinu*-plant?

2 Thompson's copy omitted the KAL sign, and hence his mistranslation of 'water' in RA 26 64.

20′ *Taramuš*, *imhur-līm*, *imhur-ešra*, *ajartu*-mussel, *ianibu*-stone, ... -stone,
21′ [.....]..., *sāpinu*-plant[?], *pallišu*-plant[?], ..., 'sea-leek'-stone,
22′ [.................................].., seed of *e'ru*, *kukru*, ...[.......................
23′–26′ ....
27′ [..........], vine/wine, 21 drugs [.................................

28′ Fig leaf, vine-leaf [.................................
29′ *ṣaṣumtu*, [...
30′ *maštakal*, *cedar*[?] [.................................
31′ *kasû*, 20 [plants ....

32′–39′ broken
40′ *ṣumlalû*, [........................

41′ Coral, [...........................

42′ *kanaktu*, *kukru*, [.......................

43′ Juniper, root of ..., [....................
44′ horned alkali, alum [...........................

45′ <new break>, *ṣaṣumtu* [..................

46′ <new break> juniper [................

47′ <new break> *baluhhu* [......
48′ [....] x *kanaktu* [..............
49′ (traces)

rev. col. iv

21′ [....................] *scales of* [...............
22′ ...., the disease will dissolve.
23′ [................]............, white plant, the name of which is Euphrates poplar-resin.
24′ its name is [......], *kanaktu*, its name is horned alkali(?) , 'cobweb' plant, 1 mana,
25′ [..............] ...., its name is ...-plant, mix the drugs
26′ [with ....]..., fat of deer horn, [you daub it with] a salve ....[............
27′ *spin* [........]......, apply fat on the nose,
28′ [..........] pig fat, deer fat, constantly.

29′ [If a man lies down and] his sleep is beneficial for him, he gets up and feels faint,
30′ [If a man's] innards hurt him prematurely.

No. 24 = **AMT 47,1** + duplicates. (plate 21–24)
diš na *ina lā simānišu* Tablet 4, see YBC 7123 + 12′ [text no. 48]

Y = K 2433 + 3989 + 4019 + 7818 + 8172 + 14216 + 14772 + 15762 + 16409 + S 357, cf. RA 26 64 f. and JSS 3,304

K 2433	=	AMT 47,1
K 3989	=	AMT 56,5
K 7818	=	AMT 53,1
K 8172	=	AMT 58,1
K 14216	=	Dream-book 364, 309[1]
K 14772	=	AMT 56,2
S 357	=	(AMT 7,7)

S 1563 (AMT 41,3) + 2061 (AMT 96,6), probably belongs to this tablet, on the basis of appearance of the tablet.
K 15453 (AMT 57,8), probably belongs to this tablet, on the basis of appearance of the tablet.

See the following tablet K 4104 (No. 25), which probably belongs to the top of rev. col. iv.

AA	=	EHE 331 + VAT 8694 + 14118 (BAM 96: 3′–9′; iii 2′–5′) [text no. 26] = ii 21′–23′ ; iv 1–3.
CC	=	VAT 10092 (BAM 104: 42–44) [text no. 28] = iv 1–3
X	=	K 6545 + 8355 + 9030 (AMT 40,5) [text no. 23] (catchline)
QQ	=	STT 100A rev. 1–7 = ll. iii 1–5.
AB	=	Ass. 13955bu (BAM 89: 8′–11′) [text no. 54]
GG	=	K 9441 = AMT 43, 5 [text no. 33 1 ff.] = iii 13–21
ff	=	K 8248 = AMT 56,1: 12 ff. [text no. 32] = iii 20–22
dd	=	S 1283 + 1947 (AMT 40,4 + 57,5) [text no. 30] = iii 18–19
EE	=	O. 194 (BAM 182) rev. 9–10 [text no. 31] (cited by Thompson, RA 26 73) = iii 18–19
VV	=	YBC 7139:8′ = No. 9d [text no. 48]

col. i

1	Y	diš na ki.ná-*ma šit-ta-šu* ugu-*šú* du$_{10}$.ga zi-*ma i-ka-šu-uš* gu[r-*ma*.......][2]
	X	[............................-*š*]*ú* ugu-*šú* du$_{10}$.ga zi-*ma i-ka-*⌜*šu*⌝-*uš*
	VV	[......... n]á-*ma šit-ta-šú* ugu-*šú* du$_{10}$.ga
2		*ana* ti-*šú* úr ^{giš}nam.tar níta ^{ú}lag.a.šà súd *ina* ì.udu hi.hi *al-la-na* d[ù-*uš ana* dúr-*šú* gar-*an*]
3	Y	diš na ki.ná-*ma* zi-*ma* ⌜*pa-nu-šú nu-pu*⌝-*hu*[3] na.bi dúr.gig [gig-*ma ana* ti-*šú*]
4	Y	*qí-lip* zú.lum.ma *qí-l*[*ip*............] *al-la-na* dù-*uš* [*ana* dúr-*šú* gar-*a*]*n*
5	Y	diš na ki.ná-*ma ši*[*t-ta-šu* ugu-*šú* du$_{10}$.ga zi-*ma i*]-*ka-šu-uš* gur-*m*[*a* ....] x
6	Y	[........] x gi [... š]u^{2}-*šú kim-ṣa-*[*a-šú* ....] x

(remainder broken)

[1] A. L. Oppenheim, *The Interpretation of Dreams in the Ancient Near East* (Philadelphia, 1956).
[2] CAD Š/3 141 cites BAM 440: 7 as parallel, but it is not.
[3] See TDP 234: 34, igi.meš-*šú nu-up-pu-hu*.

TRANSLATION

1 If a man lies down and has a good sleep, gets up and feels faint and he returns [to sleep ...],

2 to cure him, crush the root of the male mandrake and a clod of earth, mix them in fat and make a suppository [and insert it into his anus].

---

3 If a man lies down and gets up and his face is swollen, that man [suffers from] rectal disease. [To cure him],

4 [you ......] date peel with [...]-peel, you make a suppository, [you insert it into his anus].

---

5 If a man lies down and [has a good] sleep [but gets up and] feels faint and he returns [to sleep ...],

6 [......]...[....................] his hands and shins [....]..

col. ii

1 Y [diš] n[a *in-n*]*ím-me-er i-te-ni*[*k-ki-ik* i]m *ina* dúr-*šú ú-kal* ninda *u* a *tur-ra i-sil-ti* dúr gig
2 Y sa$_5$-*us-su*[1] *ul-la-ma* dugud-*šú-ma* [*la nu-u*]*h-hu-uš* kuš ur.mah *tur-ár*
3 Y ì.udu ur.mah hi.hi gur-*ma* hád.a sú[d *in*]*a* ì.giš eren hi.hi u dù-*uš ana* dúr-*šú* gar-*an*

---

4 Y diš ki.min *hi-qá* ti[2] šeg$_6$.gá [*h*]*i-qá*[3] dub.dub-*ak*
5 Y diš ki.min šum.šir.dil[4] lag mun súd *i*[*n*]*a* ì.udu hi.hi šu.si dù-*uš ana* dúr-*šú* gar-*an*
6 Y diš ki.min ^{ú}lag.a.šà illu ^{šim}buluh s[úd] *ina* ì.udu hi.hi šu.si dù-*uš ana* dúr-*šú* gar-*an*
7 Y *ina* a giš.še.nú.a šub.šub-⸢*šú*⸣ *it-qur-tú te-qé*

---

8 Y diš na dúr.gig gig-*ma i-te-nik-ki-ik* im *ina* dúr-*šú ú-kal* ^{ú}aš.⸢tál-*li*⸣[5]
9 Y [s]uhuš gi.zú.lum.ma suhuš ^{giš}nam.tar ní[t]a ⸢numun⸣ ^{ú}x [...] x ⸢numun?⸣ ^{ú}úkuš.hab [....]
10 Y [*i*]*na* ì.udu hi.hi šu.si dù-*uš* [*ina* dúr-*šú* gar-*an* a] giš.še.ná.a *ir-ta-na-haṣ*

---

11 Y ⸢^{ú}⸣igi-*lim* ^{ú}úkuš.hab ^{ú}ki.⸢kal⸣ x [.....^{ú}sum.s]ikil ^{ú}kur.kur
12 Y [níg.à]r.ra a geštin.na kala.ga im.[............] x $^{\text{gloss: u5.gar.ib.mušen ú}}$*u$_5$-ra-ni*[6]
13 Y [gazi^{s}]^{ar} ^{šim}gúr.gúr ^{šim}buluh ^{ú}[...................^{ši}]^{m}li *sah-lé-e*
14 Y [...] ^{ú}kur.ra ^{ú}*tara-muš* a.[gar].⸢gar maš⸣[.dà ....]x 23 ú.meš šeš.meš
15 Y [.] x *ta-tar-ma ina ma-suk$_x$*(TAR)-*ti*[7] *ta-pa-aṣ* [........ *t*]*a-ṣab-bat* šu.si-*ka* nigin^{mi}
16 Y [dúr-*š*]*ú ta-kar* ká dúr-*šú te-ṭè-pi šum$_4$-ma ina* x [............................. d]ù ^{šim}gír
17 Y [ì.n]un *u* illu ^{šim}buluh súd-*ma* dúr-*š*[*ú* .... s]ù-*ma ina-eš*

---

18 Y [diš ki.min ...] x *ana* ti-*šú* ^{šim}gúr.gúr ^{ú}kur.kur naga.si ú babbar [.........
19 Y [.......] ⸢^{ú}⸣gamun.ge$_6$.ki pa ú nam.ti.la še$_{10}$ u[r.gi$_7$ ....
20 Y [gaba].⸢làl⸣.[...t]i téš.bi gaz sim *ina* ì.udu hi.hi *u al*[*la-na* dù-*uš ina* dúr-*šú* gar-*an*]

---

21 Y diš na ninda gu$_7$ kaš n[ag] šà.meš-*šú* mú.meš *ú-na-paq* na.b[i ....
AA [..m]eš *ú-na-paq* [...................................
22 Y ^{ú}*šur-šur*[8] ú babbar n[ag]a.s[i] suhuš ^{giš}nam.tar níta illu li.dar ⸢^{ú}⸣[.........................
AA [^{ú}*š*]*ur-šur* ú babbar naga.si [..] ⸢^{ú}⸣gamun.ge$_6$ ⸢^{ú}⸣gamun
23 Y illu ^{šim}buluh úkuš-[*ti-g*]*i*-⸢*lum*⸣ ì.udu ur.mah hi.hi ⸢*alla-na*⸣ [dù-*uš ina* dúr-*šú* ....]
AA [.................................]-*lum-ma ina* ì.udu ur.mah hi.hi [...........................] gar-*an-ma* ti-*uṭ*

---

24 Y [di]š na dúr.gig g[ig-*ma* ì.]udu éllag udu [níta.......................

---

25 Y x x ki.a-^{d}í[d ......]
26 Y (traces)

---

1 = *samussu*, cf. Heeßel BAD 250: 2, *sīmutu*.
2 BAM 3 228: 20 and Herrero, *Thérapeutique* 59. Although a plural form *hiqāti* (see AHw 347b) is possible here, it seems preferable to have the same singular form twice within the same clause.
3 In AMT 56, 5: 4, this sign is incorrectly shown as a gloss.
4 *turû*, cf. MSL 10, 92 and 112: 147 (RS) and 118: 51, and H. Waetzoldt, *Bulletin of Sumerian Agriculture* III (1987), 35, M. Stol, *ibid.*, 57.
5 one expects aš.tál.tál.
6 The gloss = *rikibti arkabi*, see CAD R 344, an example of *Dreckapotheke*, used as a *Deckname* for the drug *urānu*.
7 The 'tar'-sign is cryptography, based upon sila(TAR) = *sūqu*, as a writing for *masūktu* (CAD M/1, 329) 'mortar' [courtesy I. L Finkel].
8 Reading F. Köcher (courtesy B. Böck), perhaps to be related to the *šuršurru*-fruit, see CAD Š/3 366.

col. ii

1 [If a] man has intestinal colic, he constantly scratches himself, he retains wind in his anus, food and fluids are regurgitated (and) he suffers from constipation of the rectum –

2 its 'redness' is *raised* and troubles him [without] giving him relief,[1] you dessicate a lion skin

3 and mix it with lion fat, you dry (it) a second time, crush and mix it in cedar oil, make a pessary and insert it into his anus.

---

4 If ditto, you take (and) boil diluted beer, you pour out the diluted beer.

5 If ditto, you crush single-clove garlic and a lump of salt, mix (them) in fat, make a pessary and insert (it) into his anus.

6 If ditto, you crush a clod of earth and resin of *baluhhu*, mix (them) in fat, make a suppository, insert (it) into his anus,

7 keep dipping it into *šunû*-juice and daub (his anus) with a salve.

---

8 If a man suffers from rectal disease and he constantly scratches himself, and he retains wind in his anus: you mix in fat *ardadillu*,

9 root of *kūru*, root of male mandrake, ... cucumber-seed, ...

10 you make a suppository and [you insert it into his rectum], and he continually bathes in *šunû*-[juice].

---

11 *Imhur-lim*-plant, cucumber, grass, [...], onion, *atā'išu*,

12 groats, strong vinegar, [........].., *urânu* (gloss: bat guano)

13 *kasû*?, *kukru*, *baluhhu*, [....], juniper, *sahlû*,

14 [...], *nīnû*, *taramuš*, gazelle-dung, [...............] these 23 drugs

15 [you ...], you repeat and you pulverise them in a mortar, you take hold of [.......] , you wrap your finger

16 and you rub his [anus], you *widen* his anal opening. If .. [..................], myrtle,

17 crush butter and *baluhhu*-resin and sprinkle his anus [with ....] and he will get better.

---

18 [If ditto ...], to cure him, *kukru*, *ata'išu*, horned alkali, 'white' plant, [..............]

19 [....], black *kamūnu*, leaf of 'health'-plant, dog excrement, [........]

20 wax, [....], pound and sieve them together, mix in fat, and [make a] suppository [and insert it into his anus].

---

21 If a man eats food (and) drinks beer, his innards are inflamed, it is stopped up, that man [suffers from ....]

22 mix *šuršurru*, 'white' plant, horned alkali, male-mandrake root, *abukkatu*-resin, black *kamūnu*, *kamūnu*,

23 *baluhhu*-resin, gourd, and lion-fat, [make a] suppository, put it [into his anus] and he will improve.

---

24 If a man suffers from rectal disease, [fat] of [male] sheep kidney, [............

---

25 ... sulphur [...]

---

26 ......

[1] Alternatively < *nahāšu*, 'does not bring good health'.

rev. col. iii

1′ Y diš na sa dú[r-*šú* ....
QQ diš na sa dúr-*šú* tag.t[ag-............................] na.bi dúr.gig *i*[*na* ......
2′ Y *ana* a giš.še.ná.⌜a⌝ [..
QQ [...] ugu šéš x [..........
3′ Y dúr-*šú ta-kar* num[un? ....
QQ dúr-*šú ta-* x numun? [...

4′ Y diš na *ki-ṣil-la-šú* g[u$_7$.meš ....
QQ diš na *ki-ṣil-*[...
5′ Y *kib-rit* im.g[ú.en.na ....
QQ [.....................................] *e-la-t*[*i* ....] x x [...............

6′ Y diš na *ki-ṣil-la-šú* gu$_7$.me[š ....
7′ Y dúr.gig gig [..................

8′ Y ^{ú}*di-šu* ^{ú}x [......................
9′ Y *nap-pi-i* x [........................

10′ Y [diš.n]a x x x [..] ⌜^{šim}gam⌝.[ma ....

11′ Y [.....................] níta ì.nun.na tuh.š[è.giš.ì ....
12′ Y [.....................] ⌜a⌝ buru$_8$ illu li.dur ú babbar x [..........

13′ Y [...................zà.hi.l]i? naga.si *qa-la-a-ti* ú [...........
GG ^{ú}kur.kur zà.[hi.li..
14′ Y [................ ^{ši}]^{m}li ^{šim}šeš mun.kù.p[ad ....
GG [.........................] ^{šim}šeš m[un...............................
15′ Y [.................]-⌜*e*⌝ gaz sim *ina* i[zi ....

16′ Y [..................] x mun naga.si *tur-á*[*r* ....
GG min zú.lum.ma mun x [..
17′ Y [.................^{š}]^{im}gam.ma il[lu ....
GG [.................] ^{šim}gam.ma ill[u ....

18′ Y [.............. g]ig gig dúr-*šú e-s*[*i-il* gar.ib.u$_5$^{mušen} suhuš ^{giš}nam.tar níta]
GG diš na dúr.gig gig dúr-*šú e-*[*sil* ....
dd diš na dúr gig-*ma* dúr-*šú e-sil* gar.ib.u$_5$^{mušen} [s]uhuš ^{giš}nam.tar níta
EE [d]iš na dúr gig-*ma* dúr-*šú e-sil* ^{mušen}u$_5$.gar.[ib su]huš ^{giš}nam.tar níta
19′ Y [.......................] *tu-kap-pat* [.................]
GG [...........] diš-*niš tu-kap-pat* [.......................
dd súd hi.hi diš-*niš tu-kap-pat ana* dúr-*šú* gar
EE súd diš-*niš tu-kap-pat ana* dúr-*šú* [..]

20′ Y [....................... ka]š nag-*ma e-si-*[*il* úh.meš *i-šal-la* šà.meš-*šú*]
GG diš na ninda gu$_7$ kaš.sag nag-*ma e-si-il* ú[h.............................]
ff [............... g]u$_7$ kaš nag-*ma e-sil* úh.meš-*šú i-šal-la* š[à.meš-*šú*]
21′ Y [*it-tan-n*]*a-bi-ṭu ir-ru-*⌜*ú-šu i-ár-ru-ru*⌝ [..]
GG [.......................] *ir-ru-šu i-ár-ru-ur* na.bi dúr.gig gig [......................]
ff [*it*]*-tan-na-bi-ṭu* [..........] ⌜*i*⌝*-ár-ru-ru ana* na.bi dúr.gig gig *ana* ti-*šú*
22′ Y [.......................... la]g mun 1/2 ma nag[a.si ..]
ff 1/3 ma.na x [..........] x ^{sar} 1/3 ma.na naga.si
23′ Y [................ ^{giš}]eren 1/2 ma ^{giš}šur.min pap 6 ú.[hi.a]

rev. col. iii

1′ If a man's rectal veins are affected [...........], that man [suffers from] rectal disease ...[...
2′ into *šunû*-juice and juice of [.........................], smear above (?) ...[....
3′ you rub his anus. *Seed* [of ....]

4′ If a man's ankles are constantly hurting[1] [............................
5′ sulphur, river mud [..............] *apart from* [........................]....[...............

6′ If a man ankles are constantly hurting [......................]
7′ he suffers from rectal disease, [..]

8′ spring grass, ... [..]
9′ a sieve [..]

10′ [If a] man ....., *ṣumlalû*, [...

11′ male [................], ghee, sesame residue, [.....................
12′ [...................] ...., *abukkatu*-resin, 'white'-plant, [........

13′ *ata'išu*, *sahlû*, roasted horned alkali, ..[..............................
14′ [................] juniper, myrrh, block-salt, [....................
15′ pound and sieve [.....].., [roast them] on a fire [...................

16′ You dessicate ditto, dates, salt (and) horned alkali, [...................
17′ [.................], *ṣumlalû*, resin [of ....

18′ If a man suffers from rectal disease, his rectum is stopped up, crush and mix together bat guano and root of male mandrake,
19′ you roll (them) up and insert it into his anus.

20′ If a man eats food and drinks (premium) beer and is constipated, he spits up his spittle, [his] bowels suffer from cramp,
21′ his intestines discharge (a putrid liquid), that man suffers from rectal disease. To cure him,
22′ one third mina [.............] lump of salt, half (var. one third) mina of horned alkali, ...]
23′ [...........................] cedar, half a mina of cypress, in total 6 drugs

[1] Painful or swollen ankles is a sign of hypertension.

24′ Y [*ina tinūri te-se*]*k-ker* e$_{11}$-*ma tu-kaṣ-ṣa* ì.giš *ana* igi šu[b]
25′ Y [..................*an*]*a* dúr-*šú* dub-*ma ina-eš*

col. iv

1′ Y [..*qer*]-*bé-nu* g[ig..........................]
AA diš na ⸢ka⸣ d[úr-*šú* ....] *um-ṣa-tu*$_{4}$ ill[u]
CC [......................-*š*]*ú* mú.mú-*hu ú-na-paq qer-bé-nu* gig *um-ṣa-tu*$_{4}$ illu
2′ Y [...] x illu li.dur numun [.......]-*tam* še$_{10}$ ur.gi$_{7}$ suhuš x [....]
AA [..] še$_{10}$ ur.gi$_{7}$ suhuš ^{giš}[..................................]
CC [...................-*t*]*u*$_{4}$ numun ^{ú}*ak-tam* še$_{10}$ ur.gi$_{7}$ suhuš ^{giš}nam.tal níta ^{ú}kur.ra^{sa}[⸢r⸣]
3′ Y [^{ú}š]um.šir.dili ^{ú}*pi-zìr* gurun ⸢^{giš}maš⸣.huš súd *ina* ì.udu hi.hi šu.si dù-*u*[*š*]
AA [.......................]^{ú}*pi*$^{!}$-*zir* gurun ^{ú}m[aš...
CC [...] šu.si dù-*uš ana* dúr-*šú* gar-*a*[*n*]

4′ Y [ki.min *ki-m*]*a* dúr-*šú* ⸢*it-ta-pú-ú*⸣[1] kuš ur.mah *ta-qàl*-[*lu*..............]
5′ Y [*ina* ì.ud]u hi.h[i š]u.si dù-*uš ana* dúr-*šú* gar-*a*[*n*]

6′ Y [.......] ⸢á$^{?}$⸣-*šú* [................................gi]g na.bi *qé-reb* dúr gi[g]
AB diš na *a-ha-šú kìn-ṣa-šú ki-ṣil-la-šú* [gig] na.bi *qé-reb* dúr.gig
7′ Y [...] ⸢šu.si⸣ dù-*uš ana* dúr-*šú* gar-*a*[*n*]
AB ^{šim}[....] ì.udu ^{šim}gig súd *ina* ì.ud[u ....] šu.si dù-*uš ana* dúr-*šú* gar-*an-m*[*a* ti]

8′ Y [.................................] ina ^{uruduu}šen.tur š[eg$_{6}$.gá]
9′ Y [....................................^{š}]^{im}gúr.gúr *sah-*⸢*lé*⸣*-e* ⸢*nu-* x⸣
10′ Y [..*ta-h*]*as-sap* nigin
11′ Y x ⸢*tu*⸣ *ki im* [..........................] x ì.nun tag
12′ Y [ì.u]du$^{?}$ *ta-za-rù t*[*a-*..................] ⸢ì⸣.nun dúr-*šú* šéš

13′ Y diš na dúr gig gi[g-*ma di-ik-š*]*á* tuku (catchline)
14′ Y dub-4-kam diš na *ina la si-ma-*[*ni-šú* murub$_{4}$.meš] gu$_{7}$.meš-*šú*
colophon = Hunger, BAK No. 329

1 Taken provisionally from *napû*, although not attested in this usage in medical texts.

24′ that you heat [in an oven], take out, and cool. Put oil into (the mixture),
25′ pour[1] [..........] into his anus and he will get better.

col. iv

1′ If a man's anal opening is inflamed and stopped up, and is ill internally; haemorrhoids: you crush
2′ *abukkatu*-resin, *aktam*-seed, dog excrement, root of male mandrake, *nīnû*,
3′ single-clove garlic, 'cobweb'-plant, the fruit of *kalbānu*, mix (them) in fat, make a pessary (var. and insert it into his anus).

4′ [If ditto] *when* his anus *acted as a sieve*, you roast lion's hide [..............],
5′ mix it [in] fat, make a suppository and insert it into his anus.

6′ If a man's arms, thighs, and ankles are sore, that man is ill within the rectum,
7′ crush [.....] and fat of *kanaktu*, [mix it] in fat of [....], make a pessary and insert it in his anus.

8′ Heat [......................................] in a small copper-dish,
9′ [..], *kukru*, *sahlû*, ...
10′ [...you] tear (and) wrap
11′ .... [..] apply ghee,
12′ you spread the fat[?], you [..........], you smear his anus with ghee.

13′ If a man suffers from rectal disease and has piercing pain (= catchline).

[1] Note the distinction in this text between drugs which are poured into the anus and the pessary or suppository which is inserted or placed in the anus. This same distinction is found in Egyptian medical texts, which call for drugs to be 'poured' (*wedeh*) into the anus, while a pessary is 'placed' (*redi*) in the anus, see J. Nunn, *Ancient Egyptian Medicine* (Norman, Oklahoma, 1996), 143.

No. 24a fragments which may belong:

Y_2 = S 1563 (AMT 31,3) + 2061 (AMT 96,6) (plate 24)

1′ [..] x ⌜gú⌝ [................

2′ [...............................] téš.bi súd *ina* a.geštin [....................................
3′ [.........................gišgi.gíd dù-*uš* túg.hi.a *tu*]-*la-ba-áš* *ana* dúr-*šú* [gar-*an*][1]

4′ [..........] ì.udu éllag udu níta [...................
5′ [................. *tu-la-ba-á*]*š* *ana* dúr-*šú* [gar-*an*]

6′ [............] ⌜-*an* *úr-né-e* súd⌝ [.................

7′ [šimgúr.gúr šiml]i šimgam.me šimb[al ....
8′ [.........]-*ṣa-a-ti* še.giš.ì zú.[lum.ma ....
9′ [.........ì.udu éllag] udu níta hi.hi *al-l*[*a-na* ....
10′ (traces)

Y_3 = K 15453 (plate 24)

1′ (trace)
2′ [...-*k*]*a-at* nu x [...]
3′ [.. *alla*?]-*na* *ana* dúr-*šú* ga[r-*an*]

4′ [... g]ig gig *ana* t[i-*šú*]
5′ [.. ga]mun.ge₆ ú [....]
6′ [...] x x [...]

[1] For the restoration, cf. text No. 28: 20.

No. 25 = AMT 58,2, diš na *ina lā simānišu* Tablet 5[1]

Z	=	K 4104 (AMT 58,2); cf. RA 26, 67; this probably belongs to K 2433+ [text no. 24], top of rev. col. iv
BB	=	VAT 10723 (BAM 88: 13′–16′) [text no. 27] = ll. 1–2
AA	=	EHE 331 + VAT 8694 + 14118 (BAM 96 iii 15′ f.) [text no. 26] = ll. 1–6;
VV	=	YBC 7126 (+) 7139 13′ [text no. 48] = l. 1

1	Z	diš na dúr gig gig-*ma di-ik-ša* t[uk-..]
	BB	[.................. g]ig-*ma di-ik-šá* tuk-*ši* [......................]-*ma-har* úh *ina*! dúr-*šú ú*-[*tab-bak*]
	AA	diš na dúr gig gig-*ma di-ik-ša* tuk ninda *u* a šà-*šú la i-m*[*a-har*] úh *ina* dúr-*šú ú-ta*[*b*]-*ba-ka*
	VV	diš na dúr [gig] gig-*ma* [..]
2	Z	*ana* ti-*šú* ^{ú}har.har ^{ú}*úr-nu-u ina* a g[azi ....]
	BB	[.......................^{ú}]*úr-nu-u ina* a gazi^{sar}[..........................] x x [........]
	AA	*ana* ti-*šú* ^{ú}har.har ^{ú}*úr-n*[*é*-.] *ina* a gazi^{sar}*ana* dúr-*šú* [d]ub-*ak* geštin.šur nag ^{šim}li
3	Z	^{šim}gúr.gúr im.gú.en.na a.gar.gar maš.dà zà.hi.l[i ....]
	AA	^{ši}[^{m}..........................] a.gar.gar maš.dà zà.hi.[l]i súd *ina* kaš ^{urudu}šen.tur *tara*-[*bak* ...]
4	Z	ì.udu ^{šim}gig ì.udu ukuš.hab numun ^{ú}si.sá [...]
	AA	^{giš}li ì.udu ^{š}[^{i}]^{m}gig ì.udu ukuš.hab num[un ....] diš-*niš* súd šu.[s]i dù-*uš ana* dúr-*šú* [gar-*an*]

5	Z	diš ki.min ^{ú}geštin.ka$_5$.a *ina* kaš nag ú babbar *ina* kaš nag [..................
	AA	diš ki.min ^{ú}geštin.⸢ka$_5$⸣.a *ina* kaš nag ⸢ú⸣ babbar *ina* [...........] x làl kur nag
6	Z	*ina* a ^{giš}še.nu *ir-ta-na-haṣ* geštin.šur.ra *ina* a gazi^{sar} *ana* dú[r-*šú* .....
	AA	*ina* a ^{giš}še.nu *ir*-[..] *ana* dúr-*šú* dub-*ak* numun ^{ú}á[b.duh]
7	Z	pa ^{giš}*šu-še* pa ^{giš}gi$_6$.pàr pa ^{ú}in$_6$.úš pa ^{giš}*pu*-[........

8	Z	diš na dúr.gig gig-*ma di-ik-ša* tuk nin[da *u* a šà-*šú la i-ma-har* úh *ina* dúr-*šú ú-tab-ba-ka*][2]
9	Z	^{ú}har.har ^{ú}*úr-nu-u ina* a ka[š ....
10	Z	^{ú}*šeš-še-ra* a.gar.gar maš.d[à ....
11	Z	ú babbar ^{šim}šeš nag[a.si ....

12	Z	diš na šà-*šú man*-g[*u* ....
13	Z	suhuš ^{giš}*šu-ši* [................................
14	Z	šu x [...

---

1 See text No. 48 (YBC 7123+) 13′.

2 Restored after l. 1.

TRANSLATION

1 If a man suffers from rectal disease and has piercing pain and his belly cannot take in food and fluids (and) he pours out mucous from his anus,

2 to cure him: pour *hašû* (and) *urnû* in *kasû*-juice into his anus, he drinks drawn wine. Crush juniper,

3 *kukru*, river mud, gazelle-dung (and) *sahlû*, decoct (it) in beer, (in) a small copper vessel,

4 crush together (var. juniper), *kanaktu*-fat, cucumber-fat, seed of *šurdunû* [...], make a pessary and [insert it] into his anus.

---

5 If ditto, he drinks fox-vine in beer, he drinks 'white' plant in beer, he drinks [... and(?)] mountain honey.

6 He continually bathes in *šunû*-juice, (and) you pour drawn wine in *kasû*-juice into his anus. [Crush] seed of *kamantu*,

7 leaf of *šūšu*-tree, leaf of *lipāru*, leaf of *maštakal*, leaf of ..[............

---

8 If a man suffers from rectal disease and has piercing pain [and his belly cannot take in food and fluids (and) he pours out mucous from his anus]

9 [Mix] *hašû* (and) *urnû* in water, beer [or ....

10 red paste, gazelle-dung, [.............

11 'white' plant, myrrh, horned alkali, [................................

---

12 If a man's innards [suffer from] paralysis [.......................

13 root of *šūšu*-tree, [........................

14 ...[...........................

No. 26 BAM 96

AA	=	EHE 331 + VAT 8694 + 14118 (BAM 96)[1]
CC	=	VAT 10092 (BAM 104: 7–8, 42–44) [text no. 28] = i 10–11; iii 2–7
Y	=	K 2433 + (AMT 47,1 +) [text no. 24] = 5′–9′; iii 2–5
AH	=	VAT 16449 (BAM 97: 9′–12′) = ii 1–4
W	=	S 36 + (AMT 43,1 and dupl.) [text no. 22] = ii 5–8
BB	=	VAT 10723 (BAM 88) [text no. 27] = iii 15–17
Z	=	K 4104 (AMT 58,2) [text no. 25] = iii 15–23

col. i

2′	AA	[..] sum^{sar}
3′	AA	[..*ina* ì.ud]u hi.hi
4′	AA	[..] gar-*an*
5	AA	[..m]eš *ú-na-paq*
	Y	diš na ninda gu$_7$ kaš n[ag] šà.meš-*šú* mú.meš *ú-na-paq*
6′	AA	[....................................... ^{ú}*š*]*ur-šur* ú babbar naga.si
	Y	na.b[i ....] ^{ú}*šur-šur* ú babbar n[ag]a.s[i]
7′	AA	[..................................] ⌜ú⌝gamun.ge$_6$ ⌜ú⌝gamun
	Y	suhuš ^{giš}nam.tar níta illu li.dar x [..............................
8′	AA	[..................................]-*lum-ma ina* ì.udu ur.mah hi.hi
	Y	illu ^{šim}buluh úkuš-[*ti-g*]*i*-⌜*lum*⌝ ì.udu ur.mah hi.hi
9′	AA	[..................................] gar-*an-ma* ti-*ut*
	Y	⌜*alla-na*⌝ [dù-*uš ina* dúr-*šú* ....]
10′	AA	[.............................]-*i* udu.níta naga.si ^{šim}buluh
	CC	[.............................] udu.níta naga.si ^{šim}bu[luh]
11′	AA	[.............................*ina* é]sir *tuš-te-mid-ma ana* dúr-*šú* gar-*an-ma ina-eš*
	CC	[.............................] ésir *tuš-te-mid ana* dúr-*šú* gar-*an-ma ina-eš*
12′	AA	[diš na.............................]-*šú* íl[2] murub$_4$.meš-*šú* tag.tag-*šú* ninda *u* kaš *ip-ru*
13′	AA	[..................................] ⌜ú<nu.>bal⌝ suhuš ^{giš}nam.tar níta x x x x x x
14′	AA	[.................................. s]úd *ina* kaš nag-*ma i-ár-ru*
15′	AA	[.................................. nag]a.si *ina* ì.udu hi.hi u dù-*uš-ma ana* dúr-*šú* gar-*an*
16′	AA	[..........................*ina*] a ra-*su-ma* en še$_{10}$-*šú i-par-ru-u*
17′	AA	[..................................] x ge$_6$ ^{ú}kur.ra
18′	AA	[..................................] x ì *ta-kar* šéš ì.giš diri *ana* igi gar-*an*
19′	AA	[..] ⌜níta⌝ *tam-kak*(?) *ina* ì.nun.na *u* ì.udu hi.hi
20′	AA	[..*ana* dúr]-*šú* gar-*an*
21′	AA	[..-*t*]*i-lu* ^{giš}kiši$_{16}$
22′	AA	[.. *a*]*na* igi dúr-*šú* šéš lá-*id*
23′	AA	[diš na ....*m*]*a-le-e si-ka-tim*
24′	AA	[..^{ú}*b*]*a-ri-ra-ta*[3] diš-*niš* gaz

[1] F. Köcher's catalogue for this text cites lines from BAM 98 and BAM 101 corresponding to ll. ii 5–8, but the texts are not close enough to be given here as duplicates.

[2] *našû*, see CAD N/2 85 f.

[3] Reading F. Köcher (courtesy B. Böck).

TRANSLATION

2′ [..] onion,
3′ mix [.. in] fat,
4′ [..] insert it [in his anus ....]

5′ If a man eats food (and) drinks beer, his innards are inflamed, it is stopped up,
6′ that man [suffers from ....]. Mix (l. 8) *šuršurru*, 'white' plant, horned alkali,
7′ root of male-mandrake, *abukkatu*-resin, black *kamūnu*, *kamūnu*,
8′ *baluhhu*-resin, gourd, and lion fat,
9′ [make a] suppository, insert it [into his anus] and he will improve.

10′ [......................................] of a male sheep, horned alkali, *baluhhu*,
11′ [..........................], you mix (it) [in] bitumen, insert it into his anus and he will recover.

12′ [If a man's ...] is tense, his groin constantly bothers him, he has thrown up food and beer,
13′ crush [..........................] *tullal*-plant, root of male mandrake, ...
14′ [..........................] he drinks it in beer and he will vomit.
15′ [....................... and] horned alkali, mix (them) in fat, make a pessary and put it into his anus.
16′ [.............................] bathe him in water until he defecates.
17′ [................................] black ..., *nīnû*,
18′ [...] you rub in and smear oil, fill it with oil (and) apply it.

19′ [................................] you make a ...., mix it in ghee and fat,
20′ [.................................] insert it [into] his [anus].

21′ [...] ...., acacia-thorn,
22′ [..........................], you rub it onto his anus and bind it on.

23′ [If a man's ... .] full of pustules,
24′ pound together *barīrātu*, [...]

25′	AA	[...] lá-*ma ina-eš*
26′	AA	[...] x *mi-iq-ta*
27′	AA	[...] hi min
28′	AA	[..]-*šú* x x -*ú*
29′	AA	(traces)

col. ii

1	AA	diš na šà.meš-*šú* ta[g.tag-*šu*] *mi-na-tu-šu* du$_8$.meš na.b[i ....]
	AH	[...........................] *mi-na-tu-šu* du$_8$.du$_8$-*ra* na.bi [..........]
2	AA	^{ú}in.uš ^{ú}kur.kur ^{ú}sumun.dar ^{ú}nu.luh.ha ⸢^{ú}⸣[.............]
	AH	[.......] *a-ta-i-šu* ^{ú}sumun.dar ⸢^{ú}⸣[
3	AA	x x x x *ina* mul$_4$ *tuš-bat ina* á.gú.zi.ga *in*[*a* ....]
	AH	[.......] *ina* mul$_4$ [...] ⸢a⸣?
4	AA	nag-*ma* [........]
	AH	nag-*ma* [........]
5	AA	ì.udu éllag gud ì.udu éllag udu.nita ì.udu ur.mah ì.nun.n[a ....]
	W	diš ki.min ⸢ì⸣.[udu gud ì.ud]u éllag udu.níta ì.nun ⸢ì⸣ [*a-si*] du.du-*ki*
6	AA	ì.giš mušen ì.giš ⸢$^{šim.giš}$⸣gír ì.giš ⸢x⸣-na ^{šim}šeš ^{giš}ere[n...
	W	ì mušen ì.giš ^{š}[^{im} ....] x ^{šim}šeš
7	AA	illu ^{šim}buluh illu li.dur ú babbar ^{ú}hab ^{šim}hab ì šé[š.meš]
	W	^{šim}bul[uh i]llu li.tar ú babbar súd diš-*niš* h[i.hi ... š]éš.meš
8	AA	ì.udu úkuš.hab gazi^{sar} *ina* ^{síg}àka *ta-lap-pap ana* dúr-*šú* gar-[*an*]
	W	[*nap-šal-ti* dú]r gig
9	AA	diš na dúr.gig.ga.kam gig ^{ú}*sah-le-e*^{sar} ^{ú}kur.ra ^{ú}gúr.gú[r]
10	AA	^{šim}li naga.si ⸢*tu*⸣-*ra-a* ^{ú}*pi-in-ze-er* zú.lum.[ma]
11	AA	téš.bi *ta-pa-aṣ ina* ì.udu hi.hi *al-la-nam* dù-*uš ana* dúr-*šú* gar-*an*
12	AA	zà.hi.li^{sar} ^{ú}kur.ra ^{ú}*kur-ka-nam er-ra*[1] *hi-il bu-*⸢*ka*⸣-[*ti*][2]
13	AA	*kib*!-*ri-tú ina* ì.udu hi.hi ú.hi.a *an-nu-ti tuš-t*[*a-bal*?]
14	AA	diš na murub$_4$.meš-*šú* ⸢gu$_7$-*šú*⸣ *iš-dú*?-*šú* ⸢du$_8$.du$_8$⸣ [na.b]i dúr gig.[ga.kam gig]
15	AA	^{ú}*ši-iz-ba-nam* x [...] x zi *sah*-[*lé-e* ....
16	AA	^{šim}gúr.gúr ^{šim}li ^{ú}*šib*-[*bur-r*]*a-tú*[3] ^{ú}[............................
17	AA	a.gar.gar maš.dà pap x [..] x ta [........................
18	AA	diš na dúr.gig gig *u* kàš-[*šú*...] x a x [...................... na.bi]
19	AA	dúr.[g]ig gig bar zú.lum.m[a ....
20	AA	diš na dúr.gig gig-*ma* hur.meš-[*šú* ....
21	AA	izi šub.šub-*su* nam.rim [................................
22	AA	^{ú}áb.duh diš-*niš* hi.hi [......................................
23	AA	diš ki.min *sah-lé-e* na$_4$ x [..........................
24	AA	^{ú}har.har ⸢^{ú}⸣[..
25	AA	^{ú}x [..
26	AA	gurun x [...

[1] spoiled? see CAD E 307 (rare), attested AMT 16,1: 2 referring to a drug.
[2] for *hīl abukkati*, see CAD A/1 81. Reading F. Köcher (courtesy B. Böck).
[3] Reading F. Köcher (courtesy B. Böck).

25′ [..] bind it on and he will recover.

26′–29′ broken

col. ii

1 If a man's innards bother him and his limbs are flaccid, that man [suffers from ...., to cure him]
2 *maštakal*, *ata'išu*, *šumuttu*, *nuhurtu*, .[....]
3 ...., leave it out over night, in the morning, ..[.........]
4 he drinks it and [he will recover].

5 Keep smearing (l. 7) fat of ox kidney, fat of male sheep kidney, lion fat, ghee, oil of creeping [myrtle],
6 bird oil, oil of myrtle, oil of ..., myrrh, cedar, [............
7 *baluhhu*-resin, *abukkatu*-resin, 'white'-plant, madder, *ṭūru*, (var. crush, mix together),
8 you wrap into a wad of wool cucumber fat and *kasû*, and insert it into his anus (var. [salve] for rectal disease).

9 If a man suffers from rectal-disease, you pulverise (l. 11) together *sahlû*, *nīnû*, *kukru*
10 juniper, horned alkali, single garlic, 'cobweb'-plant, date,
11 mix (them) in fat, you make a suppository and insert it into his anus.
12 Mix *sahlû*, *nīnû*, 'spoiled(?)' *kurkānû*, *abukkatu*-resin,
13 and sulpher in fat. You *stir* these drugs.

14 If a man has pain in his groin and his *lower extremeties* are always loose, that [man suffers from] anus-disease.
15 milk-plant, ..., *sahlû*, [.......................................]

16 *kukru*, juniper, rue, [..................
17 gazelle-dung,........... [................

18 If a man suffers from anus disease and [his] urine .... [.................that man]
19 suffers from anus disease. Date peel, [.....................

20 If a man suffers from anus disease and [his] lungs [......................
21 and fever keeps attacking him, an oath [.................................
22 Mix together [........] , *kamantu* [................................

23 If ditto, *sahlû*, ...-stone of [....
24 *hašû*, ..[....................................
25–26 (broken)

rev. col. iii

1′	AA	(traces)
2′	AA	diš na ⌜ka⌝ d[úr-*šú*..]
	CC	[......................-*š*]*ú* mú.mú-*hu ú-na-paq qer-bé-nu* gig
	Y	[...]-*bé-nu* g[ig...........]
3′	AA	*um-ṣa-tu*$_4$ ill[u ....]
	CC	*um-ṣa-tu*$_4$ illu [...........-*t*]*u*$_4$ numun ^{ú}*ak-tam*
	Y	[.................] x illu li.dur numun [..]-*tam*
4′	AA	še$_{10}$ ur.gi$_7$ suhuš ^{giš}[...]
	CC	še$_{10}$ ur.gi$_7$ suhuš ^{giš}nam.tal níta ^{ú}kur.ra^{sar}[................]
	Y	še$_{10}$ ur.gi$_7$ suhuš ^{gi}[^{š}.............................. š]um.šir.dil
5′	AA	^{ú}*pi*$^{!}$-*zir* gurun ^{ú}m[aš...]
	CC	[...] šu.si dù-*uš ana* dúr-*šú* gar-*a*[*n*]
	Y	^{ú}*pi-zìr*[1] gurun ⌜^{giš}maš⌝.huš súd *ina* ì.udu hi.hi šu.si dù-*u*[*š*]
6′	AA	diš ki.min tag-*ma* dúr-*šú il-ta-n*[*ap-pat* ....]
	CC	[............. ta]g$^{?}$ [dú]r-*šú* [..........................] x x[2] udu
7′	AA	*ina* ì.udu hi.hi šu.si [.............................
	CC	*ina* ì.udu hi.hi šu.si dù-*uš ana* dú[r-*šú* gar-*an*]
8′	AA	diš na kàš.me-*šú ina* dúr *e-te-rim* [dúr].gig [gig ......
9′	AA	*qí-lip* zú.lum.ma *ina* ì.giš [^{giš}e]ren.na hi.hi x [..........
10′	AA	diš na *qer-bé-na* gig ^{gi}[^{š}geš]tin.šur kaš.sag al.⌜ús.sa⌝ [..]
11′	AA	*tu-kaṣ-ṣa ana* dúr-*šú* dub-*ak* illu ^{šim}buluh ^{šim}buluh ^{š}[^{im}....]
12′	AA	zà.<hi.>li *ina* ì.udu hi.hi *ana* dúr-*šú* gar-*an* ^{ú}esi šu.si-*ka* m[ar-*ma ina itqi*]
13′	AA	nigin ^{ú}kur.ra ki x x naga.si *ta-sàk* šu.si-*ka* ì.n[un.na ....]
14′	AA	*ana* ugu *ta-za-ru*$_4$ *ta-kar ana* a ^{giš}še.nu šub.šub-*šú* ì.nun *tuš-t*[*e-mid* ....]
15′	AA	diš na dúr.gig gig-*ma di-ik-ša* tuk ninda *u* a šà-*šú la i-m*[*a-har*]
	BB	diš na dúr.gig gig-*ma di-ik-šá* tuk-*ši* [........]-*ma-har*
	Z	diš na dúr.gig gig-*ma di-ik-ša* t[uk-*ma*] [...]
16′	AA	úh *ina* dúr-*šú ú-ta*[*b*]-*ba-ka ana* ti-*šú* ^{ú}har.har ^{ú}*úr-n*[*é*-.]
	BB	úh *ina*$^{!}$ dúr-*šú ú*-[...^{ú}]*úr-nu-u*
	Z	[..] *ana* ti-*šú* ^{ú}har.har ^{ú}*úr-nu-u*
17′	AA	*ina* a gazi^{sar}*ana* dúr-*šú* [d]ub-*ak* geštin.šur nag ^{šim}li ^{ši}[^{m}....................]
	BB	*ina* a gazi^{sar}[..] x x [........]
	Z	*ina* a g[azi ....] ^{šim}gúr.gúr im.gú.en.na
18′	AA	a.gar.gar maš.dà zà.hi.[l]i súd *ina* kaš ^{urudu}šen.tur *tara*-[*bak* .....]
	Z	a.gar.gar maš.dà zà.hi.l[i ....]
19′	AA	^{giš}li ì.udu ^{š}[^{i}]^{m}gig ì.udu ukuš.hab num[un ....]
	Z	ì.udu ^{šim}gig ì.udu ukuš.hab numun ^{ú}si.sá [.......................
20′	AA	diš-*niš* súd šu.[s]i dù-*uš ana* dúr-*šú* [gar-*an*]

[1] correctly copied in AMT 53, 1: 3

[2] We might expect to find ì.udu éllag.

col. iii

2′ If a man's anal opening is inflamed and stopped up, and is ill internally;
3′ haemorrhoids: crush *abukkatu*-resin, seed of *aktam*,
4′ dog excrement, root of male mandrake, *nīnû*, single-clove garlic,
5′ 'cobweb'-plant, fruit of *kalbānu*, and mix (them) in fat. Make a pessary and insert it into his anus.

6′ If ditto (= in his anal opening) he is affected, and his anus is constantly [affected ....]
7′ mix (the ingredients) in fat, and make a pessary and [insert it into his] anus.

8′ If a man is *covered by his urine in the anus*, he [suffers] from [rectal] disease [.....],
9′ mix date peel in cedar oil, ..[.............][1]

10′ If a man is ill internally, you cool drawn wine, premium beer, brine of [...],
11′ pour it into his anus. Mix *baluhhu*-resin, *baluhhu*, .[.....]
12′ and *sahlû* in fat, and insert it into his anus. Rub *ušû* with your finger and
13′ wrap (it) [in a wad], you crush *nīnû* with .... and horned alkali. With your finger, you sprinkle and rub ghee [.......]
14′ over (it). Repeatedly put it into juice of *šunû*, you *mix in* ghee [...]

15′ If a man suffers from rectal disease and has piercing pain and his belly cannot take in food and fluids
16′ (and) he pours out mucous from his anus, to cure him: pour *hašû* (and) *urnû*
17′ in *kasû*-juice into his anus, he drinks drawn wine. Crush juniper, *kukru*, river mud,
18′ gazelle-dung (and) *sahlû*, you decoct (it) in beer (in) a small copper vessel,
19′ crush together juniper, *kanaktu*-fat, cucumber-fat, seed of *šurdunû* [...],
20′ make a pessary and [insert it] into his anus.

---

[1] Possibly a simplicium.

21′ AA diš ki.min ^{ú}geštin.ka$_5$.a *ina* kaš.sag nag ú babbar *ina*[..............
Z diš ki.min ^{ú}geštin.ka$_5$.a *ina* kaš nag ú babbar *ina* kaš nag [............
22′ AA [..................................] x làl kur nag *ina* a ^{giš}še.nu x [................
Z [...] *ina* a ^{giš}še.nu *ir-ta-na-haṣ*
23′ AA [......................................] *ana* dúr-*šú* dub-*ak* numun ^{ú}á[b.duh ....]
Z geštin.šur.ra *ina* a gazi^{sar} *ana* dú[r-*šú* ....] pa ^{giš}*šu-še* pa ^{giš}gi$_6$.pàr pa ^{ú}in$_6$.úš pa ^{giš}*pu*-[..............
(bottom of tablet; col. iv is uninscribed)

No. 26a BAM 102

This fragment is included here as possibly belonging to one of this group of Assur texts dealing with a sore anus (dúr.gig).
AA$_2$ = Ass. 13955/r* (BAM 102)

1 (traces)
2 ka.inim.ma dúr.gig.ga.kám

---

3 dù.dù.bi-*šú* šika *kur-ru*

4–7 Colophon = Hunger, BAK No. 200

21′ If ditto, he drinks fox-vine in premium beer, he drinks 'white' plant in beer, [......
22′ [..................................] and he drinks mountain honey, he continually bathes in *šunû*-juice,
23′ (and) you pour drawn wine in *kasû*-juice into his anus. [Crush] seed of *kamantu*, leaf of *šūšu*-tree, leaf of *lipāru*, leaf of *maštakal*, leaf of ..[............
(bottom)

TRANSLATION (BAM 102)

2 It is an incantion of the sore anus.

3 Its ritual: a *kor*(-capacity) sherd

No. 27 BAM 88

BB	=	VAT 10723 (BAM 88)
AI	=	K 2477 + (AMT 94,2 = BAM 471 ii 3′–6′ = 'Hand of the Ghost') = 18; 20–25
ff	=	K 8248 (AMT 56,1 and dupl.) [text no. 32] = ll. 1–12; 26–30
X	=	K 6545 + 8355 + 9030 (AMT 40,5: 14′ ff.) [text no. 23] = ll. –1′–2′
Z	=	K 4104 (AMT 58,2: 1–6) [text no. 25] = 13; 15 (may belong to K 2433+)
AA	=	EHE 331 + (BAM 96 iii 15 f.) [text no. 26] = 13–16
AP	=	VAT 13733 + 13738 (BAM 52: 66–71, *suālu*) = ll. 17–25
HH	=	VAT 9138 (BAM 168) [text no. 34] = ll. 17–25

–1′	BB	[..]
	X	diš na *mi-na-tu-šú* dub.dub gaba-*su u* sa.sal.meš-*šú* gu$_7$.meš-⸢*šú*⸣
	ff	[.............................. ga]ba-*su u šá-šal-la*-[*šú*] gu$_7$.meš-[*šú*......................]
0′	BB	[..]
	X	⸢á^2-*šú*⸣ *k*[*im-ṣa-a-šú u bir-ka-šú*] gu$_7$.meš-*šú* éllag *bir-ki-šú lu šá* 15 *lu šá* 150
	ff	[.................................] gu$_7$.meš-*šú* éllag *bir-ki-šú lu* šá 15 *lu šá* [15]0
1′	BB	x [..]
	X	sìg-*su-ma ina mùš-tin*-[*ni* ....] na.bi
	ff	[...............................]-*šú* múd *ú-kal-lam* na.bi
2′	BB	*hi-niq-ti* [...]
	ff	*hi-níq-ti* dúr.gig [......................................]
	X	*hi-niq-ti* dúr.gig gig *ana* ti-*šú* ^{ú}*tara-muš* ^{ú}igi-*lim*
3′	BB	[^{ši}]^{m}gúr.gúr ^{ši}[^{m}................................]
	ff	[........................... ^{giš}l]i ^{šim}man.du
4′	BB	gi.du$_{10}$.ga ^{ši}[^{m}.............]
	ff	gi.du$_{10}$.ga ^{šim}mug šim.sal
5′	BB	^{giš}eren ^{giš}e[rin.úš..........]
	ff	^{giš}eren.úš ^{giš}še.ná.a
6′	BB	^{ú}*úr-nu-u* $^{\text{⸢ú⸣}}$[.....................]
	ff	^{ú}*úr-né-e* ^{ú}har.har [^{ú}nu].luh.ha
7′	BB	^{ú}kur.ra zú.lum.m[a ....]
	ff	^{ú}kur.ra zú.lum.ma zì.munu$_4$ kaš
8′	BB	*ni-it-ku* ^{giš}geštin še [..............]
	ff	*ni-it-ku* ^{giš}geštin [.. *t*]*a-hi-it-te*
9′	BB	*i-na* nindu *te-sek-ker ana* dú[r-.......]
	ff	*i-na* nindu *te-sek-ker ana* dúr dub-*ak*

10′	BB	[.................... gi]g-*ma* dúr-*šú* gír.g[ír-..]
	ff	[diš na dú]r.gig gig-*ma* dúr-*šú* gír.gír-*su*
11′	BB	[....] ^{šim}gúr.gúr ^{šim}gam.me [....]
	ff	^{šim}li ^{šim}gúr.gúr [....................]
12′	BB	[................ h]i lagab.munu$_4$ *ina* ì.giš *u* kaš *ana* [.................]
	ff	[diš-*niš* hi.h]i ^{šim}gig lagab.munu$_4$ *ina* ì.giš *u* kaš *ana* dúr-*šú* [dub-*ak*]

TRANSLATION

−1′ If a man's limbs are *poured out*, his chest and shoulders hurt him,
0′ his arms, shins [and knees] hurt him, his testicle, either on the right side or on the left,
1′ bothers him, and he shows blood in his urethra, that man
2′ suffers from stricture of the anus. To cure him, you heat in an oven (l. 9) *taramuš*, *imhur-lim*,
3′ *kukru*, [............], juniper, *suādu*,
4′ sweet reed, *ballukku*, *šimeššalû*,
5′ cedar, *šupuhru*-cedar, *šunû*,
6′ *urnû*, *hašû*, *nuhurtu*,
7′ *nīnû*, dates, malt-flour, beer,
8′ wine-drops, ...-barley.
9′ You pour (it) into the anus.

10′ [If a man] suffers from rectal disease and his anus stings him,
11′ mix [together] juniper, *kukru*, *ṣumlalû*, [and .....]
12′ [pour] *kanaktu* and a clump of malt in oil and beer into his anus.

13′	BB	[.................... g]ig-*ma di-ik-šá* tuk-*ši*
	Z	diš na dúr.gig gig-*ma di-ik-ša* t[uk-..]
	AA	diš na dúr.gig gig-*ma di-ik-ša* tuk
14′	BB	[...................]-*ma-har* úh *ina*$^{!}$ dúr-*šú ú*-[*tab-bak*]
	AA	ninda *u* a šà-*šú la i-m*[*a-har*] úh *ina* dúr-*šú ú-ta*[*b*]-*ba-ka*
15′	BB	[.........................^{ú}]*úr-nu-u ina* a gazi^{sar}
	Z	*ana* ti-*šú* ^{ú}har.har ^{ú}*úr-nu-u ina* a g[azi..]
	AA	*ana* ti-*šú* ^{ú}har.har ^{ú}*úr-n*[*é*-.] *ina* a gazi^{sar}
16′	BB	[..............] x x [...................]
	AA	*ana* dúr-*šú* [d]ub-*ak*

17′	BB	[.........] ⸢šà-*šú*⸣ m[ú.m]ú-*hu ir-ru-šú*
	HH	[diš n]a šà.meš-*šú* mú.mú *ir-ru-šú*
	AP	diš na šà.meš-*šú* mú.meš-*hu ir-ru-šú*
18′	BB	[..] *šá* mar.gal *ma-gal* dug$_4$-dug$_4$-*ú*[1]
	AI	[..] *šá* mar.gal *ma-gal* dug$_4$-dug$_4$- x
	HH	gim *šá* mar.gal *ma-gal* d[ug$_4$]
	AP	gim *šá* mar.gal *ma-gal* dug$_4$.d[ug$_4$$^{?}$ ..]
19′	BB	[na].bi *ni-kim-ti* im *u* ud.da gig
	HH	na.bi *ni-kim-ti* im *u* ud.da gig
	AP	na.bi *ni-kim-tú* im ud.da gig
20′	BB	[ki]n-*šú* sumun-*ma* šu.gedim.ma *ana* ti-*šú* ^{ú}kur.ra
	AI	[ki]n-*šú* sumun-*ma* šu.gedim.ma ^{ú}kur.ra
	HH	kin-*šú* sumun-*ma* šu.g[edim] *ana* ti-*šú* ^{ú}kur.ra
	AP	kin-*šú i-la-bir-ma* šu.ge[dim.ma] ^{ú}kur.ra
21′	BB	^{ú}hur.sag ^{ú}har.har ^{ú}nu.luh.h[a]
	AI	^{ú}hur.sag [..............................]
	HH	^{ú}hur.sag ^{ú}har.har ^{ú}nu.[.......]
	AP	^{ú}hur.sag ^{ú}har.har ^{ú}nu.lu[h...]
22′	BB	^{ši}[^{m}l]i ^{šim}gúr.gúr ^{šim}gam.ma ^{ši}[^{m}..]
	AI	[.........].gi.du$_{10}$ ^{šim}gam.ma ^{šim}mug
	HH	^{šim}li ^{šim}gúr.gúr ^{šim}gam.ma ^{šim}bal
	AP	^{šim}li ^{šim}gúr.gúr ^{šim}gam.ma ^{šim}mug
23′	BB	*šu-luṭ* [š]im.hi.a ^{ú}lag.a.šà 11 ⸢ú⸣
	AI	*šu-luṭ* šim.hi.a [...................]
	HH	*šu-luṭ* š[im] 11 ú.hi.a šeš
	AP	*šu-lu-uṭ* šim.[...] mun ^{ú}lag.a.šà pap 11 ú.hi.a
24′	BB	*ina* kaš.s[ag š]eg$_6$-*šal ta-šá-hal* šed$_7$ ì.[giš ....]
	AI	*ina* kaš.sag šeg$_6$-*šal* ì.giš *ana* igi šub
	HH	*ina* kaš.sag šeg$_6$-*šal ta-šá-h*[*al*]
	AP	*ina* kaš šeg$_6$-[...] ì.giš *ana* igi šub-*di*

---

1 Reading courtesy J. Scurlock. CAD I/J 261 gives *išqippu* as either an earthworm or a type of bird, although rarely attested. An earthworm must be ruled out in the present context.

13′ If a man suffers from a sore anus and has piercing pain
14′ and his belly cannot take in food and fluids (and) pours out mucous from his anus,
15′ to cure him: pour *hašû* (and) *urnû* in *kasû*-juice
16′ into his anus.

17′ If a man's bowels are bloated, his intestines
18′ make a lot of noise like (that) of an *išqippu*-bird,
19′ that man suffers from flatulence and sun-fever.
20′ His condition is of long duration, (it is) the Hand of the Ghost; in order to cure him, heat in premium beer (l. 24) *nīnû*,
21′ 'mountain'-plant (*azupīru*), *hašû*, *nuhurtu*,
22′ juniper, *kukru*, *ṣumlalû*, *ballukku*,
23′ *cuttings of* aromatics[1], field-clod, – 11 plants,
24′ filter and cool them, add oil into the (mixture),

---

[1] See CAD Š/3 265; the reading is from F. Köcher, courtesy B. Böck.

25′	BB	*ana* dúr-*šú* [dub]-*ak-ma* ti
	AI	*ana* dúr-*šú* dub
	HH	šed$_7$ ì.giš *ana* igi šub-*di* *ana* dúr-*šú* dub-*ak-ma* [t]i
	AP	*ana* dúr-*šú* dub-*a*[*k*]
26′	BB	diš ki.min ^{šim}gúr.gúr ^{šim}li ⸢tuh.še.giš⸣.[ì](?)
	ff	[.........] ^{šim}li x [x x [....] x [..........................] x x x
27′	BB	^{ú}naga.si ^{ú}lag.a.šà ^{ú}[x]
	ff	[..............................^{ú}]kur.ra
28′	BB	^{ú}hur.sag 8 ú.meš šeš ina kaš x
	ff	^{ú}hur.sag 8 ú.meš kaš.l[ú.tin.n]a šeg$_6$.gá
29′	BB	(broken)
	ff	[.....] x x *ba bah-ra* ì.giš làl *ana* igi šub-*di*
30′	BB	[..] dúr-*šú* [..
	ff	*ana* dúr-*šú* dub [....] ì.[nun.na] ga ku$_7$.ku$_7$ *ana* dúr-*šú* dub-*ma ina-eš*
	BB	edge: [..].. x *u* geštin$^{!}$(text: kaš).ka$_5$.a *hi-iq* šeg$_6$-*š*[*al*....]

25′ pour it into his anus and he will recover.

26′ If ditto, ***kukru***, juniper, sesame residue,
27′ horned alkali, field-clod, ***ninû***,
28′ ***azupīru***: boil these 8 drugs in a brewer's beer
29′ [.......], *hot* ..., put oil and honey into it
30′ and pour it into his anus. Pour [.... and] ghee and sweet milk into his anus and he will get better.

---

edge: [...]... and you heat up *fox-vine* (and) thinned beer [......]

No. 28 BAM 104

CC = VAT 10092 (BAM 104)
AA = EHE 331 + VAT 8694 + 14118 (BAM 96 iii 2 f.) [text no. 26] = ll. 7–8; 42–45
Y = K 2433 + (AMT 47,1) [text no. 24] = 42–44
AJ = VAT 10649 (BAM 94): 6–8 = ll. 62–64
V = VAT 13752 + (BAM 95: 37) [text no. 21] = l. 34
AD = VAT 10170 (BAM 152 ii 11) = l. 34
AE = STT 197 iii = l. 34

1 CC [..........................]-*ma ina* [.........]
2 CC [..........................] ú.hi.a šeš *ana* x [................]
3 CC [..........................] *ta-šá-hal ina* igi [šub ....]
4 CC [..........................] ì.giš *u* kaš *ana* dúr-*šú* dub-*ak* [..]

---

5 CC [..........................ill]u li.tar ^{šim}šeš *ina* ì.u[du]
6 CC [.......................... k]a *ina* kaš.sag n[ag]

---

7 CC [..........................] udu.níta naga.si ^{šim}bu[luh]
AA [..........................]-*i* udu.níta naga.si ^{šim}buluh
8 CC [..........................] ésir *tuš-te-mid ana* dúr-*šú* gar-*an-ma ina-eš*
AA [..........................*ina* é]sir *tuš-te-mid-ma ana* dúr-*šú* gar-*an-ma ina-eš*
9 CC [.......................... -*t*]*a-'i-i* ^{šim}gig ^{šim}li
10 CC [..........................-*m*]*a alla-nu* dù-*uš ana* dúr-*šú* gar-*an*

---

11 CC [.......................... i]m.gú.en.na ^{ú}maš.tab.ba ^{ú}nu.luh.ha ^{ú}har.har
12 CC [..........................] zà.hi.li *ina* ì.udu zú.lum.ma hi.hi *ana* dúr-*šú* gar-*an* t[i]

---

13 CC [.......................... i]llu li.dur numun gi.zú.lum.[m]a ì.udu ur.mah
14 CC [..........................ú.hi.a še]š súd *ina* ì.nun hi.hi *nap-šal-tu*$_4$

---

15 CC [..........................^{ú}]igi-*lim* súd *ina* kaš.sag nag-*šú*

---

16 CC [..........................] ùz *gul-gul* nam.lú.u$_{18}$.lu *kam-mu ša* lú.ašgab
17 CC [..........................] x ra *tur-ár* súd *alla-nu* dù-*uš ana* dúr-*šú* gar-*an*

---

18 CC [.......................... ^{š}]^{im}gúr.gúr ^{ú}kur.ra ^{ú}hur.sag *sah-lé-e* ú babbar ^{ú}*ak*-[*tam*]
19 CC [.......................... nam.t]ar níta numun gi.zú.lum.ma ^{ú}šiš.ba.na[1] illu ^{šim}buluh gaz *ina* ì
20 CC [..........................d]a ^{giš}gi.gíd dù-*uš* túg.hi.a *tu-la-ba-áš ana* dúr-*šú* gar-[*an*]

---

21 CC [..........................^{ši}]^{m}li zà.hi.li ^{ú}kur.ra ^{ú}kur.kur ^{ú}*ṣa-ṣu-um-t*[*a*]
22 CC [..........................]x ^{ú}úkuš.hab zú.lum.ma *ina* ì.udu hi.hi *alla-nam* dù-*uš ana* dúr-*šú* gar-[*an*]

---

23 CC [..........................] x ^{šim}gúr.gúr ^{šim}li ^{šim}še.li ^{šim}gír gazi^{sa}[^{r}]
24 CC [.......................... ì.u]du hi.hi *ina* dè ^{giš}kiši$_{16}$ *qu-ta-r*[*u*]

---

25 CC [..........................] x ra *id-ra* súd šu.si-*ka* ^{síg}àka nigin-*mi* ú.hi.a *tu-qat-ta*[*r*$^{?}$] *ina* dúr-*šú* [gar]

---

26 CC [..........................^{ši}]^{m}gúr.gúr ^{šim}še.li ^{šim}mug ^{ú}kur.kur ^{ú}*kur-ka-nam* ^{šim}[..]
27 CC [.......................... *sa*]*h-lé-e* gazi^{sar} naga.si illu li.dur illu ^{šim}bu[luh]

---

1 Cf. CAD Š/3 147 f.l, *šizbānu*, 'milkweed', although it is likely that šiš.ba.na was a logographic rather than syllabic writing for this plant.

TRANSLATION

1 .....
2 [...........]these drugs ... [..................
3 [..................]you filter and [put] into (the mixture) [..............
4 [...............], pour oil and beer into his anus [and he will get better].

---

5 [...............................] *abukkatu*-resin (and) myrrh in fat,
6 [..............................] he drinks ... in premium beer.

---

7 [..] of a male sheep, horned alkali, *baluhhu*,
8 [.......................], you mix (it) [in] bitumen and insert it into his anus and he will get better.
9 [...............................] ...... *kanaktu*, juniper,
10 [.................................] and make a suppository, put it into his anus.

---

11 [...........................] river mud, *māštu*, *nuhurtu*, *hašû*,
12 [................] (and) *sahlû*, mix (them) in date fat, put it into his anus and he will recover.

---

13 [............................] *abukkatu*-resin, seed of *kūru*, lion fat,
14 [..........], crush these [drugs], mix (them) in ghee (as) a salve.

---

15 Crush [.......................] *imhur-lim*, he drinks it in premium beer.

---

16 [..] goat, human skull, leatherworker's fungus,
17 [.................................].., you dry out (and) crush, you make a suppository (and) insert it into his anus.

---

18 Pound (l. 19) [...............................] *kukru*, *nīnû*, *azupīru*, *sahlû*, 'white' plant, *aktam*,
19 [.............................] male mandrake, *kūru*-seed, milkweed, (and) *baluhhu*-resin, in oil,
20 [.........................].., you make a reed tube, cover it with cloth and insert it into his anus.

---

21 [.........................] juniper, *sahlû*, *nīnû*, *ata'išu*, *ṣaṣumtu*,
22 [....................].., cucumber, dates: mix (them) in fat, make a suppository, and insert it into his anus.

---

23 [.......................], *kukru*, juniper, *kikkirânu*, myrtle, *kasû*,
24 mix [................in] fat, a fumigation over coals of acacia-thorn.

---

25 Crush [.....] ..., saltpetre, wrap (them) in a wad of wool with your finger, fumigate the drugs, [insert] (them) into his anus.

---

26 [..................], *kukru*, *kikkirânu*, *ballukku*, *ata'išu*, *kurkānû*, ...
27 [...............], *sahlû*, *kasû*, horned-alkali, *abukkatu*-resin, *baluhhu*-resin,

28 CC [...............mu]n a.gar.gar maš.dà ^{šim}šeš ú.hi.a *an-nu-tu$_4$* ⸢dub$^?$⸣.me[š]

---

29 CC [..........*sah*]*-lé-e* ^{ú}*kur-ka-nam* ^{ú}nu.luh.ha ^{giš}zú.gišimmar zú.[lu]m.[ma]
30 CC [............] x ^{šim}[m]ug ^{šim}gúr.gúr ^{šim}li u$_5$.gar.ib[^{mušen}]
31 CC [............] x illu li.tar ^{šim}hab *ina* ì.udu gaba.làl hi.hi *alla-nu* dù-[*uš*]

---

32 CC [..............] x *gul-gul* nam.lú.u$_{18}$.lu *tur-ár* sú[d]
33 CC [..............] x x x *ina* a gazi^{sar} *tara-bak* lá-*i*[*d*]$^?$

---

34 CC [.............nag]a.si še$_{10}$ gud [.......] gissu hád.a gaz sim *ṭi-pu šá* dúr.gig *te-ṭe-ni-*[.....................]
V ⸢^{ú}⸣kur.ra [naga].si še$_{10}$ gud sa$_5$ *ina* gissu hád.a gaz sim *ṭà-pu šá* dúr.gig *te-ṭe-ni-pi-ma* dúr.gig zi-*hi*
AD ^{ú}kur.ra naga.si še$_{10}$ gud sa$_5$ *ina* gissu hád.a g[az] *ṭi-pu šá* dúr.gig *te-ṭ*[*e-n*]*i-pi-ma* dúr.gig [...]
AE [...........nag]a.si še$_{10}$ gud diri *ina* gissu hád.a [g]az sim [.......................] *te-ṭe-ni-pi-ma* dúr.gig zi-*hi* ti$^?$

---

35 CC [..............]ku[n]$^?$ x [n]íta *u* munus x x a a x [......] diš-*niš* hi.hi dur.gig šé[š]

---

36 CC [.......................] x [....] illu ^{šim}buluh illu li.tar [numun$^?$] g[i.z]ú.lum.ma
37 CC [.......................] x *ina* ì.u[du] x gaba.làl diš-*niš* šeg$_6$-*šal* šéš

---

38 CC [..............................] x x x[....] *šá* dúr.[gig]

---

39 CC [...........................] x *la* kúm.kúm *š*[*i-na*]*t-su*(?) šub.šub-*šú* še$_{10}$-*su* šub.šub-[*š*]*ú-m*[*a*]
40 CC [.............................]-*tu$_4$* suhuš ^{giš}nam.tar.níta suhuš ^{ú}úkuš.hab *ša* im.si.sá
41 CC [..............................] šu.si dù-*uš ana* dúr-*šú* gar-*a*[*n*]

---

42 CC [.........................-*š*]*ú* mú.mú-*hu ú-na-paq qer-bé-nu* gig *um-ṣa-tu$_4$* illu
AA diš na ⸢ka⸣ d[úr-*šú* ....] *um-ṣa-tu$_4$* ill[u]
Y [...]-*bé-nu* g[ig.................] x illu
43 CC [.......-*t*]*u$_4$* numun ^{ú}*ak-tam* še$_{10}$ ur.gi$_7$ suhuš ^{giš}nam.tal níta ^{ú}kur.ra^{sa}[⸢r⸣]
AA [...] še$_{10}$ ur.gi$_7$ suhuš ^{giš}[..............................]
Y li.dur numun [.........]-*tam* še$_{10}$ ur.gi$_7$ suhuš x [..................................]
44 CC [..] šu.si dù-*uš ana* dúr-*šú* gar-*a*[*n*]
AA [..................]^{ú}*pi*$^!$-*zir* gurun ^{ú}m[aš...
Y [š]um.šir.dil ^{ú}*pi-zìr* gurun ⸢^{giš}maš⸣.huš súd *ina* ì.udu hi.hi šu.si dù-*u*[*š*]

---

45 CC [............... ta]g$^?$ [dú]r-*šú* [.......................] x x udu *ina* ì.udu hi.hi šu.si dù-*uš ana* dú[r-*šú* gar]
AA diš ki.min tag-*ma* dúr-*šú il-ta-n*[*ap-pat* ....] *ina* ì.udu hi.hi šu.si [..............................]

---

46 CC [..] x x šub.šub-*su in*[*a* š]à$^?$-*šú* mú.mú-*hu* im *e*[*s-lu*(?)]
47 CC [...............................] x illu ^{šim}buluh súd *i*[*na* ì.u]du hi.hi *alla-nu* dù *ana* dúr-*šú* [gar]

---

48 CC [.. su]huš ^{giš}nam.tar níta suhuš ú$_5$.[gar.ib^{mušen}]
49 CC [..] še$_{10}$ ur.gi$_7$ diš-*niš* súd *alla-nu* dù-*uš ana* dúr-*šú* gar-[*an*]

---

50 CC [..............................*ina* ì].udu hi.hi *alla-nu* dù-*uš ana* dúr-*šú* gar-[*an*]

51–52 CC (traces)

28 [..........], salt, gazelle-dung, myrrh, keep pouring these drugs (into the anus).

29 [...............], *sahlû*, *kurkānû*, *nuhurtu*, palm fibre, dates,
30 [............] .., *ballukku*, *kukru*, juniper, bat guano,
31 [...........] .., *abukkatu*-resin, *ṭurû*, mix (these) in fat (and) wax, make a suppository.

32 You dry out and crush [.........] .., (and) human skull,
33 steep [...........] in *kasû*-juice, (and) bind (them on the patient).

34 Dry out in the shade *nīnû*, horned alkali, and dung of a red ox, pound and sieve, keep adding a bandage for the diseased rectum and diseases of the rectum are removed (var. and he will recover).

35 Mix together [....]..., male and female [....], ...[....], rub it on the diseased anus.

36 [..................]....., *baluhhu*-resin, *abukkatu*-resin, [seed?] of *kūru*,
37 ... [.............] in fat, heat wax together (with them) and anoint (it).

38 [..................]...... [......] of a [diseased] rectum.

39 [......................]... is always hot, his *urine spatters* him, his stools *spatter* him, ...[.....
40 [..................]..., root of male mandrake, root of cucumber from the north side (of the plant),[1]
41 [.................................] make a pessary (and) put it into his anus.

42 If a man's anal opening is inflamed and stopped up, and is ill internally; haemorrhoids: crush (l. 44)
43 *abukkatu*-resin, seed of *aktam*, dog excrement, root of male mandrake, *nīnû*,
44 single-cloved garlic, 'cobweb'-plant, fruit of *kalbānu*, mix (them) in fat, make a pessary.

45 If ditto (= a man's anal opening) is affected (lit. touched) and his anus is constantly affected [......], mix [....] in fat, make a pessary, [put it] into [his] anus.

46 [...]...afflicts him, he is inflamed *in his bowel*, flatulence is stopped [up],
47 crush [........................].. *baluhhu*-resin, mix (them) in fat, make a suppository, [put it] into his anus.

48 [..........................], crush together [..............] root of male mandrake, bat [guano],
49 [.................................] dog excrement, make a suppository and insert (it) into his anus.

50 Mix [.....................in] fat, make a suppository, insert (it) into his anus.

51–52 damaged

[1] Cf. CAD I/J 269a.

rev.

53	CC	[.. *i-t*]*a-na-áš-šá*[1] *ina sah-l*[*é-e* .....
54	CC	[..*alla-nu*] dù-*uš ana* dúr-*šú* gar-*an ina* a [.........
55	CC	[..] x dúr-*šú te-t*[*e-ne-qí-ma* ....
56	CC	[...................................... 1 gí]n naga.si 1 gín ^{šim}buluh *ši-šá-ik-*[*tu*[2]...........
57	CC	[..] x nagar dù *ana* dúr-*šú* gar-*an* en *ir-ru ú-t*[*a-áš-ru* ......
58	CC	[......................................] x hi še ^{síg}àka ì.giš sù *ana* dúr-*šú* gar-*a*[*n*]
59	CC	[..] x hi.hi <dug> *la* sáhar[3] l[i] x [........
60	CC	[...] x *-i* dúr-*šú tu-qat-tar-šú*
61	CC	[...š]ub.šub-*šú* ^{síg}àka ì.giš sù *ana* dúr-*šú* gar-[*an*]
62	CC	[.......................... *t*]*u-qa-tar-šu ina* ugu giš.šú.a tuš [...........
	AJ	[............................x] *tu-qat-tar-šú ina* giš.šú.a tuš [..................
63	CC	[..........................] x *id-ra* gim ir *um-taš-še-ra*[4] *ur-š*[*u* ....
	AJ	[.................................] x x ir <*ki-*>*ma at-tam-ši-ra ur-šu* [...............
64	CC	[..šu]b.šub-*ni* ^{síg}àka ì.giš sud *ana* dúr-*šú* gar-*a*[*n*]
	AJ	[..........................] *um-ṣa-tu*$_4$ šub.šub-*ni*
65	CC	[.......................*ina*] ⌜ì⌝.udu ^{šim}gig ^{šim}li súd *ina* ì.udu hi.hi šu.si [dù *ana* dúr-*šú* gar]
66	CC	[........................... *t*]*i* gar.gar-*an* im.gú peš$_{10}$.^{d}íd [..........
67	CC	[...........................] x *te-qí ana* dúr-*šú* gar-[*an*]
68	CC	[............................ s]úd *ina* ì.udu hi.hi šu.si dù-*uš ana* dúr-*šú* gar-[*an*]
69	CC	[...........................] *ina* ì.udu hi.hi šu.si dù-*uš ana* dúr-*šú* gar-[*an*]
70	CC	[........................] *ana* a šub šeg$_6$.gá súd lá [ti]
71	CC	[......................... ì.]udu *ina* a gazi^{sar} šid-*aš* lá [ti]
72	CC	[............................] x *qí-lip* zú.lum.ma *ina* ì.udu [.........
73	CC	[...........................] 2-*šú* 3-*šú* gar-[*an*]
74	CC	[.......................hi.]hi *ana* dúr-*šú* [gar-*an*]
75	CC	[.............................] im suhuš ^{ú}nu.luh.ha uzu *nap-šá-*[*at im-me-ri*[5]]
76	CC	[...........................] x súd *ina* ì.udu hi.hi šu.si dù-*uš* [*ana* dúr-*šú* gar-*an*]
77	CC	[.....................*s*]*i-si-*⌜*tu*$_4$⌝ *šá* gùb uzu *nap-šá-te i-*[*me-ri*]
78	CC	[..............] *in*[*a* ....] šéš x [..
79	CC	[.............................] *šá* gùb [........... *š*]*á* maš x x [..............
80	CC	[.............................] ì šu[b ....
81	CC	broken
82	CC	[.. d]úr-*šú* gar-[*an*]
83	CC	[..dú]r-*šú* gar-[*an*]
84	CC	[...] šé[š ..]
85	CC	[... *ṭ*]*i-pu-šu šá* [dúr.gig]

1 Cf. CAD N/2 103.

2 cf. CAD Š/3 126, *šiššiktu*-stone (our reference is not in CAD).

3 perhaps CAD Š/1 80?

4 or: saltpetre is released like sweat? pace CAD Z 169, citing LKU 62 rev 10, but IR is not excrement.

5 CAD N/1 304a, which only refers to the use of sheep flesh, but l. 77 appears to use donkey flesh as well.

rev.

53 [If a man's ....] heaves, in[?] *sahlû* [...
54 [...............], make a [suppository], insert (it) into his anus, in juice of [.......
55 [...] ... keep daubing his anus [and ......

56 [............................ one] shekel of horned alkali, 1 shekel *baluhhu*, *šiššiktu*-stone(?) [.......
57 [........................] make a suppository, insert (it) into his anus until the intestines *release* [....
58 [..............................] ..., sprinkle a wad of wool with oil, insert (it) into his anus.

59 Mix [..............................] .... a non-porous <pot>,
60 [...................................] ..., you fumigate his anus with it.

61 [................................] *spatters* him, sprinkle oil on a wad of wool, insert (it) into his anus.

62 [................................], you fumigate it, you have (the patient) sit upon a stool,
63 [................................] .. *saltpetre*, when he releases sweat, (and) an *uršu*-sore [........
64 [.......................(and)] haemorrhoids *break out*, sprinkle oil on a wad of wool (and) insert (it) into his anus.
65 [...............], crush *kanaktu* and juniper [in] fat, mix (them) in fat, [make] a pessary [and insert it into his anus].

66 [...................................] .... river mud, sulphur, [..........,
67 you daub [...............].., put (them) into his rectum.

68 Crush [.......................], mix (it) in fat, make a pessary, insert (it) into his anus.
69 Mix [..................] in fat, make a pessary, insert (it) into his anus.
70 You pour [.............] into water, heat it, crush (it and) bind (it) [and he will recover].
71 [.....................] fat, knead it in *kasû*-juice, bind (it) [and he will improve].

72 [Crush.........................] date peel in fat [.................
73 [.......................] put (it) twice and three times.

74 Mix [...................... put (it)] into his rectum.

75 [............................] clay, root of *nuhurtu*, flesh of [sheep's] throat,
76 crush [...................], mix (them) in fat, make a pessary, [insert (it) into his anus].

77 [...] left *joint*, flesh of donkey throat,
78 [...] in [....] you smear [.....................

79 [...................................] left [........] .... [..............

80–81 broken
82 [.. make a suppository,] insert (it) into his anus.

83 [... make a suppository,] insert (it) into his anus.

84 Smear on [...]

85 [..] his *bandage* of the [diseased anus].

86 CC [..^{ú}ku]r.ra súd gada *ta*-[........
87 CC [..] x *ana* dúr-*šú* gar-[*an*]

88 CC [..] x [................] x *ina* ì.giš súd hi.hi dúr-*šú* [gar-*an*]

89 CC [.....................................] nam.tar níta súd hi.hi *tu-kap-pat ana* dúr-*šú* gar-[*an*]

90 CC [............................ zú].lum.ma *tur-ár* súd ì.udu ^{šim}[..........
91 CC [...................................] x hi.hi *tu-kap-pat ana* dúr-*šú* gar-*an*

92 CC [............................... s]úd hi.hi *tu-kap-pat ana* dúr-*šú* gar-*an*

93 CC [................................ *ina* ì.n]un hi.hi *ana* dúr-*šú* gar-*an*

94 CC [..............................^{giš}e]ren gaz *ina* ì.nun hi.hi *al-la-nam* dù-*u*[*š*]

95 CC [....................................] x *tu-tak-kap i-na* é.gar$_8$ ⸢sahar$^?$⸣ a hu a ṣa [..
96 CC [................................. *šu*]*m-ma ta-lal* buru$_8$ man é.⸢gar$_8$ *ina*⸣ man *ta-lal ti*[*m* ...]
97 CC [...............................] x *-ak-ka ina* ì.nun hi.hi *ina* šu.si-*ka te-qí*

98 CC [.......................................*i-n*]*a* šen.tur šeg$_6$-*šal tu-kaṣ-ṣa ana* dúr-*šú* dub-*ak*
99 CC [................................. *sa*]*h-lé-e ina* ì.udu hi.hi *ana* dúr-*šú* gar-*an* ^{ú}esi
100 CC [........................ ^{giš}še.n]á.a šub-*šú* ì.nun dúr-*šú* šé[š]

101 CC [... ì.ud]u éllag udu.níta

86 Crush [...] *nīnû*, you [...] linen,
87 [...] .., insert (it) into his anus.

---

88 Crush [..] in oil, mix (it), [insert it] into his anus.

---

89 Crush (and) mix [.........................] ... male mandrake, you make a pill (and) insert (it) into his anus.

---

90 Dry out (and) pound [................], dates, mix fat, .. [..................
91 [..] you make a pill, insert (it) into his anus.

---

92 Crush (and) mix [.......................], you make a pill, insert (it) into his anus.

---

93 Mix [.................... in] ghee, insert (it) into his anus.

---

94 Pound [..................and] cedar, mix (it) in ghee, make a suppository.

---

95 [...........................], you prick, in a wall (?) ....
96 [........................] .... a second wall(?) of the bandage(?)
97 [.............................] ....., mix in ghee, daub (it) with your finger.

---

98 Heat up [............................in a small] dish, you cool (and) pour (it) into his anus.
99 Mix [.....................] *sahlû* in fat, insert (it) into his anus,
100 Add to it *ušû*? [....................] *šunû*, smear his anus with ghee.

---

101 [...] fat of a male sheep kidney.

No. 29 AMT 44,5 = RA 26, 74.

CD	=	S 1587 (AMT 44,5)
AK	=	K 2417 (AMT 31,4: 7–9) = ll. 6–9

1′	CD	(traces)
2′	CD	[diš na ....] x *-a ši-hat* uz[u] [gig ....
3′	CD	[.....................] ⸢ki x⸣ *ana* dúr-*šú* dub *ina* a.meš ra.meš na[ga.si ....
4′	CD	[...............] x x *tu-qat-tar-šú* ^{giš}*si-hu* ^{giš}*ár-gan-na* ^{giš}*ba-r*[*i-ra-tu* .....
5′	CD	[...... ì.udu] gud šeg$_6$-*šal* zì.gig *tel-li-ih ina* kuš [sur-*re* ...]
6′	CD	[diš.na .... *šit-t*]*a-šú*[1] *ina* šà-*šú i-ta-na-bal* 14 še *si-ik-ti* [........
	AK	[diš na dú]r gig-*ma šit-ta-šú ina* šà-*šú i-ta-na-bal* mun em[e.sal.la .....
7′	CD	[.......... *l*]*u* ì.giš ì.udu gud [...............
	AK	[................ *lu*] ⸢ì⸣.udu. [...] *lu ina* ì.giš [š]ub-*di ina* mul$_4$ *tuš-*[*bat* .
8′	AK	[diš ki.min] ⸢*šit-ta-šú i-ta*⸣*-na-bal* 15 še *si-ik-ti* ^{giš}kiši$_{16}$ 15 še *sik-*[*ti* ....
9′	AK	[....] 1/2 gín ì.[u]du [g]ud téš.bi *tu-sa-mah ana* dúr-*šú* gar-*an* [.......
10′	CD	[............ š]im.hi.a dù.a.bi-*šú-nu* ^{ú}har.har[................
11′	CD	[............] x x súd
12′	CD	(traces)

[1] his excrement? cf. CAD Š/3 142 (*šittu* C), although not citing this passage.

TRANSLATION

2′ [If a man ...]... [suffers from] 'peeling flesh'-disease [......,
3′ pour [........................] ... into his rectum, keep washing him in water, horned alk[ali ....
4′ fumigate him [with.........]..., *sīhu*, *argannu*, *barīrātu*, [.......
5′ Boil [...........fat of an] ox, sprinkle wheat flour, [smear it] on leather [and tie it on..].

6′ [If a man is] ill in the anus and his stools are dried out in his bowels, 14 grains of powder (var. gourmet salt), [............
7′ put (them) [in ....] or oil/fat[1] of an ox or in oil, leave it out over night [.........

8′ [If a man, ditto] his stools are dried out, 15 grains of powder of reeds, 15 grains of powder of [.....
9′ [...] half a shekel of ox fat, you mix (them) together and insert (them) into his anus [....

10′ [................] the aromatics, all of them, *hašû*, [....................
11′ crush [................]............

---

[1] It appears as if ì.giš and ì.udu are alternatives (i. e., either oil or fat).

No. 30 **AMT 40,4 + 57,5** (plates 25–26)

dd	=	S 1283 + 1947 (AMT 40,4 + 57,5) (Bab. script)
EE	=	O. 194 (BAM 182 rev. 9–10) [text no. 31] = 12–13
GG	=	K 9441 (AMT 43, 5: ll. 5–6, 11–12) [text no. 33] = 9–13
Y	=	K 2433+ (S 357 = AMT 7,7: 9′–10′) [text no. 24] = ll. 12–13

1′	dd	nu[mun ....
2′	dd	zì.á[š.àm ....
3′	dd	*ina* kuš.e[din sur ....
4′	dd	diš na múd *ina* d[úr$^{?}$-*šú ú-tab-ba-ka* ....
5′	dd	^{giš}eren.sig[1] š[im ....
6′	dd	zú.lum.ma *tab-k*[*a*] x [..... ....
7′	dd	9 ú.meš *an-nu-ti ina* g[a ....
8′	dd	*ana* dúr-*šú t*[*a-šap-pak* ....
9′	dd	diš na dúr.gig gig-*ma lìb-ba-šu* d[ab-..]
	GG	[..] na dúr.gig gig-*ma* šà-*šú* dab-*su*
10′	dd	*it-te-nen-sil* ^{ú}igi-*līm* ^{ú}<nam>.tar nita ⸢^{ú}⸣[..]
	GG	*it-te-nen-s*[*il* ....]
11′	dd	^{ú}igi-*ešra* ú.meš *an-nu-ti* diš-*niš* súd *ina* kaš nag-*ma ina-eš*
	GG	[^{ú}]igi-*ešra* ú.hi.a *an-nu-ti* téš.bi sú[d ....]
12′	dd	diš na dúr gig-*ma* dúr-*šú e-sil* gar.ib.u$_5$^{mušen}
	EE	[.. n]a dúr gig-*ma* dúr-*šú e-sil* ^{mušen}u$_5$.gar.[ib]
	GG	diš na dúr.gig gig dúr-*šú e*-[.........................
	Y	[........... gi]g gig dúr-*šú e-s*[*i-il* ....
13′	dd	[s]uhuš ^{giš}nam.tar níta súd hi.hi diš-*niš tu-kap-pat ana* dúr-*šú* gar
	EE	[su]huš ^{giš}nam.tar níta súd hi.hi diš-*niš tu-kap-pat ana* dúr-*šú* [..]
	GG	[...] diš-*niš tu-kap-pat* [...............]
	Y	[..] *tu-kap-pat* [...............]

rev.

14′	dd	[diš ki.min] *šit-ta-šú ina lìb-bi-šú i-ta-nab-bal*
15′	dd	[na.b]i *zi-zi-na* gig *ana* ti-*šú* 1/3 sìla ^{giš}naga.si
16′	dd	1/3 sìla a ^{giš}geštin.kala.ga 5 gín *ṭa-ab-ti*
17′	dd	5 gín ^{ú}kur.ra^{sar} *ina* kaš.sag šeg$_6$-*šal* ì.giš
18′	dd	*ana* igi šub.šub *ana* dúr-*šú* dub-*ak*
19′	dd	^{ú}*ni-nu-ú* ^{ú}*úr-nu-ú* ^{ú}nu.luh.ha
20′	dd	^{ú}*ka-si-i sah-lé-e* ^{ú}úkuš.hab mun
21′	dd	naga.si ú babbar ì.udu éllag udu níta 10 ú.meš
22′	dd	al.la.an ⸢dù$^{?}$⸣-*u*[*š*$^{?}$ ....]
23′	dd	^{šim}gúr.gúr ^{šim}li ^{ši}[^{m}...........
24′	dd	^{ú}har.har ^{ú}nu.[luh.ha ....
25′	dd	^{giš}naga.si [....................
26′	dd	zú.lum.⸢ma⸣ 12 ú.meš gab[a.làl ....

[1] Perhaps a phonetic variant to giš.eren.síg // *lukšu*, see CAD L 240.

TRANSLATION

ll. 1′–3′ fragmentary

4′ If a man [pours out] blood from his anus[?] [...............
5′ pine-needles[?] ... [..
6′ *poured out* date, .[..
7′ [Mix] these nine plants in milk [and ....
8′ and you [pour them] into his anus [............

9′ If a man suffers from rectal disease and his bowel is affected, [.............
10′ he is continually constipated – *imhur-līm*, male mandrake, [..], (and)
11′ *imhur-ešra*: crush these plants together, he drinks (them) in beer and he will get better.

12′ If a man is ill in the rectum and his anus is stopped up: crush (and) mix bat guano,
13′ (and) root of male mandrake, roll them together (in a pill) and insert it into his anus.

14′ [If ditto], his stools keep drying up inside him,[1]
15′ that [man] is ill with *zēzēnu*-disease; to cure him, heat up 1/3 sila of horned alkali,
16′ 1/3 sila of strong vinegar, 5 shekels of salt,
17′ and 5 shekels of *nīnû* in premium beer, keep putting oil
18′ into it[2] and pour it into his anus.

19′ *Nīnû*, *urnû*, *nuhurtu*,
20′ *kasû*, *sahlû*, cucumber, salt,
21′ horned alkali, 'white'-plant, fat of a male sheep: 10 drugs (with which)
22′ you make a suppository, [.....................

23′ *Kukru*, juniper, ...[...................
24′ *hašû*, *nuhurtu*[?], [......................
25′ horned alkali, [..............................
26′ and dates: 12 drugs. Wax [.................................

---

[1] *ina lìb-bi-šú* could refer to 'his belly' or simply adverbially to the middle, referring to his rectum.

[2] See AHw 822a, 'darauf(?)', referring to our phrase.

27′	dd	[*a-na u*]*m-ṣa-a-ti* zi-*hi* še [...........[1]
28′	dd	[$^{\text{na4}}$*g*]*a-bé-e* ⸢šika⸣ ^{giš}*nu-úr-m*[*u-ú* ....
29′	dd	⸢diš⸣-*niš* súd ì.g[iš$^{?}$ ....] x *um-ṣa-*[*a-ti* ....

30′	dd	diš na ninda gu$_7$ kaš [n]ag-*ma* na.[bi ....][2]
31′	dd	gi.gíd hur.meš gig ⸢ú⸣[......
32′	dd	ka-*šú ta-kap-par* [.................
33′	dd	^{giš}geštin.šur.ra x [...............
34′	dd	[..] x ⸢uš ú⸣[.....................
35′	dd	(trace)

---

1 cf. BAM 182 rev. 7′–8′, although not a duplicate to these lines.

2 For ll. 30′–35′, cf. BAM 566, 7′–18′, dealing with problems of the windpipe, as here.

27′ [To] remove haemorrhoids, crush together (l. 29) barley [..........
28′ alum, pomegranate-rind, [..............................
29′ [put] oil [into it], ... haemorrhoids [.......................

30′ If a man eats food and drinks beer and [that] man [..............
31′ he is ill in the windpipe; .[...
32′ you wipe down his mouth [.................................
33′ drawn wine ..[..
34′–35′ (broken)

No. 31 BAM 182

EE	=	O. 194 (BAM 182)
XX	=	A. 198 (BAM 159: 9–11) = l. 6
AL	=	CT 23 10 26 ff. = ll. 18–20
SS	=	K 2428 + 2458 (AMT 82,2) + 6728 [text no. 45] = 7′–10′
Y	=	K 2433+ [text no. 24] = rev. 9–10
dd	=	S 1283 + 1947 (AMT 40,4 + 57, 5) [text no. 30] = rev. 9–10
ff	=	K 8248 (AMT 56,1: 8–9) [text no. 32] = rev. 11–12
H	=	K 9441 (AMT 43,5) [text no. 33]

obv.

1′	EE	⸢gú⸣.níg.àr.⸢ra⸣ ^{na4}*ga*$^{?!}$-[*bu-u*.........................
2′	EE	diš na gìš-*šú ú-zaq-qa-ta-šú* numun ^{ú}[.................
3′	EE	diš na gìš-*šú ú-kàs-sa*<*-as-su*> *hi-níq-ti* é[llag ....
4′	EE	*ana* ti-*šú* ú babbar súd *ina* ì hi.hi *ina* x [................
5′	EE	[d]iš na gìš-*šú ú-zaq-qat-su* numun gada x [......*ina* ^{urudu}šen.t]ur$^{?}$ ⸢*tara*⸣-*bak ina* kuš sur-*re*
6′	EE	[diš n]a *ina* gìš-*šú* múd *ú-tab-ba-kam* gim munus ^{gi}[^{š}..............................g]al ^{ú}nu.luh.ha naga.si *ina* kaš.lú.tin.na
	XX	diš na *ina* gìš-*šú* múd *ú-tab-ba-ka* gim munus ^{giš}tukul *ma-hi-iṣ an*[*a* t]i-*šú* gú.gal ^{ú}nu.luh.ha naga.si diš-*niš* súd [......] *ina* mul$_{4}$ *tuš-bat ina še-rim* nu *pa-tan* nag-*ma* ti
7′	EE	[diš n]a *maš-ka*$_{15}$(kak)-*dù* dab$_{5}$-*su* ^{giš}še$^{!}$.ná$^{!}$.a[1] ^{ú}ku$_{6}$ numun ⸢^{ú}*qut*⸣-*ri*[2] pa ^{giš}kiri$_{6}$ dù.a.bi
	SS	diš na *maš-k*[*a-*...].a.bi
8′	EE	[g]azi^{sar} ^{giš}šinig ^{ú}*túl-lal* ^{giš}gišimmar.tur gi.šul.hi ^{giš}*kam-u*$_{5}$[3]
	SS	gazi^{sar} ^{giš}š[inig ....]-⸢*u*$_{5}$⸣
9′	EE	suhuš ^{giš}dìh suhuš ^{giš}kiši$_{16}$ téš.bi *ta-har-ra-aṣ ina* šà útul *u* a.geštin
	SS	suhuš ^{giš}dìh su[huš ....] x te
10′	EE	a pú *ina* nindu úš-*er gi-na-am* ra.meš-*su*
	SS	esir *ina* nindu ú[š ....-*a*]*ṣ*
11′	EE	diš na *maš-ka*$_{15}$-*dù* gig úkuš-*ti-gil-li* numun ^{giš}ma.nu
12′	EE	^{ú}*ka-zal-la* nag.nag ^{ú}lagab.a.šà.ga ^{ú}*zu-qa-qí-pa* [súd]
13′	EE	zì.gig *ina* kaš.sag h[i.h]i gim ^{dug}utul$_{7}$ *tara-bak* [ti]

---

1 The signs are gud du$_{10}$.gam ku$_{7}$.hi.a, emended by Köcher. The line requires collation, since the signs gud = *alpu*, du$_{10}$.gam = *kimṣu* and ku$_{7}$ = *matqu* are clear as drawn, with the possibility of the latter sign being a logogram for *marû*, 'fattened', see CAD M/1 306 lex. Irving Finkel suggests an alternative reading of *alappānu matqu* for gud.umun$_{10}$$^{?}$.ku$_{7}$.hi.a, a type of sweet beer, cf. CAD A/1 335.

2 Reading Franz Köcher, courtesy B. Böck.

3 See CAD K s. v. *kam'atu* (120, 'truffle') *kammu* (125, 'a fungus'), and *ka'u* (309 'mushroom').

TRANSLATION

1′ Vetch (*kiššēnu*), alum, [...............

2′ If a man's penis stings him: seed of [...................

3′ If a man's penis hurts (lit. gnaws at) him, [he suffers from] stricture of the kidney[?] [.....
4′ To cure him, crush 'white'-plant and mix (it) in oil and in ... [.............

5′ If a man's penis stings him: seed of flax ...., steep [it] in a small vessel[?] and spread it on leather.

6′ If a man's penis drips blood, he is 'struck with a weapon' like a (menstruating) woman, to cure him, crush together pea, *nuhurtu*, and horned alkali in brewer's beer, you leave it out over night and in the morning he drinks it on an empty stomach, and he will recover.

7′ If a man has been seized by *maškadu*, you cut up together (l. 9) *šunû*[?], *urânu*, seed of *qutru*, any garden leaf,
8′ *kasû*, tamarisk, *tullal*, young date-palm, *šalālu*-reed, truffle,
9′ root of the *baltu*-thorn, root of acacia-thorn into a bowl, and you heat vinegar and
10′ well water (var. bitumen) in an oven and regularly bathe him.

11′ If a man suffers from *maškadu*, he keeps drinking (in a potion) gourd, *e'ru*-seed,
12′ and *kazallu*, [crush] 'field-clod'-plant, 'scorpion'-plant;
13′ mix flour in premium beer, when you make a concoction, [he will improve].[1]

[1] See CAD R 9, *kīma rabīki tarabbak*.

14′ EE én *maš-ka$_{15}$-dù iš-tu ṣe-er*<*-ret*> *šá-ma-me ur-dam*$^{!}$ *u mi-šil im-tú šá* muš [*il-qé*][1]
15′ EE [*ša*] gír.tab *i-mat-sa al-qé-ma* dumu *im-ta a-tar mi-šìr-*[*ti* ....
16′ EE [*pa*]*-a la* gar*-in šin-na ṣa-bit* gar *kal giš-šá kim-ṣa ki-ṣal-la* : murub$_4$ [giš.kun *u šá-šal-li* tu$_6$.én]

17′ EE [k]a.inim.ma *maš-ka$_{15}$-*[*dù*]

18′ EE [én] *a-re-eh-hi ra-ma-ni a-ra-ah-hi zu-u*[*m-ri* ....[2]
AL én *a-ra-ah-hi ra-ma-ni a-ra-hi pag-ri* gim ur.gir$_7$ *u* mí.ur šah mí.šah ⸢*ir-tak*⸣*-bu-u*
19′ EE [gi]m ^{giš}apin *ina* edin *er-ṣe-tú ir-hu-u* ki*-tú im-hu-ru* [..........]
AL *ina* edin*-šú* : gim ^{giš}apin *er-ṣe-tú ir-hu-ú er-ṣe-tú im-hu-ru* [numun]*-šú*[3]
20′ EE [*a-n*]*am-di* én *ana ra-ma-ni-ia u* su*-ia lim-hu*<*-ru*>*-ma*
AL *lim*^{im}*-hur ra-ma-ni li-ir-hi ra-ma-ni* t[u$_6$ én]
21′ EE [*ra*]*-ma-ni-šu li-ir-ʾ-ú zu-um-ri-*[*šu lišēṣi lumna*][4]

22′ EE [k]a.inim.ma *maš-k*[*a-du*]

23′ EE [diš ki.min] x ^{ú}*kur-ka-nam* ^{ú}*kam.u$_5$* giš.še.ná.a *ana* ì [.........
24′ EE [én é.n]u.ru šid*-ma* gìri^{2}*-šú* gig šu^{2} *tu-maš-šá-aʾ* [.........

25′ EE [én ......] x *bu-uh-ru bu-ha-ru šu-ú maš-*[*ka-du*]
26′ EE [*mi-šil im-t*]*ú ša* ^{d}*a-nim* mul.meš *šá-ma-mi* [...............
27′ EE [..................] x *šá* muš *il-qé šá* gír.tab *i-mat-sa* [*al-qé* ....
28′ EE [...............] x in$^{?}$ *šin-na* : *šun-na ul šá-kin* x [.............
29′ EE [............................ mu]rub$_4$ giš.kun [......................
30′ EE [............................. *a*]*t-*[*t*]*a maš-k*[*a-du* ....
(broken)

rev.
1′ EE [............................] hi x [......................

2′ EE [..................................] šid [........................
3′ EE [..................] *u* ì.udu hi.hi *ina* [......................

4′ EE [diš na múd] dúr*-šú i-te-ez-zi* <zi> *ur-ši ina* x [...........[5]
5′ EE [........... z]ú.lum.ma ^{šim}li ^{šim}gúr.gúr [...........
6′ EE [........] ni ú.hi.a *an-nu-ti* diš*-niš* súd šu.si dù*-uš ana* dú[r*-šú* gar*-an*]

7′ EE [diš na d]úr gig*-ma um-ṣa-ti šu-ti* ^{ú}kur.ra x [............
8′ EE [*u* d]úr*-šú* šéš.meš *ur-še* gaz.meš *um-ṣa-a-ti u*[*q-ṭa-ta-pa*...........[6]

---

1 See. ll. 27′–29′ below. Köcher gives these lines as duplicates to K 2453 + (= CT 23 5–14 i 4′–8′), but I cannot find the parallels. Cf. however, the unpublished dissertation of Collins, *Natural Illness*, 238 (editing these lines) and 243 (*maškadu* 5 and 8). Parallel (but not duplicate) passages to this three-line extract can be found in BAM 124 iv 12–15 and BAM 127: 9–13.
Collins (op. cit. 239) suggests the emendation *ṣe-er*<*-ret*>, but his interpretation of l. 15′ differs considerably, reading: *i-mat-sa il*$^{!}$*-qé ut*$^{!}$*-tur im-ta a-tar mi-hir-*[....

2 This incantation has been edited by A. Cavigneaux, apud *Mesopotamian Magic*, ed. T. Abusch and K. van der Toorn (Groningen, 1999), 265–267.

3 Restored after Maqlû VII 26, see A. Cavigneaux, op. cit. 266.

4 Restored after Maqlû VII 28, see A. Cavigneaux, op. cit. 266.

5 see BAM 152 iii 16–18; AHw 1434 suggests *ṭīb*(zi) *ur-ši*, but BAM 152 has no zi sign before *ur-ši*.

6 See text No. 34: 51. Cf. CAD Š/3 191.

14′ Incantation. *Maškadu* has descended from the 'halter' of heaven, and [took] half the poison of a snake
15′ (and) I took the poison [of] a scorpion. The child [*took*] poison and excess *of the sea*,
16′ (although) not provided with a mouth (but) with teeth, – seizing all of the hip, shin, and ankle: hips, [buttocks, and *backside*; incantation].[1]

17′ Incantation for *maškadu*.

18′ Incantation. I impregnate myself, I impregnate my body, like a dog and bitch or pig and sow
19′ have sex in the steppe; like a plow that has seeded the earth and the earth has received its [seed],
20′ I cast the spell so that I should receive (it) in myself and in my body, and [may (the patient) receive (it)]
21′ himself and impregnate [his] body and [cause the evil to depart].

22′ Incantation for *maškadu*.

23′ [ditto] [put] .. , *kurkānû*, truffle, and *šunû*-shrub into oil, [.................
24′ recite the incantation and massage his ailing feet and hands [...........

25′ [Incantation. ....].., while kept hot, it is *maškadu*,
26′ [half of the] spittle of Anu, the stars of heaven [..........
27′ he took [half of the venom] of the snake, [I took] the poison of the scorpion [...
28′ [......................] .... he is not provided with a tooth(?) (var. *šunnu*-vessel) .....[..............
29′ [..] the hips and groin [....................
30′ [.................................], 'you are *maškadu*' [................
(rest broken)

rev.

1′–2 (broken)
3′ mix [...........] in sheep fat and in [......................

4′ [If a man's] anus excretes [blood] and a [he has] a sore on [...............................
5′ [..........], dates, juniper, *kukru*, [...
6′ [........].., crush these plants together and make a pessary and [insert it] into [his] anus.

7′ [If a man] is ill in the rectum and is ... with haemorrhoids, *nīnû*, .. [.........
8′ [and] keep smearing his anus (so that) the sores are *smashed* and haemorrhoids are plucked [off .....

---

[1] See BAM 124 iv, 18–19, which is the basis for our restoration. The line is corrupt, and our assumption is that the line should read *šin-na* gar *ṣa-bit*, see l. 29′ of this same text.

9′	EE	[diš n]a dúr gig-*ma* dúr-*šú* *e-sil* u$_5$.ib.gar[^{mušen}]
	Y	[................g]ig dúr-*šú* *e-s*[*i*-.........................]
	dd	diš na dúr gig-*ma* dúr-*šú* *e-sil* u$_5$.ib.gar^{mušen}
10′	EE	[su]huš ^{giš}nam.tar níta súd *tu-kap-pat ana* dúr-*šú* [gar-*an*]
	Y	[................................] diš-*niš tu-kap-pat* [............................]
	dd	[s]uhuš ^{giš}nam.tar níta súd hi-hi diš-*niš tu-kap-pat ana* dúr-*šú* gar
11′	EE	diš na dúr gig dúr-*šú ú-zaq-qat*^{2}-*su* šà.meš-*šú in-n*[*i-bi-ṭu*]
	ff	[diš na dúr.g]ig gig-*ma* dúr-*šú ú-zaq-qat-su* šà.meš-*šú it-ta-nin-b*[*i-ṭ*]*u*
12′	EE	*ú-ta-sal* a geštin.a kaš.sag šeg$_6$-*šal tu-kaṣ-ṣa ana* dúr-[*šú* ....]
	ff	*ú-ta-as-sal* [..........] x kaš.sag šeg$_6$-*šal* šed$_7$ *ana* dúr-*šú* dub-[*ak*]
13′	EE	diš na dúr.gig gig-*ma e-sil* ^{šim}li ^{ú}hab súd *ana* dúr-[*šú* gar-*an*]
14′	EE	^{ú}kur.ra súd *ina* gada nigin-*mi* ì *ina* x ra x *ana* dúr-*šú* [gar-*an*]
15′	EE	^{ú}kur.ra gaz šeg$_6$-*šal ana* dúr-*šú* gar-*an kal* x [..]
16′	EE	ú.hi.a *an-nu-ti ina* a.gazi^{sar} šub-*šú-ma* [ti]
17′	EE	[diš na dú]r g[i]g [................] x gur *lu u ina* a tar x x [..]
18′	EE	[..] x ri$^?$ x x x ú
19′	EE	[........] x [..................................] x bar giš x x nu [..] diš-*niš*
20′	EE	[...] x [.......................................] x – x -*šú* gar-[*an*]
21′	EE	[diš n]a dúr gig [..
22′	EE	^{šim}buluh a ^{šim}[..
23′	EE	diš na dúr gig gig-[*ma* ....
24′	EE	na.bi x x [..
25′	EE	diš [n]a [...

(rest broken)

9′ [If a] man is ill in the rectum and his anus is blocked up, crush bat guano
10′ (and) root of male mandrake together, roll it up (into a pill) and insert it into his anus.

11′ If a man is ill in the rectum and his anus stings him and his innards are bloated,
12′ he is suffers from constipation, boil vinegar and premium beer, cool (it) and pour it into his anus.

13′ If a man is ill in the rectum and it is blocked up, crush juniper and madder and [insert it] into his anus,
14′ crush *nīnû*, wrap it in linen, [insert] oil in ... into his anus.
15′ Pound *nīnû*, boil (it) and insert (it) into his anus. All the ..[....
16′ put these drugs in *kasû*-juice and [he will recover].

17′ (remainder broken)

No. 32 AMT 56,1

ff	=	K 8248 (AMT 56,1)
X	=	K 6545 + 8355 + 9030 (AMT 40,5) [text no. 23] = ll. 1–4
TT	=	K 6056 (AMT 69,8): 11–16 [text no. 46] = rev. 5–8; 10–11
EE	=	0. 194 (BAM 182 rev. 11′–12′) [text no. 31] = ll 8–9
AI	=	K 2477 + (AMT 94,2) = BAM 471 i 9′–11′ = 7–9
BB	=	VAT 10723 (BAM 88 1′–9′) [text no. 27] (collated) = 4–7; 10–11; rev. 1–4
GG	=	K 9441 (AMT 43,5) [text no. 33] = ll. 12–16
Y	=	K 2433 + (S 357 = AMT 7,7) [text no. 24] = ll. 12–13

1	ff	[.. ga]ba-*su u šá-sal-la*-[*šú*] gu$_7$.meš-[*šú*]
	X	diš na *mi-na-tu-šú* dub.dub gaba-*su* u sa.sal.meš-*šú* gu$_7$.meš-*šú*
2	ff	[..] gu$_7$.meš-*šú* éllag *bir-ki-šú lu* šá 15 *lu šá* [15]0
	X	á^2-*šú k*[*im-ṣa-a-šú u bir-ka-šú*] gu$_7$.meš-*šú* éllag *bir-ki-šú lu šá* 15 *lu šá* 150
3	ff	[......................................]-*šú* múd *ú-kal-lam* na.bi *hi-níq-ti* dúr gig
	X	sìg-*su-ma ina mùš-tin*-[*ni* ....] na.bi *hi-niq-ti* dúr.gig gig
	BB	[..] *hi-niq-ti* [.........]
4	ff	[.. ^{giš}l]i ^{šim}man.du gi.du$_{10}$.ga ^{šim}mug šim.sal
	X	*ana* ti-*šú* ^{ú}*tara-muš* ^{ú}igi-*lim* ^{ú}[..............................
	BB	[...................^{ši}]^{m}gúr.gúr ^{ši}[^{m}..........................] gi.du$_{10}$.ga ^{ši}[^{m}...............]
5	ff	[^{giš}eren] ^{giš}eren.úš ^{giš}še.ná.a ^{ú}*úr-né-e* ^{ú}har.har
	BB	^{giš}eren ^{giš}e[rin.úš......................] ^{ú}*úr-nu-u* $^{⸢ú⸣}$[.................]
6	ff	[^{ú}nu].luh.ha ^{ú}kur.ra zú.lum.ma zì.munu$_4$ kaš *ni-it-ku* ^{giš}geštin
	BB	[..................] ^{ú}kur.ra zú.lum.m[a ....] *ni-it-ku* ^{giš}geštin
7	ff	[.. *t*]*a-hi-it-te i-na* nindu *te-sek-ker ana* dúr dub-*ak*
	BB	še [...............] *i-na* nindu *te-sek-ker ana* dú[r-........]
8	ff	[diš na dúr.g]ig gig-*ma* dúr-*šú ú-zaq-qat-su* šà.meš-*šú it-ta-nin-b*[*i-ṭ*]*u ú-ta-as-sal*
	EE	diš na dúr.gig gig-*ma* dúr-*šú ú-zaq-qat^2-su* šà.meš-*šú in-n*[*i-ib-ṭu*] *ú-ta-sal*
9	ff	[...........] x kaš.sag šeg$_6$-*šal* šed$_7$ *ana* dúr-*šú* dub-[*ak*]
	EE	a geštin.na kaš.sag šeg$_6$-*šal tu-kaṣ-ṣa ana* dúr-[........]
10	ff	[diš na dú]r.gig gig-*ma* dúr-*šú* gír.gír-*su* ^{šim}li ^{šim}gúr.gúr [.........................]
	BB	[..............] gig-*ma* dúr-*šú* gír.g[ír ....] ^{šim}gúr.gúr ^{šim}gam.me [....]
11	ff	[diš-*niš* hi.h]i ^{šim}gig lagab.munu$_4$ ì.giš *u* kaš *ana* dúr-*šú* [dub-*ak*]
	BB	[......................... gi]g lagab.munu$_4$ *ina* ì.giš *u* kaš *ana* [...............]
12	ff	[diš na ninda g]u$_7$ kaš nag-*ma e-sil* úh.meš-*šú i-šal-la* š[à.meš-*šú it*]-*tan-na-bi-ṭu*
	GG	diš na ninda gu$_7$ kas.sag nag-*ma e-si-il* ú[h...]
	Y	[...................... ka]š nag-*ma e-si*-[...-*n*]*a-bi-ṭu*
13	ff	[.........] ⸢*i*⸣-*ár-ru-ru* <*ana*> na.bi dúr.gig gig *ana* ti-*šú* 1/3 *ma-na* ì.giš$^?$
	GG	*ir-ru-šu i-ár-ru-ur* na.bi dúr.gig gig [..
	Y	*ir-ru-⸢ú-šu i-ár-ru-ru⸣* [..
14	ff	[1/3 ma.na] x^{sar} 1/3 ma.na naga.si 1/3 ma.na ^{šim}gúr.gúr 1/3 ma.na ^{šim}li
	GG	1/3 ma ^{šim}gúr.gúr 1/3 ma ^{šim}li 1/3 ma ^{giš}eren 1/3 ma x [.......................
15	ff	[...........] x x x [.....] x x x ú.hi.a šeš.meš *ina* kaš.tin.na
16	ff	[..] šub-*di ana* dúr-*šú* dub-ma *ina-eš*
	GG	[*i*]*na* im.šu.rin.na *te-sek-ker* e$_{11}$-*ma tu-kaṣ-ṣa* ì.giš *ana* igi š[ub ....

TRANSLATION

1 If a man's limbs are flaccid (lit. poured out), his chest and shoulders hurt him,
2 his arms, shins [and knees] hurt him, his testicle, either on the right side or on the left,
3 bothers him, and he shows blood in his urethra, that man suffers from stricture of the anus.
4 To cure him, you heat in an oven (l. 7) *taramuš*, *imhur-lim*, juniper, *suādu*, sweet reed, *ballukku*, *šimeššalû*,
5 cedar, *šupuhru*-cedar, *šunû*, *urnû*, *hašû*,
6 *nuhurtu*, *nīnû*, dates, malt-flour, beer, wine-drops(?),
7 and ...-barley, and you pour (it) into the anus.

8 If a man suffers from rectal disease and his anus stings him and his bowels are cramped and he is constipated,
9 boil vinegar and premium beer, cool it and pour it into his anus.

10 [If a man] suffers from rectal disease (and) it stings him: mix [together] juniper, *kukru*, *ṣumlalû*, [.....
11 <boil> *kanaktu* (and) clump of malt in oil and beer and [pour it] into his anus.

12 If a man eats bread and drinks beer and is constipated, he spits up his spittle, and [his] bowels are constantly cramped,
13 his intestines discharge (a putrid liquid), that man suffers from rectal disease. To cure him, one-third mina oil,
14 one-third mina of ..., one third mina of horned alkali, one-third mina *kukru*, one-third mina juniper (var. differs in order),
15 [................................], heat these drugs in tavern-beer
16 in an oven, remove and cool it, put it into (the mixture), pour it into his anus and he will get better.

rev.

1′ ff [.........] ^{šim}li x [x x [....] x [....................................] x x x
BB diš ki.min ^{šim}gúr.gúr ^{šim}li ⌜tuh.še.giš⌝.[ì...........]
2′ ff [.......................... ^{ú}].kur.ra ^{ú}hur.sag 8 ú.meš *ina* kaš.l[ú.tin.n]a šeg$_6$.gá
BB ^{ú}naga.si ^{ú}lag.a.šà ^{ú}[.....] ^{ú}hur.sag 8 ú.meš šeš ina kaš. x [................
3′ ff [.....] x x *ba bah-ra* ì.giš làl *ana* igi šub-*di ana* dúr-*šú* dub
BB [...] dúr-*šú* [....]
4′ ff [....] ì.[nun.na] ga ku$_7$.ku$_7$ *ana* dúr-*šú* dub-*ma ina-eš*

5′ ff [*ana* murub$_4$.meš] *áš-ṭa-a-te lu-ub-bu-ka* lagab.munu$_4$ numun $^{\text{giš.šim}}$man.du
TT diš *a-na* murub$_4$ *áš-ṭa-a-ti l*[*u-*...]
6′ ff [..........^{šim}]bal gi.du$_{10}$.ga šim.šeš *sik-ka-ti ina* ì *u* kaš šeg$_6$-*šal ana* dúr dub
TT [..................] gi.dug$_4$.ga ^{šim}šeš *si*[*k-*...]

7′ ff [ki.min ^{šim}]šeš gazi^{sar} ^{ú}nu.luh.ha ^{šim}gúr.gúr naga.si lag.a.šà
TT ^{šim}šeš gazi^{sar} ^{ú}nu.luh.ha [..]
AI [1 g]ar ^{šim}šeš gazi^{sar} ^{ú}nu.luh.ha ^{šim}gúr.gúr naga.si lag.a.šà
8′ ff [.........r]a$^{?}$ ^{ú}hur.sag *ina* kaš *u* ga *ta-sàk bu-uh-ru-s*[*u*] ì *ina* igi šub
TT [.........................] *ina* kaš *u* ga súd *bu-uh-ru* è ì.giš *ana* [................]
AI [^{ú}kur.r]a ^{ú}hur.sag *ina* kaš *u* ga *ina* im.šu.rin.na *te-sek-ker*[1] *tu-še-lam-ma*
9′ ff [..] x egir-*šú* ga *mat-qa ana* dúr-*šú* dub
AI [.....] x x è ì.giš *ana* igi šub-*di ana* dúr-*šú* dub egir-*šú* ga *mat-qa ana* dúr-*šú* dub-*ma* *ina-eš*

10′ ff [*ana* sa murub$_4$ *lu-u*]*b-bu-ka* numun $^{\text{giš.šim}}$man.du ^{šim}gi.du$_{10}$.ga
TT *ana* sa murub$_4$ *lu-ub-bu-ki* numun.gada ^{šim}[............................
11′ ff [................].ra gig.ba *ina* ì.giš *u* kaš šeg$_6$-*šal*
TT gazi^{sar} níg.àr.ra gig.ba ina ì.[.........................]
12′ ff [...........................] x -*ma* ti

13′ ff [ki.min .... ^{ši}]^{m}buluh ^{šim}man.du zú.lum.ma
14′ ff [...............................] šeš.meš *ina* kaš šeg$_6$-*šal ana* dúr-*šú* dub

[1] Reading F. Köcher, courtesy B. Böck.

rev.

1′ If ditto, *kukru*, juniper, sesame residue, [................

2′ horned alkali, 'field-clod'-plant, *nīnû*, *azupīru*, boil these 8 drugs in a brewer's beer,

3′ [.......], ... while steaming, put oil and honey into it and pour it into his anus.

4′ Pour [...], ghee and sweet milk into his anus and he will get better.

5′ In order to make the stiff groin supple, clump of malt, seed of *suādu*,

6′ [........] *ballukku*, sweet reed, myrrh and *sikkatu*, boil them in oil and beer and pour them into his anus.

7′ [Ditto], you crush (var: you heat and remove from the oven), myrrh, *kasû*, *nuhurtu*, *kukru*, horned alkali, field-clod,

8′ *nīnû*? (and) *azupīru* in beer and milk, and while it is hot you add in oil, (var. you heat it in an oven and remove it)

9′ take out [....] and add in oil and pour it into his anus; afterwards pour sweet milk into his anus and he will get better.

10′ In order to make the tendons of the groin supple: boil flax seed, *suādu*, 'sweet-reed',

11′ *kasû*, groats, (and) wheat in oil and beer,

12′ [.......................................] and he will recover.

13′ [Ditto, ...], [crush] *baluhhu*, *suādu*, dates

14′ [.................]; boil these [plants] in beer and pour them into his anus.

No. 33 AMT 43,5

GG = K 9441 = AMT 43,5
Y = K 2433 + (S 357 = AMT 7,7 = iii 13–21) [text no. 24] = ll. 1–8
ff = K 8248 = AMT 56,1: 12 ff. [text no. 32] = ll. 7–10
dd = S 1283 + 1947 (AMT 40,4 + 57,5) [text no. 30] = ll. 5–6; 11–12
EE = O. 194 (BAM 182) rev. 9–10 [text no. 31] (cf. RA 26 73) = ll. 5–61

1	GG	^{ú}kur.kur zà.[hi.li..
	Y	[............ zà.hi.l]i? naga.si *qa-la-a-ti* ú [..^{ši}]^{m}li
2	GG	^{šim}šeš m[un..
	Y	^{šim}šeš mun kù x [...............................]-*e* gaz sim *ina* dè [.....................
3	GG	min zú.lum.ma mun x [...
	Y	[................m]a mun naga.si *tur-á*[*r* ....
4	GG	^{šim}gam.ma ill[u ....
	Y	^{šim}gam.ma ill[u ....
5	GG	diš na dúr.gig gig dúr-*šú e*-[*sil* ....
	Y	[........gi]g gig dúr-*šú e-si*[*l*..
	dd	diš na dúr gig-*ma* dúr-*šú e-sil* gar.ib.u$_5$^{mušen} [s]uhuš ^{giš}nam.tar níta súd hi.hi
	EE	[d]iš na dúr gig-*ma* dúr-*šú e-sil* ^{mušen}u$_5$.gar.[ib su]huš ^{giš}nam.tar níta súd
6	GG	diš-*niš tu-kap-pat* [......................
	Y	[...] *tu-kap-pat* [........................
	dd	diš-*niš tu-kap-pat ana* dúr-*šú* gar
	EE	diš-*niš tu-kap-pat ana* dúr-*šú* [..]
7	GG	diš na ninda gu$_7$ kas.sag nag-*ma e-si-il* ú[h.................[1]
	Y	[...................... ka]š nag-*ma e-si*-[...-*n*]*a-bi-ṭu*
	ff	[............... g]u$_7$ kas nag-*ma e-sil* úh.meš-*šú i-šal-la* š[à.meš-*šú it*]-*tan-na-bi-ṭu*
8	GG	*ir-ru-šu i-ár-ru-ur* na.bi dúr.gig gig [...
	Y	*ir-ru*-⸢*ú-šu i-ár-ru-ru*⸣ [..
	ff	[........] ⸢*i*⸣-*ár-ru-ru ana* na.bi dúr.gig gig *ana* ti-*šú* 1/3 ma.na x [..........] x ^{sar} 1/3 ma.na naga.si
9	GG	1/3 ma ^{šim}gúr.gúr 1/3 ma ^{šim}li 1/3 ma ^{giš}eren 1/3 ma x [...........
	ff	1/3 ma.na ^{šim}gúr.gúr 1/3 ma ^{šim}li [.................................] (traces) ú.hi.a šeš.meš *ina* kaš.tin.na
10	GG	[*i*]*na* im.šu.rin.na *te-sek-ker* e$_{11}$-*ma tu-kaṣ-ṣa* ì.giš *ana* igi š[ub ....
	ff	[..š]ub-*di ana* dúr-*šú* dub-*ma ina-eš*
11	GG	[diš] na dúr.gig gig-*ma* šà-*šú* dab-*su it-te-nen-s*[*il* ....]
	dd	diš na dúr.gig gig-*ma lìb-ba-šu* d[ab-..] *it-te-nen-sil* ^{ú}igi-*līm* ^{ú}<nam>.tar nita ⸢^{ú}⸣[..]
12	GG	[^{ú}]igi-*ešra* ú.hi.a *an-nu-ti* téš.bi sú[d ....]
	dd	^{ú}igi-*ešra* ú.meš *an-nu-ti* diš-*niš* súd *ina* kaš nag-*ma ina-eš*

1 See var. K 11317 (AMT 44,6), cf. RA 26, 80.

TRANSLATION

1 Pound and sieve *ata'išu*, *sahlû*, roasted horned alkali, [............], juniper,
2 myrrh, pure salt, [......], and [.................................] on coals [......].

---

3 Ditto. Dry out dates, salt, horned alkali, [....................
4 *ṣumlalû*, resin of [..

---

5 If a man suffers from rectal disease and his anus is blocked up,[1] crush and mix bat-guano and the root of male mandrake,
6 roll them together in a pill and put it into his anus.

---

7 If a man eats bread and drinks premium beer and is stopped up, he spits up his spittle and his bowels are constantly cramped,
8 his bowels discharge (a putrid liquid), that man suffers from rectal disease. To cure him, one third mina of ... [.......], one third mina of horned alkali,
9 one third mina of *kukru*, one-third mina of juniper, one-third mina of cedar, one-third mina of ....,
10 you heat these drugs in tavern beer in an oven, remove and cool it, and add oil into it and insert it into his anus and he will get better.

---

11 If a man suffers from rectal disease and his bowel is affected, he is continually constipated – *imhur-līm*, male mandrake, .[..], (and)
12 *imhur-ešra*: crush these plants together , he drinks it in beer and he will get better.

---

[1] Note that the anus being blocked up is seen as the cause of constipation.

13 GG [diš na] dúr.gig gig-*ma e-sil ù ú-nap-paq i-* x [..........................

14 GG [....] *ina* ì.giš *ù* kaš nag ^{šim}li ^{šim}gúr.gúr hi.[hi ....

15 GG [...] *ana* dúr-*šú* gar-*an ina* a ^{giš}še.ná.a ra-*su* [........................

16 GG [...] x sù *ana* dúr-*šú* gar-*an* x [................................

13 [If a man] suffers from a sore anus and is constipated and stopped up,[1] ....,
14 he drinks [....] in oil and beer, mix juniper and ***kukru*** [.......
15 [...], insert it into his anus and bathe him in ***šunû***-juice [........
16 sprinkle [....] and insert it into his anus ..[..............................

---

[1] See Thompson, RA 26, 74, translating 'breaks wind', and although CAD N/1 277 avoids translating the term.

No. 34 BAM 168

HH	=	VAT 9138 (BAM 168)
BB	=	VAT 10723 (BAM 88: 17–25) [text no. 27] = ll. 1–6
AE	=	STT 97 ii 6–13 (= ll. 33–39); iii 29–37 = ll. 40–41, 46–52
AF	=	VAT 8027 (BAM 54 18–19, text mostly *suālu*) = ll. 78–79
AI	=	K 2477 + (AMT 94,2 = BAM 471 ii 3′–6′) = ll. 1–6
AG	=	A 250 (BAM 108: 1–14) = ll. 62–72
AQ	=	VAT 7822 (BAM 49 rev. 24′–31′) = ll. 54–61
AR	=	VAT 14082 (BAM 50 rev. 1–6) = ll. 57–61
AP	=	VAT13733 + 13738 (BAM 52: 27–38, *suālu*) = ll. 1–5; 7–17
AS	=	VAT 11203 (BAM 53: 7–10) = ll. 33–36
AO	=	K 5834 + (BAM 579 ii 54′-64′, *suālu*) = ll. 18–32.
V	=	VAT 13752 + (BAM 95) [text no. 21] = ll. 70–75; 78–81.
W	=	S. 36 + (AMT 43,1 and duplicates) [text no. 22] = ll. 70–77.

1	HH	[diš n]a šà.meš-*šú* mú.mú *ir-ru-šú* gim *šá* mar.gal *ma-gal* d[u$_{11}$]
	BB	[.........] šà-*šú* m[ú.m]ú-*hu ir-ru-šú* [...] *šá* mar.gal *ma-gal* du$_{11}$.du$_{11}$-*ú*
	AI	[.. *š*]*á* mar.gal *ma-gal* du$_{11}$.du$_{11}$.-⸢*ú*⸣
	AP	diš na šà.meš-*šú* mú.meš-*hu ir-ru-šú* gim *šá* mar.gal *ma-gal* dug$_{4}$.d[ug$_{4}$$^{?}$ ..]
2	HH	na.bi *ni-kim-ti* im *u* ud.da gig kin-*šú* sumun-*ma* šu.g[edim]
	BB	[..] bi *ni-kim-ti* im *u* ud.da gig [ki]n-*šú* sumun-*ma* šu.gedim.ma
	AI	[..ki]n-⸢*šú*⸣ sumun-*ma* šu.gedim.ma
	AP	na.bi *ni-kim-tú* im ud.da gig kin-*šú i-la-bir-ma* šu.ge[dim.ma] ^{ú}kur.ra
3	HH	*ana* ti-*šú* ^{ú}kur.ra ^{ú}hur.sag ^{ú}har.har ^{ú}nu.[luh.ha]
	BB	*ana* ti-*šú* ^{ú}kur.ra ^{ú}hur.sag ^{ú}har.har ^{ú}nu.luh.h[a]
	AI	^{ú}kur.ra ^{ú}hur.sag [.......................................]
	AP	^{ú}hur.sag ^{ú}har.har ^{ú}nu.lu[h...]
4	HH	^{šim}li ^{šim}gúr.gúr ^{šim}gam.ma ^{šim}bal *šu-luṭ* š[im]
	BB	^{š}[^{im}l]i ^{šim}gúr.gúr ^{šim}gam.ma ^{ši}[^{m}..] *šu-lu*[*ṭ* ši]m.hi.a
	AI	[.................] gi du$_{10}$ ^{šim}gam.ma ^{šim}mug *šu-luṭ* šim.hi.a
	AP	^{šim}li ^{šim}gúr.gúr ^{šim}gam.ma ^{šim}mug
5	HH	mun 11 ú.hi.a šeš *ina* kaš.sag šeg$_{6}$-*šal ta-šá-h*[*al*]
	BB	^{ú}lag.a.šà 11 ⸢ú⸣.[...] *ina* kaš.sa[g š]eg$_{6}$-*šal ta-šá-hal*
	AI	x x x x x [...] x *ina* kaš.sag šeg$_{6}$-*šal*
6	HH	šed$_{7}$ ì.giš *ana* igi šub-*di ana* dúr-*šú* dub-*ak-ma* [t]i
	BB	šed$_{7}$ ì.[..] *ana* dúr-*šú* [...] -*ak-ma* ti
	AI	ì.giš *ana* igi šub *ana* dúr-*šú* dub

7	HH	numun gada ^{ú}*ak-tam* ^{ú}a.zal.lá ^{ú}hab ^{giš}*si-hu* ^{ú}*á*[*r-gan-nu*]
	AP	[......................]-*tam* ^{ú}a.zal.lá ⸢^{ú}⸣[...........................]-*nu*
8	HH	^{giš}lum.ha ^{ú}*áp-ru-šá* ^{im}sahar.babbar.kur.ra ^{im}sahar.g[e$_{6}$.kur.ra]
	AP	^{ú}⸢lum.ha⸣ [..................]sahar.babbar.kur.ra ^{im}sahar.[.............]
9	HH	^{im}sahar.na$_{4}$.kur.ra naga.si níg.àr.ra še.gig.ba x [....]
	AP	[..................................].si gig.sig$^{?}$ [...]
10	HH	lagab.munu$_{4}$ gazi^{sar}*sah-lé-e* ^{ú}sumun.dar ^{ú}kur.r[a]
	AP	[lag]ab.munu$_{4}$ gazi^{sar}[.......................................r]a
11	HH	^{ú}*úr-nu-u* ^{ú}hur.sag ^{ú}kur.zi ^{ú}*zi-bu-*[*u*]
	AP	^{ú}⸢*úr*⸣-*nu-u* ^{ú}*a-zu-pi-ru* ⸢^{ú}⸣[..........]

TRANSLATION

1 [If a] man's bowels are bloated, his intestines make a lot of noise like an *išqippu*-bird,
2 that man suffers from bloating and 'sun-fever', his condition is of long duration, it is the Hand of the Ghost-disease.
3 To cure him – *nīnû*, *azupīru*, *hašû*, *nuhurtu*,
4 juniper, *kukru*, *ṣumlalû*, *ballukku*, *cuttings of* aromatics,
5 salt (var. 'field-clod'-plant): you boil and filter these 11 drugs in premium beer,
6 cool them, add oil to it pour them into his anus, and he will improve.

---

7 Flax seed, *aktam*, *azallû*, madder, *sīhu*, *arganu*,
8 *barīrātu*, *aprušu*, *alluharu*(-mineral dye), black dye,
9 alum, horned alkali, groats, wheat, ..[...]
10 clump of malt, *kasû*, *sahlû*, *šumuttu*, *nīnû*,
11 *urnû*, *azupīru*, *samīnu*, black cumin,

12	HH	^{ú}har.har ^{ú}nu.luh.ha ^{ú}*si-bir-rù* ^{ú}*ti-[iá-tú]*
	AP	^{ú}*zi-*[..........]nu.luh ^{ú}*sip-pi-ru* ⌜^{ú}⌝[............]
13	HH	^{ú}*kám-ka-du* ú nam.ti.la ^{ú}geštin.ka$_5$.a ^{ú}*ṣa-ṣu[m-tú]*
	AP	^{ú}*kam-ka-d[u* ....k]a$_5$.a ^{ú}[.............]
14	HH	^{ú}še.ná.a $^{ú.d}$*šá-maš* ^{ú}*tara-muš*$_8$ ^{ú}igi-*lim* ^{ú}igi-*eš[ra]*
	AP	^{ú}še.ná.a ⌜^{ú}⌝[........................] ^{ú}igi.[..................]
15	HH	^{ú}kur.kur ^{ú}*kur-ka-nam* ^{ú}maš.tab.ba ^{ú}lag.a.šà
	AP	[...........] ^{ú}*kur-ka-nam* ⌜^{ú}⌝[.........................]
16	HH	zú.lum.ma dilmun^{ki}mun pap 1 *šu-ši* 3 ú.hi.a *mar-ha-ṣu*
	AP	[.............................] mun pap 1 *šu* 3 ú.hi.[.................]
17	HH	*rubbû*(gal-*u*) *ina* kaš.kala.ga a níg.àr.ra šeg$_6$-*šal ana* dúr-*šú* dub
	AP	*šim-mat ri-mu-tú šá-áš-šá-ṭu* ⌜šu gud.ma⌝ [šu nam.érim dúr.gig]
	AP	*u kal* gig *bul-lu-ṭu ina* kaš.kala.ga a níg.⌜àr.ra x⌝ [...........]
	AP	šeg$_6$-*šal ta-šá-hal tu-kaṣ-ṣa* 1/2 sìla ì.giš *ana* igi šub-*di ana* dúr-*šú* d[ub]
18	HH	diš na tab ud.da *ši-biṭ* im *šim-ma-tú ri-mu-tú šá-áš-šá-ṭu*
	AO	diš na *ši-bit* im *hi-mit* ud.d[a ....
19	HH	šu gud.ma šu nam.érim dúr.gig dù.gig *ana* ti-*šú*
	AO	[.............] šu nam.érim dúr.gig *u* [....................]
20	HH	10 gín ú nam.ti.la 10 gín ^{ú}*ti-iá-tú* 10 gín ^{ú}kur.kur
	AO	[........................] 10 gín ^{ú}*ti-ia-tu* 10 gín ⌜^{ú}⌝[........]
21	HH	10 gín ^{ú}har.har 10 gín ^{ú}nu.luh.ha 10 gín ^{ú}kur.ra
	AO	[...] 10 gín ^{ú}kur.ra
22	HH	10 gín *úr-nu-u* 10 gín mun.kù.pad 10 gín ^{ú}hur.sag
	AO	10 gín *ú[r-*...]
23	HH	10 gín ^{ú}luh.mar.tú 10 gín ú babbar 10 gín ^{na4}*ga-bi-i*
	AO	10 gín *šib-bur-ra-tu*$_4$ [..]
24	HH	10 gín ^{giš}li 10 gín ^{giš}gúr.gúr 10 gín *ak-tam* 10 gín mun
	AO	[..............] 10 gín ⌜^{šim}gúr⌝.[.......................................]
25	HH	10 gín numun ^{giš}hab 10 gín ^{šim}gam.ma 10 gín ^{šim}man.du
	AO	[..] 10 gín ^{šim}man.du
26	HH	10 gín ^{šim}buluh 10 gín ^{giš}eren 10 gín ^{šim}šeš
27	HH	10 gín gi.du$_{10}$ 5 gín ^{giš}*si-hu* 5 gín ^{giš}*ár-gan-nu*
	AO	10 gín gi.du$_{10}$ 5 gín ^{giš}*si-hu* [....................]
28	HH	5 gín lum.ha 5 gín $^{ú.d}$utu 25 ú.hi.a.meš
	AO	[...................................] 25 ú.hi.a
29	HH	*u* šim.hi.a šeš diš-*niš* gaz sim kaš.sag a gazi^{sar}
	AO	šim.hi.a šeš diš-*niš* g[az ....]
30	HH	*u* a.geštin.na kala.ga ti-*qé* zì.da.meš *an-nu-ti ina* šà! (text: sikil) šub-*di*
	AO	a.geštin.na *dan-na-ti* ti-*qé* z[ì...]
31	HH	*ina* nindu úš-*ir ina še-rim* e$_{11}$ šed$_7$ làl *u* ì *hal-ṣa ana* igi šub-*di*
	AO	[........................] *ina še-rim* e$_{11}$-*ma* šed$_7$ *ta-šá-hal* ì *hal-*[.........]
32	HH	1-*šú* 2-*šú* 3-*šú ana* dúr-*šú* dub-*ak*
33	HH	^{giš}eren ^{giš}šur.mìn ^{giš}*dap-ra-nu* ^{šim}gír ^{šim}bal! gi.du$_{10}$
	AE	[......................] ^{giš}*dap-ra-nu* ^{šim}gír ^{šim}bal ^{ši}[^{m}....]
	AS	[..] ^{ú}gír ^{šim}bal ^{šim}sal

12 *hašû*, *nuhurtu*, *šibirru*(-plant), *tiātu*,
13 *kamkadu*, 'health'-plant, fox-vine, *ṣaṣumtu*
14 *šunû*, sun-plant, *taramuš*, *imhur-līm*, *imhur-ešra*,
15 *ata'išu*, *kurkānû*, *maštu*, field-clod-plant,
16 Dilmun-date (and) salt. Total: 63 drugs; boil a lotion
17 soaked in strong beer and water of groats, and pour (it) into his rectum. (other mss. differ)

---

18 If a man suffers from 'sun-fever', flatulence, paralysis, lameness, *šaššaṭu*-disease,
19 Hand of the Ghost(-disease), Hand of the Oath, disease of the rectum, (or) any disease, in order to cure him,
20 10 shekels of 'health'-plant, 10 shekels of *tiātu*, 10 shekels of *ata'išu*,
21 10 shekels of *hašû*, 10 shekels of *nuhurtu*, 10 shekels *nīnû*,
22 10 shekels of *urnû*, 10 shekels of clump of salt, 10 shekels of *azupīru*,
23 10 shekels of rue, 10 shekels of 'white' plant, 10 shekels of alum,
24 10 shekels of juniper, 10 shekels of *kukru*, 10 shekels of *aktam*, 10 shekels of salt,
25 10 shekels of madder seed, 10 shekels of *ṣumlalû*, 10 shekels of *suādu*,
26 10 shekels of *baluhhu*, 10 shekels of cedar, 10 shekels of myrrh,
27 10 shekels of 'sweet reed', 5 shekels of *sihu*, 5 shekels of *argannu*,
28 5 shekels of *barīrātu*, 5 shekels of 'sun'-plant: pound and sieve these 25 drugs
29 and aromatics together. Take premium beer, *kasû*-juice
30 and strong vinegar, add this powder (of ground up ingredients) to it,
31 heat (it) in an oven, take it out in the morning, cool (it), add honey and pressed oil to it,
32 pour (it) once, twice, and three times into his anus.

---

33 You should prepare equal amounts of ingredients (l. 35) of cedar, *šurmēnu*, *daprānu*, thorn, *ballukku*, sweet reed,

34 HH ^{šim}gam.ma ^{ú}*tara-muš* ^{ú}igi-*lim* ^{ú}igi-*ešra* ^{ú}*kur-ka-nam*
AE [............] ^{ú}*tara-muš* ^{ú}igi-*lim* ^{ú}igi-*ešra* ^{ú}[..............]
AS [.............................] $^{⸢ú⸣}$igi-*lim* ^{ú}igi-*ešra* [..............]
35 HH ^{giš}man.du *mal-ma-liš tu-šam-⸢ṣa* téš⸣.bi *ta-ka-sim* a.meš
AE [.........] x *mal-ma-liš tu-šam-ṣa* diš-*niš* [.......... *ina* igi š]ub-*di*
AS [....................-*m*]*a-liš tu-šam-ṣa* [..]
36 HH ^{giš}li 15.meš sù *ina* igi ^{d}*gu-la* gub-*an*
AE [..........................*ina* igi ^{mul}ù]z *tuš-bat*
AS $^{⸢šim⸣}$li 15.meš x [..............................] (+ traces)
37 HH níg.na ^{giš}li ^{ú}kur.kur *ta-šá-rak ina še-rim* šeg$_6$-*šal*
38 HH *ta-šá-hal* 10 gín làl 12 sìla ì *hal-ṣa ana* šà š[ub-*di*]
AE [*t*]*a-šá-hal* [.. šub-*d*]*i*
39 HH *ana* dúr-*šú* dub-*ak ana* dúr-*šú* si.sá-*ma*[1] [ti]
AE [.. t]i

---

40 HH a ^{giš}li a zú.lum.ma a ^{giš}še.ná.a a ^{š}[^{im}...]
AE diš *e-sil-ti* šà-*šú šu-šu-ri* [... *ana* t]i-*šú* a $^{šim⸢}$li⸣ a zú.lum.ma a [...........] x a a ú
41 HH ⸢a⸣ *ṣa*$^{!}$-*ṣu-un-tú* a gaz[i^{sar}]
AE a *ṣáh-ṣu-te* a gazi[^{sar}]

---

42 HH x har ì.giš ^{ú}igi-*lim* 7 še [.............]
43 HH 7 še ^{ú}úkuš.hab diš-*niš* súd *ina* ⸢ì⸣[....]
44 HH *u* kaš gaz nu *pa-tan* nag-*ma* ti-*uṭ*

---

45 HH diš na *hi-niq-ti* bun gig 2 gín ^{šim}šeš 2 gín illu ^{šim}buluh
46 HH a ^{ú}har.har a ^{ú}nu.luh.ha a mun a šim.hi.a dù-*šú-nu*
AE [.............a ^{ú}]nu.luh.ha a mun a šim.hi.a dù.a [....]
47 HH a.meš *šú-nu-ti* 1/2 sìla ta.àm ti-*qé* diš-*niš* gaz šeg$_6$-*šal*
AE [..........-*n*]*u-ti* 1/2 sìla ta.àm ti-*qé* [........................]
48 HH *ta-šá-hal* šed$_7$ 1/2 ì.giš ki-*šú-nu* hi.hi 7 še ú nam.ti.la
AE [..-*š*]*á-hal* šed$_7$ ì.giš ki [..l]a
49 HH súd *ana* šà šub-*di* a.meš *ana* 3-*šú ta-za-az-ma*
AE súd *ana* šà šub a.meš *ana* ⸢3⸣-*šú ta*-[.............]
50 HH 1-*šú* 2-*šú* 3-*šú ana* dúr-*šú* dub-*ak e-sil-ti* šà-*šú* si.sá[2]
AE [.......... -*š*]*ú* 3-*šú ana* dúr-*šú* dub *e-sil-ti* šà-*šú* s[i.....]
51 HH *šum-ma ur-še* gaz.meš *šum-ma um-ṣa-a-tú uq-ṭa-ta-pa*
AE [..................] gaz.meš-*šú* [......] *um-ṣa-a-ti* ⸢*uq-ṭa*⸣-[......]
52 HH gig *up-ta-šah* dúr-*šú ur-tap-pa-áš*[3] *mar-ha-ṣu an-nu-u*
AE [...........-*ša*]*h* [..]
53 HH *ša* nam.ri.búr.da gig dù.a.bi

---

54 HH ^{giš}eren ^{giš}šur.mìn ^{giš}*dap-ra-nu* ^{šim}gír gi.du$_{10}$ ^{šim}bal
AQ [*ana* t]i-*šú* ^{giš}eren ^{giš}šur.mìn ^{giš}*dap-ra-nu* $^{šim⸢}$gír gi.du$_{10}$⸣ ^{šim}bal
55 HH ^{šim}sal ^{šim}gam.ma ^{šim}man.du ^{šim}gúr.gúr ^{giš}li
AQ ^{šim}sal ^{šim}gam.m[a] ^{šim}man.[..] ^{šim}gúr.gúr ^{šim}li
56 HH ^{ú}kur.kur ^{ú}har.har naga.si ^{ú}nu.luh.ha
AQ ^{ú}kur.kur ^{ú}har.ha[r] naga.[..] ^{ú}nu.luh.ha

---

1 Cf. AMT 80,1:7, *ú-šeš-še-ram-ma*.
2 = *šūšuru*, see Goltz, *Heilkunde*, 54, for an edition and translation of these lines.
3 CAD R 158, II/2 of *rapāšu*, 'the sick person(?) will find relief, his anus will be widened', and see also CAD Q 165.

34 *ṣumlalû*, *taramuš*, *imhur-līm*, *imhur-ešra*, *kurkānû*,
35 (and) *suādu*, you chop them together, sprinkle water
36 (and) juniper 15 times?? and set (them) before Gula (var. you leave it out under the Goat-star),
37 you sprinkle a brazier with juniper and *ata'išu*, boil (it) in the morning,
38 you filter (it). Put into (it) 10 shekels of honey and 12 sila of pressed oil,
39 pour it into his anus, administer an enema into his anus and he will improve.

---

40 Juniper juice, date juice, *šunû*-juice, juice of [....],[1]
41 juice of *ṣaṣuntu*, *kasû*-juice.

---

42 Crush together ..., oil, *imhur-līm*, 7 grains of [...........]
43 7 grains of cucumber, pound it together in oil
44 and beer, he drinks (it) on an empty stomach and he will recover.

---

45 If a man suffers from stricture of bladder, 2 shekels of myrrh, 2 shekels of *baluhhu*-resin,
46 juice of *hašû*, juice of *nuhurtu*, salt-water, the juice of all of these aromatics:
47 take a half sila of each of these juices, pound them together, boil (it),
48 you filter (it), cool (it), mix a half (sila) of oil with them. Crush 7 grains of 'health'-plant,
49 add (it) into (the mixture), divide the fluids into 3 parts and
50 pour (it) into his anus once, twice, and three times, to relieve his constipation (lit. to cause the stopping up of his bowel to pass through).
51 If *uršu*-sores are smashed (or) if the haemorrhoids are plucked off,
52 the illness will be relieved, his anus will be widened; this lotion
53 (is) for releasing from an oath (and) for all kinds of disease.

---

54 Cedar, *šurmēnu*, *daprānu*, thorn, sweet-reed, *ballukku*,
55 *šimeššalû*, *ṣumlalû*, *suādu*, *kukru*, juniper,
56 *ata'išu*, *hašû*, horned alkali, *nuhurtu*,

[1] Ms. AE differs, see Köcher's note, BAM II xvii.

57 HH ^{šim}šeš ^{šim}hab ^{šim}buluh.hi.a[1] 18 ú.hi.a šeš
AQ ^{šim}šeš ^{šim}hab ^{šim}buluh.hi.a ⸢18⸣ ú.hi.a šeš
AR ^{šim}šeš [...............................] 18 ú.meš š[eš.meš]
58 HH *mal-ma-liš* diš-*niš ta-ka-sim ina* kaš *u* a.geštin.na
AQ *mal-ma-liš* diš-*niš t*[*a*]-*ka*-AD [.....] ⸢*u*⸣ a.geštin.na
AR [....................................] *ina* kaš *u* a.geš[tin....]
59 HH *tu-lab-bak ina a-tu-gi* úš-*ir ina še-rim* e$_{11}$-*ma*
AQ *tu-lab-bak ina* ⸢*a-tu*⸣-*gi te-sek-ker* [........................] e$_{11}$-*a*
AR [.................................] *te-sek-ker i*[*na* ....]
60 HH *ta-šá-hal* làl *u* ì *hal-ṣa ana* šà dub *bah-ru-su*
AQ *ta-šá-hal* làl *u* ì *hal-ṣa ana* šà gaz [........]-*su*
AR [..........] làl *u* ì [...........................] *bah-ru-su*
61 HH *ana* dúr-*šú* dub-*ak ina* dúr-*šú* si.sá-*ma* ti
AQ *ana* dúr-*šú* dub-*ak ina* dúr-*šú* si.sá-*ma* ti
AR [..]

---

62 HH diš na šà-*šú* kúm tuk-*ši* kúm šà *šá-ha-ṭi* ^{ú}úkuš.hab
AG diš na šà-*šú* kúm tuk-*ši* kúm šà *šá-ha-ṭi* ^{ú}úkuš.hab
63 HH ^{šim}buluh ^{ú}nu.luh.ha ^{ú}har.har diš-*niš* súd *ina* kaš šub
AG ^{šim}buluh ^{ú}nu.luh.ha ^{ú}har.har diš-*niš ina* kaš šub-*di*
64 HH *ina* mul$_{4}$ *tuš-bat*! *ina še-rim* šeg$_{6}$-*šal ta-šá-hal* làl *u hal-ṣa ana* igi šub-*di*
AG *ina* [mu]l$_{4}$ *tuš-bat ina še-rim* šeg$_{6}$-*šal ta*-[..]-*hal* làl *u* <ì> *hal-ṣa ana* igi šub-*di*
65 HH *bah-ru-su ana* dúr-*šú* dub-*ak* si.sá-*ma* ti
AG *bah-ru-su ana* dúr-*šú* dub-*ak* si.sá-*ma* ti-*uṭ*

---

66 HH diš na *e-sil-ti* šà-*šú šu-šu-ri u ur-še* gaz.meš *um-ṣa-a-te qut-tu-pi*
AG [*ana*] *e-sil-ti* šà-*šú* si.sá-*ri* [*u*]*r-ši* gaz.meš *um-ṣa-te qut-tu-pi*
67 HH ^{šim}li ^{šim}gúr.gúr ^{ú}nu.luh.ha naga.si ú nam.ti.la
AG ^{šim}gúr.gúr ^{giš}li naga.si ⸢^{ú}⸣nu.luh.ha ú nam.ti.la
68 HH *mal-ma-liš* lá *ina* kaš *u* a.geštin.na šeg$_{6}$-*šal ta-šá-hal*
AG *mal-ma-liš* lá *ina* kaš *u* a.geštin.na šeg$_{6}$-*šal ta-šá-hal*
69 HH šed$_{7}$ ì.giš *ana* igi šub *ana* dúr-*šú* dub-*ak*
AG šed$_{7}$ làl *u* ì *ana* igi šub *ana* dúr-*šú* dub

---

70 HH diš na *ina la si-ma-ni-šú* murub$_{4}$.meš-*šú* gu$_{7}$.meš-*šú kim-ṣa-a-šú*
W diš na *ina la si-ma-ni-šú* ⸢murub$_{4}$-*šú*⸣ gu$_{7}$.meš-*šú kim-ṣa-a-š*[*ú* ...... -*š*]*ú*
V diš na *ina* [.....-*m*]*a-ni-šú* murub$_{4}$.meš-*šú* gu$_{7}$.meš-*šú* gìri^{2}.meš-*šú i-ta-á*[*r-raṣ*]
AG [......] *ina la si-ma-ni-šú* murub$_{4}$.meš-*šú* gu$_{7}$.meš-*šú* [........]-*a-šú*
71 HH *i-za-qata-šú* úr.meš-*šú i-tan-na-ah*[2] *bur-ka-šu i-kaṣ-ṣa-a-šú*
AG *i-za-qata-šú* úr.meš-*šu* [.................]-*ah bur-ka-šú i-kaṣ-ṣa-ṣa-šú*
W *bur-ka-šu i-kaṣ-ṣa-ṣa-šú*
V *kim-ṣa-a-šú i-ka-ṣa-a*-[*š*]*ú*
72 HH diš na *ina meṣ-hi-ru-ti-šú* dúr.gig *ana* ti-*šú*
AG [............] *meṣ-hi-ru-te-šú* dúr.gig gig
W na.bi *ina meṣ-hi-ru-ti*-⸢*šú*⸣ [.. g]ig *ana* ti-*šú*
V na.bi *ina meṣ-hi*-⸢*ru-ti*⸣ dúr.gi[g] *ana* t[i-.]

---

1 The same orthography appears in BAM 579 iv 17.
2 CAD B 255 translates 'his loins become weak', but it seems likely here that úr.meš refers to the thigh (*pēmu*) rather than the lap (*sūnu*).

57 myrrh, *ṭurû*, *baluḫḫu*: you should cut up (l. 58) these 18 drugs
58 together in equal parts, you steep (them) in beer or vinegar.
59 Heat (it) in a kiln, remove (it) in the morning and
60 you filter it, add (var. pound) honey and pressed oil into it, while it is hot
61 pour (it) into his anus, administer an enema in his anus and he will recover.

---

62 If a man's bowel has a temperature, to alleviate the internal fever: crush together cucumber,
63 *baluḫḫu*, *nuḫurtu*, *ḫašû*, put it into beer,
64 leave (it) out over night, boil (it) in the morning, you filter it, put honey and pressed oil into (the mixture),
65 while it is hot pour it into his anus, administer an enema and he will get better.

---

66 If a man's bowels need to relieve constipation (lit. cause a stoppage to pass) or crush sores and pluck out haemorrhoids,
67 weigh out juniper, *kukru*, *nuḫurtu*, horned alkali, 'health'-plant,
68 in equal measure, boil (them) in beer or vinegar, you filter it,
69 cool it, put oil into it (var. honey or oil), pour (it) into his anus.

---

70 If a man's groin hurts him at an inappropriate time, and his shins
71 cause him a stinging pain (var. he stretches out his feet), he is weak in his thighs and his knees (var. shins) gnaw at him with pain (var. are cold for him),
72 that man suffers in the rectum (already) during his youth. To cure him:

73	HH	^{ú}gamun.ge$_6$ ^{ú}kur.ra ^{šim}gig ú nam.ti
	W	^{ú}kur.ra ^{šim}li ^{šim}gig ^{šim}gúr.gúr ú nam.⸢ti⸣.la
	V	^{ú}kur.ra ^{šim}li ^{šim}gúr.gúr ^{šim}gig ú nam.ti.la
74	HH	gazi^{sar}*mal-ma-liš* súd *ina* ì.udu hi.hi *alla-nu* dù-*áš*
	W	*mal-ma-liš* súd *ina* ì.udu hi.hi al.la.na dù-*uš*
	V	*mal-ma-liš* súd *ina* ⸢ì⸣.[u]du [.... nag]ar-*nu* dù-*uš*
75	HH	ì.giš ^{giš}šur.mìn sù *ana* dúr-*šú* gar-*an-ma* ti
	W	ì.giš šur.min sù *ana* dúr-*šú* gar-*an-ma ina-eš*
	V	ì.giš šur.min sù *ana* dúr-*šú* gar-*an-ma* ti

76	HH	diš ki.min u$_5$.níg.ib^{mušen} ^{ú}kur.ra illu ^{šim}buluh ú babbar
	W	[diš ki.mi]n ⸢u$_5$⸣.gar.ib^{mušen} ^{ú}kur.ra illu ^{šim}buluh
77	HH	zú.lum.ma ^{mun}*eme-sal-lim* ì.udu gud 7 ú.meš *alla-nu* [..]
	W	zú.lum.ma dilmun^{ki}[an.dah.šu]m mun 6 ú.hi.a *an-nu-tim alla-nu šam-ru*

78	HH	zú.lum.ma dilmun^{ki} naga.si *tur-ár* ì.udu éllag udu.ní[ta]
	V	[z]ú.lum.ma dilmun^{ki} naga.si ì.udu éllag udu.níta
	AF	[.............] dilmun^{ki} naga.si ì.udu éllag udu.níta
79	HH	^{šim}gúr.gúr ^{giš}li ^{šim}gam.ma illu ^{šim}buluh
	V	^{šim}gúr.gúr ^{giš}l[i ^{šim}gam.ma illu ^{šim}buluh]
	AF	^{šim}gúr.gúr [................................]
80	HH	illu li.tar 8 ú.meš *alla-nu* im kud-[*si*]
	V	illu li.t[ar .... *all*]*a-nu lat-ku šá* im kud-*si*
81	HH	*ana* dúr-*šú* gar-*an bul-ṭu lat*-[*ku*]
	V	[..............] gar-[*an*]

colophon: *ana ṣa-bat epēši*(dù-*ši*) ^{m}*Ki-ṣir-*^{d}*Nabû* a ^{md}*Šamaš*-[*ib-ni*] *ha-an-ṭiš ana is-su-*[*uh*]

73 crush in equal amounts black *kamūnu*, *nīnû*, *kanaktu*, 'health'-plant',
74 *kasû*, mix them in fat and make a suppository,
75 sprinkle (on it) cypress oil, insert it into his anus and he will improve.

---

76 If ditto, bat guano, *nīnû*, *baluhhu*-resin, 'white' plant,
77 dates (var. of Dilmun), gourmet-salt, ox fat, these 7 (var. 6) drugs for a *powerful* suppository.

---

78 You dry out Dilmun dates, horned alkali, fat of the kidney of a male sheep,
79 *kukru*, juniper, *ṣumlalû*, *baluhhu*-resin,
80 *abukkatu*-resin – 8 drugs – insert a suppository
81 into his anus to stop flatulence; a proven remedy (var. a proven suppository which stops wind).

No. 35 BAM 99 diš na *ina lā simānišu*

II	=	VAT 13726 (BAM 99)
AD	=	VAT 10170 (BAM 152) iii 8–12; 27–29
AM	=	JRL 10, 74: 13–15 = ll. 27–29
JJ	=	A 254 (BAM 100 rev. 2–8) [text no. 36] = ll. 19–24
W	=	S. 36 + (AMT 43,1 +) [text no. 22] = ll. 42–54
V	=	VAT 13752 + (BAM 95: 27–28) [text no. 21] = ll. 25–26
YY	=	A 239 (BAM 161 vi 1–6) = ll. 21–24

1	II	[diš na] dúr-*šú* múd *ú-tab-ba-ka* na.bi *qer-bé-nu* gig *ana* ti-[*šú*]
2	II	[........................] ì.giš kaš.sag *ana* dúr-*šú* dub-*ak* ^{giš}gúr.gúr ^{giš}li
3	II	[..........................^{ú}nu.luh.].ha šum.šir.dili naga.si illu ^{šim}buluh
4	II	^{šim}an [..............................] x téš.bi *ta-sàk ina* ì.udu gaba.làl *u* ^{šim}hab
5	II	hi.hi-*m*[*a* šu.si] dù-*uš ana* dúr-*šú* gar-*ma ina-eš*
6	II	[diš na ....] x ^{ú}har.har
7	II	[..] *ina* kaš nag *i-ár-ru*[1]
8	II	[.. g]ìr.pad.du nam.lú.u$_{18}$.lu[2]
9	II	[...] *ina* ì.udu hi.hi šu.si dù-*uš*
10	II	[..................................] *ina* a gazi^{sar} *ina* kaš.sag [..............]
11	II	[...] ^{ú}esi šu.s[i dù-*uš*]
12	II	[.....................] *an-ni-tu*$_4$ [..]
13	II	[diš na ....] a [....................................
14	II	x[..
15	II	illu ^{šim}buluh ⌜numun zi x x x⌝ [............................
16	II	šu.si dù-*uš ana* dúr-*šú* gar-*an* ^{ú}geštin.ka$_5$.a x [...........]
17	II	diš na múd *i-te-zi qé-reb* dúr-*šú i-za-qat-su* gi[m ....
18	II	*ina* ì.udu hi.hi šu.si dù-*uš ana* dúr-*šú* [gar-*an* .....]
19	II	diš na múd *ina* dúr-*šú* gim munus *ša na-ah-ša-te* šub.šub-*a t*[*a*-..........][3]
	JJ	diš na múd *ina* dúr-*šú* gim munus *ša na-ah-ša-te* šub-*a ta-hi-is-su-ma*
20	II	dúr.gig.ga.kám nu tuk-*ši ter-di-it ir-ri* gig n[a$_4$...........]
	JJ	dúr.gig.kám nu tuk-*ši ter-di-it ir-ri* gig na$_4$ zú.lum.ma
21	II	*ina* ^{síg}hé.med nigin-*mi* ì.giš šéš sù.sù *ana* dúr-*šú* gar-[*an*]
	JJ	*ina* ^{síg}hé.med nigin-*mì* ì.giš šéš sù *ana* dúr-*šú* gar
	YY	*ina* ^{síg}hé.med nigin-*mi* ì.giš šéš sù *ana* dúr-*šú* gar-*an*
22	II	^{im}sahar.na$_4$.kur.ra ^{im}kal.la ^{ú}nu.luh.ha súd *ina* kaš [...]
	JJ	^{im}sahar.na$_4$.kur.ra ^{im}kal.la ^{ú}nu.luh.ha súd *ina* kaš nag
	YY	^{im}sahar.na$_4$.kur.ra ^{im}kal.la ^{ú}nu.luh súd *ina* kaš nag
23	II	^{ú}sumun.dar súd *ina* kaš nag ^{ú}*úr-né-e* súd *ina* kaš n[ag]
	JJ	^{ú}sumun.dar súd *ina* kaš nag ^{ú}*úr-*⌜*né*⌝*-e* súd *ina* kaš ⌜nag⌝
	YY	^{ú}sumun.dar súd *ina* kaš nag ^{ú}*úr-né-e* súd *ina* kaš nag
24	II	*ina* a.meš šed$_7$ *ir-ta-na-h*[*aṣ*]
	JJ	a.meš šed$_7$ *ir-ta-na-h*[*aṣ*]
	YY	a.meš šed$_7$ *ir-ta-na-haṣ*

1 note use of emetic here.

2 Dreckapotheke.

3 See ll. 42 f. below.

TRANSLATION

1 [If a man] passes blood [from] his anus, that man suffers internally; to cure [him],
2 pour [......................] oil (and) premium beer into his anus; *kukru*, juniper,
3 you crush together [................................] *nuhurtu,* single cloved garlic, horned alkali, *baluhhu*-resin,
4 ...[..........................], mix wax or *ṭūru* in fat,
5 and make a [pessary], insert it into his anus and he will get better.

6 [If a man ....] .. *hašû,*
7 he drinks [....................] in beer . He vomits,
8 [..], human bone,
9 [..................] mix it in fat, make a pessary,
10 [................................] in *kasû*-juice, in premium beer,
11 ..... [...], *ušû,* [make] a pessary,
12 [.........................] this [...]

13–14 (broken)
15 *baluhhu*-resin, seed of ..... [...................................
16 make a pessary, insert it into his anus, fox-vine .. [........

17 If a man excretes blood, the middle of his rectum stings him like [........]
18 mix in fat, make a pessary and [insert (it)] into his anus [......]

19 If a man passes blood from his anus like a haemorrhaging woman, ...
20 and he does not have (symptoms) of rectal disease (but) suffers from diarrhoea,
21 wrap date-stone in red wool, smear (and) spatter with oil, insert (it) into his anus.
22 Crush alum, yellow *kalû*-ochre, *nuhurtu,* he drinks (it) in beer,
23 crush *šumuttu,* he drinks (it) in beer. Crush *urnû,* he drinks (it) in beer,
24 he should keep bathing in cold water.[1]

[1] This recipe appears to consist of a series of simplicia.

25	II	diš na dúr.gig gig múd *i-te-ez-zi qé-reb* dúr-*šú i-ha-áš ana* [ti-*šú*]
	V	diš na dúr.gig gig múd *i-te-ez-zi qé-reb* dúr-*šú i-ha*-[...............]
26	II	^{šim}buluh ^{šim}gig bar ú.lum.ma *ina* ì.udu hi.hi *ana* dúr-*šú* gar-*an-ma* t[i]
	V	$^{ši]m}$buluh ^{šim}gig bar zú.lum.ma *ina* ì.udu hi.hi u dù-*uš* [.....]-*šú* gar-*an*
27	II	diš na *ina* dúr-*šú* múd *ú*-[*tab*]-*ba-ka* gim munus ^{giš}tukul *ma-hi-iṣ ana* ti-[*šú*]
	AD	diš na *ina* dúr-*šú* múd *ú-tab-ba-ka* gim munus ^{giš}tukul sìg-*iṣ ana* ti-*šú*
	AM	[.. $^{g]iš}$tukul sìg-*iṣ ana* ti-[..]
28	II	numun ^{giš}kiši$_{16}$.hab [u]gu.súh.ha téš.bi súd *ina* geštin al.še[g$_6$].gá
	AD	numun ^{giš}kiši$_{16}$.hab[1] ugu.súh.ha diš-*niš* súd *ina* geštin *ba-áš-li* nu *pa-tan*
	AM	[..] súd *ina* geštin al.šeg$_6$.g[á]
29	II	[n]ag.meš-*ma* ti-*uṭ*
	AD	nag-*ma* ti
	AM	[....-*m*]*a* ti
30	II	[diš na *ina* dúr-*šú* múd *ú-ta*]*b-ba-ka* na.bi *qer-bé-nu* gig
31	II	[*ana* gig-*šú* nu][2] gíd.⌈da⌉ múd gud *ina* geštin al.šeg$_6$.gá
32	II	[..................*b*]*a-lu pa-tan* nag.meš-*ma* ti-*uṭ*
33	II	[diš ki.min ....] im.kal.la nu.luh.ha *ina* kaš nag
34	II	[...b]i kaš nag
rev.		
35	II	[...] kaš nag
36	II	[....] x x [... h]i.hi nag
37	II	1/3 kisal a ^{giš}nu.úr.ma ku$_7$.ku$_7$ igi.5.gál.la ^{šim}hab nag
38	II	^{ú}har.har súd *ina* kaš nag
39	II	^{ú}ina.úš súd *ina* kaš [n]ag
40	II	$^{[he]-pí\ eš-šú}$súd *ina* kaš šub-*di ina* mul$_4$ *tuš-bat* nu *pa-t*[*an ina* kaš nag]
41	II	*e-ma* nag *ina* a.meš *ir-s*[*u*]-*nu*
42	II	diš na *ina* dúr-*šú* gim munus *ša na-ah-ša-te* šub.šub-*a ta-hi-su-ma*
	W	[diš na ú]š *ina* dúr-*šú* gim munus *ša na-a*[*h-šá-tú* šub.šub-*a t*]*a-hi-is-su-ma*
43	II	dúr.gig.ga.kám nu tuk *ter-di-it ir-ri* gig
	W	dúr.gig.ga.kam [..-*š*]*i ter-di-it ir-ri* g[ig]
44	II	^{im}kal.la ^{im}sahar.na$_4$.kur.ra nu.luh.ha súd
	W	[...................................^{ú}nu.l]uh.ha súd
45	II	*ina* kaš nag KU.KU[3] ^{na4}kur-*nu* dib.ba *ina* ^{síg}hé.me.da
	W	*ina* kaš nag [..K]U ^{na4}ka.gi.na.dib.ba *ina* s[íg$^?$ ....]
46	II	nigin-*mi* ì.giš ^{giš}eren sù *ana* dúr-*šú* gar-*an ur-né-e*
	W	[...................ere]n sù *ana* dúr-*šú* gar-*an* [.....-*n*]*é-e*
47	II	*ina* kaš nag illu ^{šim}buluh *ina* a šed$_7$ *ir-ta-na-haṣ*
	W	*ina* kaš nag illu ^{šim}buluh *ina* a šed$_7$ *ir-ta-na-haṣ*

1 order of ingredients differs.
2 See Herrero, *Thérapeutique*, 41 for restoration.
3 see CAD Q 208.

25 If a man suffers from a diseased rectum, defecates blood and the middle of his rectum 'hastens' (has diarrhoea), in order [to heal him], mix *baluhhu, kanaktu* and date peel in fat,
26 (var. make a pessary,) insert it into his anus and he will improve.

27 If a man passes blood from his anus, (as if) struck by a weapon like a (menstruating) woman, to cure him,
28–29 crush together seed of *dadānu*-carob and ..., he drinks (it) continually in boiled wine on an empty stomach and he will improve.

30 [If a man] passes [blood from his anus], that man suffers internally,
31 [in order for his illness not] to be prolonged, he keeps drinking bull's blood in boiled wine
32 [..........................] on an empty stomach and he will improve.

33 [If ditto], he drinks [.......], yellow ochre and *nuhurtu* in beer.

34 [..]., he drinks beer.

rev.

35 [..], he drinks beer.
36 Mix [..], he drinks (it).

37 He drinks one-third *kisal* of sweet pomegranate juice, (and) a fifth (measure) of *ṭūru*.

38 Crush thyme and he drinks (it) in beer.[1]

39 Crush *maštakal* (and) he drinks (it) in beer.[2]

40 Crush (broken original), put it in beer, leave it out over night and [he drinks it in premium beer] on an empty stomach.
41 Whatever he drinks, they soaked in water.

42 If a man passes blood from his anus like a woman haemorrhaging, ...
43 and he has no (symptom) of rectal disease, (but) he suffers from diarrhoea,
44 crush yellow ochre, alum, and *nuhurtu*,
45 in premium beer. Wrap powders and magnetite in red wool,
46 and sprinkle cedar oil and insert it into his anus. He drinks *urnû*
47 in beer and constantly soaks *baluhhu* resin in cold water.

[1] Simplicium.
[2] Simplicium.

48	II	pa ^{giš}gi$_6$.pàr pa ^{giš}*šu-še* pa ^{giš}eme.ur.gir$_7$ pa ^{giš}kiši$_{16}$-*ha-ah*
	W	[.. ^{g}]^{iš}gi$_6$.pàr pa ^{giš}*šu-ši* [..................] eme.ur.gir$_7$ pa ^{giš}kiši$_{16}$-*h*[*a*-....]
49	II	pa ^{ú}gìr.naga.ga^{mušen} pa ^{giš}ma.nu pa ^{giš}úr.tál.tál
	W	[..] ^{ú}<gìr.>naga.ga^{mušen} pa ^{giš}ma<.nu> [... ú]r.tál.tál
50	II	gaz *ina* kaš *ta-la-aš* gur-*ma* è ga[z]
	W	gaz *ina* kaš [...............] ⸢è⸣ gaz
51	II	*ina* ì.udu hi.hi *ina* kuš *te-ṭer-re* [..]
	W	*ina* ì.udu hi.hi *ina* kuš *te-ṭer-re* lá
52	II	diš n[a ....] x x [....]
53	W	diš na x [....gu$_7$$^{?}$-*s*]*u* : 1/3 sìla a *u* ì.giš [.................
	II	(broken)
54	II	⸢1 sìla zì.gig⸣ sim ^{dug}bur.zi a diri *ana* šà du[b ....
	W	1 sìla zì.gig sim ^{dug}bur.zi a diri [.............
55	II	*ina* mul$_4$ *tuš-bat ina še-rim tu-kaṣ-ṣa ana* dúr-*šú* dub-[.....]
56	II	(colophon): 7 *nis-hu* gaba.ri é.sa.bad *šá* bal.ti^{ki}
		(For the rest of the colophon see, Hunger BAK No. 202, copied by Kiṣir-Assur.)

48 Pound (l. 50) *lipāru*-leaf, *šūšu*-leaf, 'dog's tongue'-leaf, and leaf of 'thorny plant',
49 leaf of ...., *êru*-tree leaf, leaf of *uzun lalî*,
50 you soften it in beer and again take it out and pound it,
51 mix it in fat and spread it on leather and bind it on.

52 If a man [..]...

53 If a man ..[.......]... one third *sila* of water or oil [...........

54 Sieve 1 *sila* of emmer-wheat, fill a stone-jar with water, [.................
55 leave it out over night, you cool it in the morning (and) pour it into his anus [and he will improve].
56 (colophon): 7th extract of a copy of the Esabad-temple of Assur.

No. 36 BAM 100

JJ = A 254 (BAM 100)
II = VAT 13726 (BAM 99) [text no. 35] = ll. 2–9
YY = A 239 (BAM 161 vi 1–6) = ll. 5–9

1′	JJ	[.......................................] x *sah-*⸢*lé-e*⸣ naga.si *ina* ì.udu hi.h[i]

rev.

2′	JJ	diš na múd *ina* dúr-*šú* gim munus *ša na-ah-ša-te* šub-*a*
	II	diš na múd *ina* dúr-*šú* gim munus *ša na-ah-ša-te* šub.šub-*a*
3′	JJ	*ta-hi-is-su-ma* dúr.gig.kám nu tuk-*ši*
	II	*t*[*a*-..........] dúr.gig.ga.kám nu tuk-*ši*
4′	JJ	*ter-di-it ir-ri* gig $^{\text{na4}}$zú.lum.ma
	II	*ter-di-it ir-ri* gig ^{na}[^{4}...........]
5′	JJ	*ina* ^{síg}hé.med nigin-*mì* ì.giš šéš sù *ana* dúr-*šú* gar
	II	*ina* ^{síg}hé.med nigin-*mi* ì.giš šéš sù.sù *ana* dúr-*šú* gar-[*an*]
	YY	*ina* ^{síg}hé.med nigin-*mi* ì.giš šéš sù *ana* dúr-*šú* gar-*an*
6′	JJ	^{im}sahar.na$_4$.kur.ra ^{im}kal.la ^{ú}nu.luh.ha súd
	II	^{im}sahar.na$_4$.kur.ra ^{im}kal.la ^{ú}nu.luh.ha súd
	YY	^{im}sahar.na$_4$.kur.ra ^{im}kal.la ^{ú}nu.luh súd
7′	JJ	*ina* kaš nag ^{ú}sumun.dar súd *ina* kaš ⸢nag⸣
	II	*ina* kaš [...] ^{ú}sumun.dar súd *ina* kaš nag
	YY	*ina* kaš nag ^{ú}sumun.dar súd *ina* kaš nag
8′	JJ	^{ú}*úr-*⸢*né*⸣*-e* súd *ina* kaš ⸢nag⸣
	II	^{ú}*úr-né-e* súd *ina* kaš n[ag]
	YY	^{ú}*úr-né-e* súd *ina* kaš nag
9′	JJ	a.meš šed$_7$ *ir-ta-na-h*[*aṣ*]
	II	*ina* a.meš šed$_7$ *ir-ta-na-h*[*aṣ*]
	YY	a.meš šed$_7$ *ir-ta-na-haṣ*

TRANSLATION

see above, text No. 35 ll. 19–24.

1′ Mix[....................................].., *sahlû* and horned alkali in fat.

2′ If a man passes blood from his anus like a haemorrhaging woman,
3′ ..[.....] and he does not have (symptoms) of rectal disease
4′ (but) suffers from diarrhoea,
5′ wrap date-stone in red wool, smear (and) spatter with oil, insert (it) into his anus.
6′ Crush alum, yellow ochre, *nuhurtu*,
7′ he drinks (it) in beer. Crush *šumuttu*, he drinks (it) in beer.
8′ Crush *urnû*, he drinks (it) in beer.
9′ He should keep bathing in cold water.

No. 37 AMT 95,3 + (plate 27)

K 8182 (AMT 95,3) + 11102 (AMT 50,6) + 13404 (AMT 53,11), see RA 26 74 f.

col. i

1′ [...]-*šú*
2′ [...] *tara-bak* / *muš*$_8$
3′ [...] ti

4′ [...] x šeg$_6$-*šal*
5′ [...] x *ina-eš*

6′ [...] *ina-eš*

7′ [...] làl ì *hal-ṣa*
8′ [..] x *ina-eš*

9′ [...] x ka làl ì *hal-ṣa*
10′ [...] dub-*ma ina-eš*

11′ [diš na kàš.meš-*šú ut-ta-na-tak*][1] *ka-la-a* nu zu *mut-qí-ta ša*
12′ [.....................................] x *ša* ^{giš}lam.gal ^{giš}hašhur hád.a
13′ [................................] x ^{giš}*nu-úr-ma* ku$_7$.ku$_7$ ^{giš}*ur-zi-in-ni*
14′ [................................] àr-*en* sim
15′ [...............................] x zì.kum *ana* šà šub-*di* ì.udu gaba.làl
16′ [............................] ⸢ú⸣.hi.a *an-nu-ti ana* šà *ta-šá-pa-ah*
17′ [............................. g]u$_7$.meš-*ma* šà.meš-*šú ik-ka-ṣa-ru*

18′ [diš na uzu-*šú*(?)] ⸢*i-šah*⸣-*hu-uh* šà.meš-*šú em-ru*[2]
19′ [....................... *lì*]*b-bi-šú i-te-ek-ke-ek*
20′ [..........................] x *i-ha-a-ru* dúr-*šú ú-zaq-qat-su*

---

col. ii.

1′ (traces)
2′ 10$^?$ ud.meš lá-*m*[*a* ....

3′ diš na *i-kab-bít* sa [.......................
4′ na.bi dúr.gig giš [............................
5′ 1 ma.na ì.udu éllag udu 4 [ma.na ....
6′ diš-*niš* gaz sim *ina* ^{kuš}edin s[ur-*re*....................
7′ *qí-lip* zú.lum.ma gaz *al-la-n*[*u* dù-*uš ina* dúr-*šú* gar-*an ina-eš*]

---

1 Restored from BAM 111 ii 21, see Text No. 3.

2 phrase cited CAD Š/1 76. The term *šahāhu* usually refers to hair falling out or dissolving of a kidney stone but it can refer to 'flesh' in general.

TRANSLATION

col. i

1′–2′ ....

3′ [..] he will improve.

4′ Boil [..]
5′ [.......................................] and he will get better.

6′ [.......................................] and he will get better.

7′ [.......................................] honey (and) pressed oil,
8′ [.......................................] ... he will get better.

9′ [....................................]... honey (and) pressed oil,
10′ [.........................] pour (it) [into his anus] and he will get better.

11′ [If a man constantly drips urine (and)] he cannot retain (it), a sweet cake of
12′ [.....................], dry out [.....] of pistachio (and) apple,
13′ [...............................].. sweet pomegranate, *urzīnu*,
14′ mill and sieve [.........................],
15′ put into (the mixture) [............].. (and) *išqūqu*-meal, fat, wax,
16′ [............................], sprinkle these drugs into it,
17′ have him keep eating [....................] and his bowels will be made binding.[1]

18′ [If a man's flesh(?)] is wasting away and his bowels are colicky,
19′ [..] he scratches his stomach,
20′ [...................................] he *vomits*(?) and his anus stings him.

col. ii

1′ (broken)
2′ bind for 10$^{?}$ days and [.......................................

3′ If a man is troubled (lit. heavy) ...[............................
4′ that man is diseased in the anus, ... [....................
5′ 1 mina of sheep fat, 4 [mina ....
6′ pound and sieve together, spread (it) on a leather-strip [..................
7′ pound date peel, [make] a suppository, [insert it into his anus and he will get better].

[1] presumably against diarrhoea.

8′ diš ki.min *qí-lip* zú.lum.ma *ur-ru-*⸢*ru*?⸣ ti⸣-[*qé*..............
9′ mun *ina* ì udu hi.hi *al-la-na* dù-[*uš ina* dúr-*šú* gar-*an ina-eš*]

10′ diš ki.min *sum-ma-tiš la-áš-at qí-lip* zú.lu[m.ma ....]
11′ mun ^{ú}naga *ina* ì udu hi.hi *alla-nu* dù-[*uš ina* dúr-*šú* gar-*an ina-eš*]

12′ diš ki.min gazi^{sa}[⸢ à]r-*en* sim *ina* a.meš gim *kib-ri-*[*ti* ..][1]
13′ *ina* ^{urudu}šen.tur $šeg_6$-*šal* e_{11}.a *al-la-n*[*a* dù-*uš ina* dúr-*šú* gar-*an ina-eš*]

14′ diš ki.min 5 sìla ⸢numun⸣ gada àr-*en* sim *ina* ga *ta-*[*rab-bak*][2]
15′ gaba *u* maš.sìla ud.14.kám lá-*ma* ti *maš-ka-an-t*[*u lat-ku*]

16′ u_4-*ma* lál.meš *an-na-a-te* lá-*uš* 1/3 sìla a zú.[lum.ma]
17′ 10 kisal ì.giš nag egir-*šú* ú nu nag
18′ ud.6.kám a.rá ud.8.kám nag.nag.meš-*ma* [ti]

19′ diš ki.min 1/3 sìla *si-ik-ti* tuh.še.giš.ì 1 sìla z[ì ..]
20′ gaba *u* maš.sìla lá-*su* 1/3 sìla ^{ú}igi-*lim* [....]
21′ *ana* dúr-*šú* si.sá-*ma buh-ri-tú* [....]

22′ u_4-*ma* lá.meš *an-na-a-ti* lá-*uš ina* ^{iti}zíz.à[m ...]

23′ *a-di* lál.meš *an-na-a-ti sum*<*mu-*>*ha-t*[*ú*............
24′ *ina* a gazi$^{⸢sar⸣}$x x x.......[..........]
(bottom)

---

[1] Simplicium.
[2] Simplicium.

8′ [If] ditto, take *dried* date peel [....................
9′ mix salt in fat, make a suppository and [insert it into his anus and he will get better].

10′ If ditto, *whispers like a dove*[1], date peel [.......
11′ mix salt (and) horned alkali-plant, make a suppository [and insert it into his anus and he will get better].

12′ If ditto, mill *kasû*, sieve, boil it in water like sulphur,
13′ in a small copper dish, remove it, [make] a suppository, [insert it into his anus and he will get better].

14′ If ditto, grind up 5 sila of flax seed, sieve, and you steep it in milk,
15′ bind (it) for 14 days on the chest and shoulder and he will improve; the ingredients [are checked].

16′ When you have tied these poultices on him, he drinks (l. 18) 1/3 *sila* of date-juice,
17′ 10 *kisal*-weight of oil, afterwards he should not drink a drug,
18′ he keeps drinking it for six to eight days[2] and [he will improve].

19′ If ditto, 1/3 *sila* of powder of sesame bran, 1 *sila* of ...-flour,
20′ bind it on the chest and shoulder. Administer (as an enema) 1/3 *sila* of *imhur-līm* plant [....]
21′ into his anus and a hot dish [..................].

22′ When you have tied on these poultices on him, in the month of Šebaṭ [....]

23′ As long as these *assorted* poultices [.........]
24′ in *kasû*-juice [..............................]

---

[1] Analagous with *summiš*, 'like a dove', see CAD S 380. The word *la-âš-at* is uncertain, perhaps a form of *lahāšu*, 'to whisper', referring to a sound made by part of the body.

[2] or 'from the sixth to the eighth day'.

No. 38 AMT 101,3

K 8369 (AMT 101,3), collated, see RA 26, 86[1]

col. i

1′ [.............]-*ṣa* àr-*e*[*n* ....
2′ [...........] ú.hi.a *an-nu-ti* [..........................
3′ [.......] ⌜ì⌝ *a-si mut-tal-li-ki t*[*e-te-ne-eq-qí-ma ina-eš*][2]

4′ [diš na ... *u*]*r-ši* sa$_5$ *ana ur-eš* gaz.meš ^{šim}gúr.gúr ^{šim}li
5′ [.......] x ^{ú}áb.duh numun ^{giš}gi.zú.lum.ma 7 ú.hi.a *an-nu-ti*
6′ [.........]-*ṣa* àr-*en* sim ki illu ^{šim}buluh ú.hi.a *an-nu-ti*
7′ [....... *al-l*]*a-na* dù-*uš* ì ^{giš}eren sù *ana* dúr-*šú* gar-*an-ma ina-eš*

8′ [.... *ina* $^{\text{n]a4}}$zú *zaq-te sal-te* ugu *lam-ṣa-te-šú tu-kak*
9′ [........] a.bára diš-*niš* súd *ina* ì hi.hi dúr-*šú te-te-né-eq-qí-ma ina-eš*

10′ [.......*i*]*na* a ^{giš}še.ná.a ra-*su* dabin *ina* dè *tu-qat-tar-šú*
11′ [...... ^{ú}ku]r.kur 4 ú.hi.a *an-nu-ti* téš.bi ti-*qé*
12′ [........ gaz s]im *ina* $^{\text{na4}}$zú *zaq-te sal-te* ugu *lam-ṣa-te-šú tu-kak*
13′ [...... dè ^{giš}]kiši$_{16}$ *tu-qat-tar* ú babbar súd
14′ [dúr-*šú*] mar.meš-*ma ina-eš*

15′ [...............] súd *ina* šu a.zu gur-*ti* gig tuk-*ši*[3]
16′ [............a] ^{giš}še.ná.a ra-*su* dabin.meš *ina* dè *tu-qat-tar-šú*
17′ [......... ^{ú}k]ur.kur ^{ú}kur.gi.rín.na *šá* kur-*e* ^{ú}*hab-šal-lu-ur-hu*
18′ [........$^{\text{gi]š}}$*mar-gu-ṣa* 7 ú.hi.a téš.bi gaz sim
19′ [ì.udu él]lag udu níta zú.lum.ma hi.hi *ina* dè *tu-qat-tar-šú*
20′ [....... mur]ub$_4$.meš-*šú ra-pal-te-šú* lá gig *lu-uš-ši-pa* tuk

---

21′ [diš na *ina* dúr-*šú* múd *ú-tab-ba-ka* n]a.bi *qer-be-ni* dúr gig *ana* gig-*šú* nu gíd.da
22′ [................a ^{giš}še.n]á.a *ina* dè *tu-qat-tar-š*[*ú* ....]

col. ii

1′ šu.si *tu-l*[*a-am-mi* ....
2′ luh-*si* ^{šim}gúr.gúr ⌜súd⌝ [.........................
3′ *i-lík-šú-ma*[4] ú babbar [.........................

4′ diš ki.min ^{šim}gúr.gúr ^{šim}l[i ....
5′ pa ^{giš}*nu-úr-ma* pa x [....................

---

[1] Thompson's suggestion that this tablet may belong to K 13738 (AMT 61, 2) is not possible since column markings do not match.
[2] See l. 9′ below.
[3] See the parallel in text K 1847 (No. 15): 4.
[4] *ilku* = posterior, CAD I 81, a rare word.

TRANSLATION

1′ [...........] ..., you grind up [...........................

2′ [.........], these [x] drugs [.................

3′ you keep smearing [on his anus] the oil of creeping[1] myrtle [and he will get better].

4′ [.....] a red blister: In order to break up the blisters, *kukru*, juniper,

5′ [.........], *kamantu*, seed of date-reed, these seven drugs

6′ [.......]..., you grind up and sift together with *baluhhu*-resin, (of) these drugs

7′ [.....], you make a suppository, sprinkle cedar oil, insert it to his anus and he will get better.

8′ [....], you scrape the top of his *lamṣātu*-sore [with] a sharp pointed flint,

9′ crush [.....] lead together, mix them in oil, you continually daub (it) into his anus and he will get better.

10′ [........], bathe (him) in juice of *šunû*-shrub, you fumigate him (with) *tapinnu*-flour over coals,

11′ [and with ... and] *ata'īšu*, take these 4 drugs together,

12′ [pound (and)] sift [...], you scrape the top of his *lamṣātu*-sore [with] a sharp pointed flint,

13′ you fumigate [... on coals] of acacia-thorn, crush 'white'-plant,

14′ continually rub (it) [into his anus] and he will get better.

15′ Crush [................]. (The patient) has a relapse of the illness despite being in the care of the healer:

16′ bathe him [in ... and in juice] of *šunû*-shrub, you fumigate him with *tapinnu*-flour over coals.

17′ [....,] *ata'īšu*, mountain-*kurkānû*-plant, *habšallurhu*,

18′ [... and] *marguṣu* – pound and sift these seven drugs together,

19′ mix (them) [with the fat of] the kidney of a male sheep (and) dates, you fumigate him over coals,

20′ bind [...] his groin (and) haunches; he has *lūššipu*-disease.[2]

21′ [If a man pours out blood from his anus], that man is ill in his anus internally; in order for his illness not to be prolonged,

22′ fumigate him with [.... and juice of] *šunû*-shrub over coals [and he will get better].

---

col. ii

1′ You wrap a pessary [.......................

2′ wash (it), crush *kukru* [.........................

3′ [....] his posterior (with) 'white'-plant [...............

4′ If ditto, *kukru*, juniper, [...................................

5′ pomegranate-leaf, leaf of [.....................

---

[1] See CAD A/1 326, in which the verb can refer to the motion of liquids, hence potentially 'flowing oil of myrtle'.

[2] Perhaps, 'let me exorcise'-disease, assuming a derived form from *wašāpu*, which is rare.

6′ pa ^{ú}*tu-lal* pa [.......................................
7′ a.gar.gar maš.dà zì *tu-* x [[1]..............
8′ *ina* ì.udu hi.hi *ina* hád.d[a ....
9′ sim zì.kum zì.gig [............................
10′ *ur-ri u* ge$_6$ *šu-hi-š*[*ú* ....
11′ 10 ud.meš lá-*su* maš x [.................
12′ diš-*niš* gaz nu *pa-tan* [.........................

13′ diš ki.min šu.si a.bára *ina* [...................
14′ šu.si *tu-la-am-m*[*i*[2]...............................
15′ *ina* a $^{\text{⌜šim⌝}}$ x [...
16′ *u*$_4$*-ma* šum x [.......................................

---

[1] perhaps *tu-q*[*at-tar*], 'you fumigate'.

[2] <*lamû*, 'wrap', not attested in the D-stem. in med. contexts, and otherwise rare, but it matches similar expressions elsewhere in this corpus, cf. šu.si-*ka mu-šá-ṭi talammi* (nigin) (No. 24, S 36+ ii 3). Alternatively on can read *tu-lam* (< *lummu*), 'you moisten' [courtesy R. Biggs].

6′ leaf of *tullal*, leaf of [..........
7′ gazelle droppings,[1] flour .....[.......................
8′ mix it in fat, in drying out [..........................]
9′ sift (them), *isqūqu*-flour, wheat, [........................
10′ day and night [on] his buttocks [and ....]
11′ bind him for 10 days, ... [........................
12′ Pound together [........, he drinks it] on an empty stomach [.....

13′ If ditto, [....] a lead pessary in [............................
14′ wrap [.......] the pessary [.................
15′ in the juice of ..[.....................................
16′ the day .....[..

[1] Dreckapotheke.

Drugs for anus desease

No. 39 BAM 431

MM = K 9684 + 9999 + S 341 + Rm 328 (BAM 431) v 7′–10′ [text no. 18]
NN = K 4164 + 11691 + Rm 352 (+) K 4176 (BAM 430) v 13′–16′ [text no. 40]

7′ MM numun ^{giš}ha.lu.úb ^{ú}eme.ur.gi_{15}
NN [............] ha.lu.úb ^{ú}eme.ur.gi_{15}
8′ MM ^{ú}*tara-muš*$_8$ *kam-ka-du*
NN [..*t*]*ara-muš*$_8$ *kam-ka-du*
9′ MM ^{ú}har.har ^{ú}kur.ka.na-*ú*
NN [.ha]r.har ^{ú}kur.ka.na-*ú*
10 MM 6 *maš-qit* dúr.gig
NN [.. *ma*]*š-qit* dúr.gig

No. 40 BAM 430

NN = K 4164 + 11691 + Rm 352 (+) K 4176 (BAM 430) v 3′–8′

3′ [........ n]umun ^{ú}eme.ur.gi_{15}
4′ $^{⸢ú⸣.zì}$nu.luh.ha
5′ $^{⸢ú⸣}$har.har
6′ [*šib-bur-ra-t*]*u*$_4$ ^{ú}*ha-hi-in*
7′ ú babbar ^{ú}$sila_{11}$.gá
8′ ⸢ú⸣ níg.lá[1] dúr.gig

See No. 9 ii 34′–36′.

[1] *naṣmattu*, see note on Text No. 2 (Ms. B) ii 6.

No. 41 BAM 98

OO = A 223 (BAM 98)

This list of drugs corresponds generally to a similar list of drugs in text No. 22 11–13, although the two lists are not duplicates.

ì él[lag ....
ì mušen x [.........
ì udu é[llag ....
ì udu él[lag ....
gaba.làl [.............
^{šim}buluh [............
⸢15 ú⸣.[hi.a ....
x x [..............
rev. x *šá* dù x [..........
nap-šal-ti dúr.gig

No. 42 BAM 101

PP = Ass. 13955/k* (BAM 101)
V = VAT 13752+ (BAM 95) [text No. 21]

1	PP	TA *lìb-bi* dub.m[eš] meš-[*tim*]
2	PP	*ú-na-as-si-ha-* x
3	PP	*a-na a-ha-meš ú-qa*[*r-rib*]
4	PP	ì.udu éllag gud níta : ⸢ì⸣. [...]
	V	[ì].udu éllag gud ì.udu éllag udu.níta
5	PP	ì.nun.na gaba.[làl]
	V	ì.nun gaba.làl
6	PP	ì. a[z] du.du x [...]
	V	[ì] az du.du
7	PP	ì *hal-ṣu* úš ^{giš}er[en]
	V	ì *hal-ṣa* úš ^{giš}e[ren]
8	PP	^{šim}šeš ^{šim}hab ^{šim}[.]
	V	$^{[ši]m}$šeš ^{šim}hab ^{šim}buluh
9	PP	[i]llu [..................]
	V	illu ^{šim}buluh illu li.tar
10	PP	ú [.........................
	V	ú babbar diš-*niš* súd dúr-*šú* eš.meš
11	PP	*nap-šal-t*[*i* d]úr.g[ig]
	V	*nap-šal-t*[*i*]
12	PP	*a-na ṣa-bat e-pe-*[*ši*] (= Hunger BAK No. 208, see BAM 168 colophon, above)
13	PP	^{m}*Ki-ṣir-*^{d}*Nabû* [*šá* ^{δ}*Nabû tuklat-su*]
14	PP	A ^{md}*Šamaš-ibni* ^{lú}[maš.maš *bīt Aš-šur*]
15	PP	[*ha-an*]*-ṭiš* [*is-su-uh*]

TRANSLATION

1–3 I excerpted (the following recipe) from among many tablets (and) I collected (them) together:

---

4 Crush together (l. 10) fat of the kidney of a male ox, fat ... (var. of the kidney of a male sheep)

5 ghee, wax,

6 oil of creeping myrtle, ...

7 pressed oil, 'blood' of cedar,

8 myrrh, *ṭūru*, *baluḫḫu*,

9 *baluḫḫu*-resin, resin of *abukkatu*,

10 white' plant, smear (the patient's) anus

11 (as a) salve for a sore anus.

(colophon)

Note: l. 11 should be compared with BAM 105, which is an incantation to be recited in conjunction with providing treatment for rectal disease. BAM 105: 7–8 reads, dù.dù.bi *ina al-la-ni nap-šal-ti maš-qí-ti* dúr.gig šid-*nu*, 'its ritual: recite (the incantation) over a pessary, salve, or potion for a sore anus'.

No. 43 STT 100

1′ [...............................] x -*šú* ^{ú}kur.ra^{sar}[....................
2′ [.......................] x hi.hi *ana* dúr-⸢*šú* gar⸣-*a*[*n* ....]

3′ [diš na im *ina* šà-*šú* nigin-*ma ú*]-*na-pih ma-la i-kal-la* na.bi dúr g[ig]
4′ [gig ....] x *ana* ti-*šú* ^{ú}kur.ra súd *ina* ì.udu hi.hi
5′ [*alla-nu* d]ù-*uš* ì.giš *dap-ra-ni-in ana* dúr-*šú* gar-*an*[1]

6′ [..................] ^{ú}nu.luh.ha sum.šir.dili illu buluh zú.lum.ma
7′ [......................ú].meš šeš.meš súd *alla-nu* dù-*uš ana* dúr-*šú* gar-*ma ina-eš*
8′ di[š ki.min ....^{šim}]gúr.gúr ^{šim}buluh.hi.a šu.bi.aš.àm
9′ diš ki.min *sah-lé-e* ^{ú}[ku]r.ra ^{šim}gúr.gúr ^{šim}li naga.s[i]
10′ ^{ú}úkuš.hab ^{ú}*ṣa-ṣ*[*u-u*]*n-tú* zú.lum.ma *šu*-[*p*]*u*-[*uh-ru*]

11′ diš na im *ina* šà-*šú* nigin [...] x *ú*-⸢*na-pih*⸣ [*ma-la i-kal-la*] (see l. 3)
12′ na.bi dúr.gig gi[g ....
13′ *ina* kaš.sag nu *pa-tan* [...
14′ 1/3 sìla a.geštin.na *tu*-[.......................................
15′ 1/2 sìla ì *hal-ṣa ana* š[à šub ....

16′ (trace)

---

[1] Simplicium.

TRANSLATION

1′ [.........................], ... *nīnû*, [...................

2′ Mix [.......................], insert (it) into his anus [....]

3′ [If a man has wind circulating in his bowel (and)] made (it) swell up, as much as (his bowel) retains, that man [suffers] from rectal disease,

4′ [..................]. To cure him, crush *nīnû*, mix it in fat,

5′ make [a suppository], insert *daprānu*-oil into his anus.

6′ [....................], *nuhurtu*, single-cloved garlic, *baluhhu*-resin, date,

7′ [.............], crush these [drugs], make a suppository, insert it into his anus and he will get better.

8′ If ditto, [.......] *kukru*, *baluhhu*-aromatics, ditto.

9′ If ditto, *sahlû*, *nīnû*, *kukru*, juniper, horned alkali,

10′ cucumber, *ṣaṣuntu*, dates, *šupuhru*.

11′ If a man has wind circulating in his bowel (and) made (it) swell up, as much as [(his bowel) retains],

12′ that man suffers from a rectal disease, [..............

13′ [he drinks ....] in premium beer on an empty stomach,

14′ you [....] one-third *sila* vinegar [..

15′ [put] into [it] one-half *sila* of pressed oil [..........................

No. 44 AMT 58,9 + 81,9 (plate 28)

K 10567 + 13901 (AMT 58,9 + 81,9) = RA 26, 85; (NB script)

1′ [....] ⸢numun⸣ x [..
2′ [.............................. *saḫ*]-*le-e as-*⸢*né -e*⸣ x [..]
3′ [..............................ga]ba.làl ú nam.ti.l[a]
4′ [............] 3 ú.meš *al-la-nu* ⸢dúr.gig⸣

5′ [...................... ^{š}]^{im}gúr.gúr ^{šim}li
6′ [..........................] ^{ú}naga.si ú nam.ti.la
7′ [..........................] x *al-*⸢*la*⸣*-nu* dúr.gig

8′ [..................................] x *dan-nu-ti*
9′ [..........................*al-la*]-*nu* dúr.gig

rev.

1′ [..] dú[r ...]

2′ [..................................] ⸢ú kù⸣ ú x sar x
3′ [..................................^{gi}]^{š}*še-nu-ʾu* [tu]ḫ.še.giš.ì
4′ [......................................gar]-*an*

5′ [..................................^{ú}k]ur.ra ^{ú}*nam-ruq-qu*
6′ [.................................. ḫi].ḫi ki.min

7′ [..] x gal nu gaz *ina* kaš 3 u_4*-me* gar-*an*
8′ [..................................] x tuk za.gìn.n[a] ki.min

---

9′ [..] x x x x ⸢sù šà šub⸣- *di*

TRANSLATION

1′ [........] seed of [...

2′ [.............................], *sahlû*, Dilmun date palm,

3′ [..........................], wax, 'health'-plant,

4′ [1]3 drugs (for) a suppository for a sick anus.

5′ [.............................], *kukru*, juniper,

6′ [..............................], horned alkali, 'health'-plant,

7′ [... drugs for] a suppository for a sick anus.

8′ [.................] strong ... [.......]

9′ [.. drugs for a] suppository for a sick anus

rev.

1′ [..] anus [.......

2′ [................................], pure plant, ...

3′ [..............................] *šunû*, sesame residue,

4′ put [..............................].

5′ Mix [...........................], *nīnû*, *namruqqu*,

6′ [..] ditto.

7′ Pound [......................] ... place it in beer for 3 days,

8′ [.............................]....., lapis, ditto.

9′ Put into it [..................]........................

No. 45 K 2428 + 2548 + 6728 (plates 29–30). Recipe for *maškadu*-disease which may be associated with renal disease

SS	=	K 2428 + 2548 + 6728
EE	=	O. 194 (BAM 182) [text no. 31]

1′	SS	⌜ú$^{?}$⌝ [..
2′	SS	*ina* x [..
3′	SS	diš na si[g$_{7}$...]-*šú*
4′	SS	^{giš}šu k[u ....-*m*]*a*
5′	SS	pa ^{giš}nam.[tar .... *ta*]-*sàk*
6′	SS	*ina* im.šu.[rin.na *te-sek-ker* .... ^{šim}b]uluh
7′	SS	*ina* šà ra x [..]-*su*
8′	SS	diš na *maš-k*[*a*-..].a.bi
	EE	[diš n]a *maš-ka$_{15}$*(kak)-*dù* dab$_{5}$-*su* ^{giš}še$^{!}$.ná$^{!}$.a ^{ú}ku$_{6}$ numun ⌜^{ú}*qut*⌝-*ri* pa ^{giš}kiri$_{6}$ dù.a.bi
9′	SS	gazi^{sar} ^{giš}š[inig ....]-⌜*u$_{5}$*⌝
	EE	[g]azi^{sar} ^{giš}šinig ^{ú}*túl-lal* ^{giš}gišimmar.tur gi.šul.hi ^{giš}*kam-u$_{5}$*
10′	SS	suhuš ^{giš}dìh su[huš .... g]eštin
	EE	suhuš ^{giš}dìh suhuš ^{giš}kiši$_{16}$ téš.bi *ta-har-ra-aṣ ina* šà tu$_{7}$ *u* a.geštin.na
11′	SS	esir *ina* nindu ú[š ....-*a*]*ṣ*
	EE	a pú *ina* nindu úš-*er gi-na-am* ra.meš-*su*
12′	SS	diš na *maš-ka-da* da[b-*su* ....
13′	SS	^{ú}hab ^{giš}*bi-nu* [..................................
14′	SS	suhuš ^{giš}*šu-š*[*e* ....
15′	SS	*tu-la-*⌜*ap*⌝-[*pat*..............................
16′	SS	e$_{11}$.a x [................................

rev.

1′		(traces)
2′	SS	[ka.inim.ma *m*]*aš-ka-du*
3′	SS	[.....................] *la* šu.ti *šum-ma* gìri lú *šá* 15
4′	SS	[....................] šu.ti *šum-ma* gìri lú *šá* gùb
5′	SS	^{ú}nam.t[i.la ....] šu.ti ki síg mí.aš.gàr gìš nu zu
6′	SS	nu.nu én 7.k[am$^{?}$ šid-*n*]*u ina* úr-*šú* kéš-*ma* ti *la-at-ki*
7′	SS	diš na maš.sil$_{7}$.lá[1] da[b-*s*]*u* ^{ú}kur.gi.rín.na súd
8′	SS	*ina* ì.giš šéš.[š]éš-*su-ma* ti
9′	SS	diš ki.min ^{ú}⌜eme⌝.zal.lá buluh *ina* ì du$_{10}$.ga šéš-*su*
10′	SS	diš ki.min ^{ú}*kur-ka-nam* [*i*]*na* ì šéš-*su*$^{!}$(text me)-*ma ina-eš*

[1] interpreted here as phonetic for maš.sìla.

TRANSLATION

1′–2′ (broken)

3′ If a man, yellow [................................] his [.....],
you crush ...., [...]..
5′ mandrake leaf, [.......................................],
[you heat it] in an oven ....] *baluḫḫu*,
steep into it ....[...]..

8′ If a man has been seized by *maškadu*-disease, you cut up together (l. 10′) *šunû*, *urânu*, *qutru* seed, leaf of any garden,
9′ *kasû*, tamarisk, *tullal*, young date-palm, *šalālu*-reed, truffle,
10′ root of the *baltu*-thorn, root of acacia-thorn, in a bowl and in vinegar
11′ your heat up bitumen (var. well water) in an oven and regularly bathe him.

12′ If a man [has been] seized by *maškadu*-disease, [..............
13′ madder, tamarisk, [..
14′ *šūšu* root, [...
15′ you smear [...
16′ take (it) out [..

rev.

2′ [Incantation] for *maškadu*-disease.

3′ Take ... [..................], if the right foot of a man,
4′ take [......................], if the left foot of a man,
5′ take 'health'-plant, [................], spin (it) (l. 6′) with the wool of a virgin kid,
6′ [recite] the incantation seven [times?], bind (it) to his lap and he will recover; proven.

7′ If a man *is seized in the shoulder*: crush *kurkānû*,
8′ keep rubbing him in oil and he will improve.

9′ If ditto, rub him with gourmet-plant, *baluḫḫu*, (and) sweet oil.

10′ If ditto, rub him with *kurkānû* in oil and he will get better.[1]

[1] Lines 7′–10′ = Simplicia.

11′ SS én *maš-ka-du maš-ka-d*[*u man-za-a*]*s-su nar-ba-as-su*
12′ SS *man*!(text kur)-*za-az* anše *man-za-as-s*[*u* .....] x -*ma* en ti.la en dingir
13′ SS *iz-za-az e-li-šu* [*ir-ru-u*]*b maš-ka-du*
14′ SS *ar-ki bu-lim* [*lam i*]*k-šu-du-nik-ka*
15′ SS ^{na4}zú *u* ⸢gír.šu.i⸣ [*šá* ^{d}gu].la tu$_6$.én

16′ SS ka.in[im.ma *maš-ka-d*]*a*-kam

17′ SS kìd.k[id.b]i sahar ⸢šub⸣ [........................] *hu-šah ta-šab-ba-aš*
18′ SS *ana* šà ⸢na$_4$⸣.bur šub-*di* én *ana* šà ⸢šid-*nu*⸣ [..] x ⸢gi *tu*⸣-*maš-šá-*'*-šú*

19′ SS én *lib-li* ^{d}girra *li*-[*nu-uh qab-l*]*i*[1]
20′ SS *ka-šu-uš-ta*(?) *li-ṣi* [*šá* šu-*ka* é]n

21′ SS én en én *u* ti.la ^{d}é.a [lugal abzu]
22′ SS *lid-di-ka ti-a-šú šá* ti.la ^{d}marduk maš.maš dingir.meš [*ši-pat* TI.LA *lid-di-ka*][2]

23′ SS min ka.inim.ma *maš-ka-du* : kìd.kìd.bi za.gá.mug[3] gal [.........

24′ SS diš na *maš-ka-du* gig ^{ú}úkuš.ti.gil.la [....................
25′ SS ú babbar hád.du súd *ina* kaš.sag šeg$_6$-*š*[*al* ....

26′ SS diš k[i.min ....

27′ SS diš k[i.min ....

28′ SS giš [...

29′ SS diš [...

---

1 This incipit occurs in CT 23 11: 33–34.
2 Restored from K 2453 iii : 32–33, and STT 275 ii 25′, courtesy B. Böck.
3 For zag.mug.

11′ Incantation. *maškadu, maškadu,* his [usual place is] his lair,
12′ his usual place is the abode of the ass, [....] and the lord of life, the divine priest
13′ stands over him, *maškadu* enters
14′ behind the herd, [before]
15′ the flint and scalpel [of] Gula reach you. Incantation.

16′ It is an incantation of *maškadu.*

17′ Its ritual: you gather dust [.............] ......,
18′ put it into a stone vessel, recite the incantation onto it [...]..., you massage him.

19′ Incantation. May the fire be extinguished, may [the battle abate]
20′ may ..... go out [of your control]. Incantation.

21′ Spell. Lord of the incantation and life, may Ea [lord of the Apsû]
22′ cast for you his spell of life, let Marduk, exorcist of the god, [recite for you a life-bestowing incantation].

23′ Second incantation (of) *maškadu*: its ritual: the great *new year* .... [......

24′ If a man suffers from *maškadu*, dry and crush gourd, [..............
25′ 'white' plant, boil it in premium beer [..................................

26′ (remainder damaged)

No. 46 AMT 69,8

TT	=	K 6056 (= AMT 69,8), cf. JRAS 1937, 275 f.
ff	=	K 8248 = AMT 56,1 rev. 5′–8′ [text no. 32] = ll. 11–16
AI	=	BAM 471 i 9′–10′ = ll. 13–14
AP	=	VAT 13733 + 13738 (BAM 52 5–7) = ll. 13–14

1′–6′	TT	broken
7′	TT	*ina* ⌜kaš x x x⌝ [....................................
8′	TT	diš ki.min a.gar.gar udu.níta x [......................
9′	TT	diš ki.min hénbur ^{giš}lagab.mu[nu$_4$ ....
10′	TT	*ina* túg.hi.a sur [....................................
11′	TT	diš *a-na* murub$_4$ *áš-ṭa-a-ti l*[*u-*..]
	ff	[.....................] *áš-ṭa-a-te lu-ub-bu-ka* lagab.munu$_4$ numun $^{\text{giš.šim}}$man.du [.... ^{šim}]bal
12′	TT	gi.dug$_4$.ga ^{šim}šeš *si*[*k-*...]
	ff	gi.du$_{10}$.ga ^{šim}šeš *sik-ka-ti ina* ì *u* kaš šeg$_6$-*šal ana* dúr dub
13′	TT	^{šim}šeš gazi^{sar} ^{ú}nu.luh.ha [...]
	ff	[diš ki.min ^{šim}]šeš gazi^{sar} ^{ú}nu.luh.ha ^{šim}gúr.gúr naga.si lag.a.šà [....r]a$^{?}$ ^{ú}hur.sag
	AI	[diš] ⌜6⌝ ^{šim}šeš gazi^{sar} ^{ú}nu.luh.ha ^{šim}gúr.gúr naga.si lag.a.šà [^{ú}kur.r]a ^{ú}hur.sag
	AP	[diš k]i.min ^{šim}šeš gazi^{sar} ^{ú}nu.luh.ha ^{šim}gúr.gúr naga.si [...] ⌜^{ú}⌝kur.ra ^{ú}hur.sag
14′	TT	*ina* kaš *u* ga súd *bu-uh-ru* è ì.giš *ana* [..]
	ff	*ina* kaš *u* ga *ta-sàk bu-uh-ru-s*[*u*] ì *ina* igi šub [... du]b egir-*šú* ga *mat-qa ana* dúr-*šú* dub
	AI	*ina* kaš *u* ga *ina* im.šu.rin.na *te-sek-ker tu-še-lam-ma* [........] x x è ì.giš *ana* igi šub-*di ana* dúr-*šú* dub egir-*šú* ga *mat-qa ana* dúr-*šú* dub-*ma ina-eš*
	AP	*ina* kaš *u* kàš *ina* nindu úš-*er* e$_{11}$-*ma* [......................] ì.giš *ana* igi šub-*di-ma ana* dúr-*šú* dub-*ak* egir-*šú* ga *mat-*[..................................]
15′	TT	*ana* sa murub$_4$ *lu-ub-bu-ki* numun.gada ^{šim}[...........................
	ff	[..........................-*u*]*b-bu-ka* numun $^{\text{giš.šim}}$man.du ^{šim}gi.du$_{10}$.ga
16′	TT	gazi^{sar} níg.àr.ra gig.ba ina ì.[.......................]
	ff	[...............].ra gig.ba *ina* ì.giš *u* kaš šeg$_6$-*šal*
17′	TT	diš <ki.min> ^{šim}gúr.gúr ^{šim}li ^{šim}bal ^{šim}man.[du ....]

rev.

1	TT	diš na gìri^{2}-*šú* gar x [.......................
	TT	KU.KU *uš* x [...............................
	TT	e$_{11}$ a ga[zi^{sar} ....
	TT	diš bu uš[1] [.......................................

[1] *būšu* 'stench'?

TRANSLATION

7′ in beer ..... [..

8′ If ditto, male sheep droppings, .. [..............

9′ If ditto, a stalk of malt [............
10′ spread it on cloth [....................................

11′ If, to make a stiff groin supple, lump of malt, seed of *suādu*, [........] *ballukku*,
12′ sweet reed, myrrh, and *sikkatu*, boil them in oil and beer and pour it into his anus.

13′ (var. If ditto), crush myrrh, *kasû*, *nuhurtu*, *kukru*, horned alkali, field-clod, *nīnû* (and) *azupīru*,
14′ in beer and milk (var. urine), (var: you heat and remove from the oven), and remove it while hot, put oil in it, pour it into his anus; afterwards pour sweet milk into his anus and he will get better.

15′ In order to make the sinews of the groin supple: boil flax seed, *suādu*, 'sweet-reed',
16′ *kasû*, groats (and) wheat in oil and beer.

17′ If <ditto>, *kukru*, juniper, *balukku*, *suādu* [........

---

rev.

1 If a man, his feet ....
2 powder ...
3 remove, juice of *kasû* [..............

---

4 If .... [..............................

TT diš na sa [...

TT ^{ú}i[n.nu.uš ....

TT a ^{giš}[...

TT pa ^{giš}[...

TT pa ^{g}[^{iš} ....

TT pa ^{g}[^{iš} ....

TT ú[...

If a man, the sinews [...................
maštakal, [............................
juice of [.............................
leaf of [............................
leaf of [..........................
leaf of [........................
....[..................................

No. 47 AMT 57,1

81-7-27, 72 = AMT 57,1

obv.

1′ geštin.⸢šur *ana* dúr-*šú* dub-*ak*⸣ [..........

2′ *ina* a ^{giš}še.nu ra.meš x [..................

3′ diš ki.min ú babbar *ina* ì.giš hi.hi ⸢*ana*⸣ x [...........

4′ ^{šim}gúr.gúr ^{šim}li pa ^{giš}*bi*-[*ni* ....

5′ diš ki.min ^{ú}*an*-x x ^{ú}gamu[n ....

6′ *ina* ì.udu hi.hi *alla-nu* d[ù-*uš* ....

7′ [diš] k[i.m]in a.geštin.na kala.ga šeg$_6$.gá *ana* š[à ....

8′ [............................. š]è.^{d}iškur[1] *ina* ì.giš x [........

(bottom of tablet)

rev.

1 (traces)

2 [na.bi$^?$ dú]r.gig g[ig-*ma* ....

3 [^{ú}]kur.kur ^{ú}igi-*l*[*im* ....

---

4 [diš n]a dúr.gig g[ig-*ma* ....

5 [.......... -*t*]*i lu* ⸢^{ú}⸣[..................

---

[1] Presumably a plant name, like šè.^{d}nisaba, see CAD Z 151.

TRANSLATION

1′ Pour drawn wine into his anus [............
2′ keep bathing (him) in *šunû*-juice... [...............

3′ If ditto, mix 'white' plant in oil, into .. [.......
4′ *kukru*, juniper, tamarisk leaf, [......................

5′ If ditto, ..., *kamūnu*, [................
6′ mix in fat, make a suppository [and insert it into his anus .....

7′ [If] ditto, boil strong vinegar, [put ....] into (it),
8′ [...............................]..... in oil [.............

---

rev.

2 [that man] suffers from a rectal disease [and ....
3 *ata'išu*, *imhur-līm*, [.....................

---

4 [If a] man suffers from rectal disease [and ....
5 either [............ or ....

Miscellaneous texts

Assur catalogue of medical incipits

No. 48 YBC 7123+ and 7126 (+) 7139 (ed. F. Köcher)

See *Sachs Memorial Volume* pp. 11–13

diš na u[r-[1]..
diš na *šá* múd$^?$ [..
diš na zi x [..] x [......

---

en 8 dub.me[š ....] da [........
7′ en én *ú-š*[*á*$^?$-*an-ni*(?)[2]....................... *š*]*ú re-hu-su* [šub-*a*][3]
diš na éllag-*su* g[u$_7$-*su* : diš na .... mú.m]ú$^?$.meš-*h*[*u*$^?$
diš na dab éllag-*su* [...] x.lá gig

10′ nígin 3 dub.meš diš [na éllag-*su* gu$_7$-*su* ....] *šá mu-ṣa*

---

diš na *ina la si*-[*ma-ni-šú* murub$_4$.meš-*šú* gu$_7$.meš-*šú*]
[..........] x na kúm ud.da en.te.na im *u ša-ra* apin nu íl
diš na *li*-[*diš* na *li-kis* dúr.gig šà.meš ....
[diš na ki.n]ú-*ma šit-ta-šú* ugu-*šú* dùg.ga
diš na dúr.[gig] gig-*ma*

---

nígin 5 du[b.meš diš na *ina la si-ma-ni-šú*] murub$_4$.meš-*šú* gu$_7$-*šu šá* dúr.gig.ga.kam
15′ en diš n[a..] x x ud.da buru$_8$[4] diri-*ú*

---

diš x [.................................. diš na sa] úr.meš-*šú* diš-*niš* gu$_7$.meš-*šú* diš na *bur-ka-šú*
mun-ga diri
[nígin 3 dub.meš ....] x su (rasur) íl

---

1 Köcher suggests *urbatu*, but *uršu* is just as likely, see BAM 95: 10
2 Alternatively one could read ú(*šammu*) *šá* [.........
3 cf. BAM 111: 16 (text No. 3).
4 These signs are given on the copy (*Sachs Memorial Volume*, p. 14 No. 9d 11′) as partially erased.

Diagnostic handbook

No. 49 (plates 31–35)

ww = VAT 303 + 404 + 579 + 589 + 1751 = Labat TDP XIV (p. 129 ff.); SBH 148[1]

w$_2$ = BM 38655 (for restorations of col. iv) [see Heeßel, BAD, p. 145] (plate 35)

col. i

1′ [diš gu.du.meš-*šú* sa$_5$.meš sìg nu.tuk diš gu.du 15-*š*]*u* sig$_7$-*át* gig-*su* man-*ni*

2′ [diš gu.du 150-*šú* sig$_7$-*át* gig-*su* dugud : diš gu.du.me]š-*šu* sig$_7$.meš *na-hi-id*

3′ [diš gu.du 15-*šú* sig$_7$-*át* gig-*su* dugud : diš gu.du 1]50-*šu* ge$_6$-*á*[*t*] *na-hi-id*

4′ [diš gu.du.meš-*šú* ge$_6$.meš ...... : diš gu.d]u 15-*šu* *tar-kat ú-zab-bal-ma* ug$_6$ (=TDP 130: 41)

5′ [diš gu.du 15-*šú* *tar-kat*............: diš gu].du.meš-*šu* *tar-ku* gam

6′ [diš gu.du 15-*šú* *du-*'*-ú-mat* .... : diš gu].du 150-*šu* *du-*'*-ú-mat* gig-*su* man-*ni*

7′ [diš gu.du.meš-*šú* *du-*'*-ú-ma* .... : diš] gu.du 15-*šu* *nap-hat* gig-*su* man-*ni*

8′ [diš gu.du 150-*šú* *nap-hat* .... : diš] gu.du.meš-*šu* *nu-up-pu-hu* gig-*su* man-*ni*

9′ [diš gu.du 15-*šú* *muq-qú-ta-át* .... : di]š gu.du 150-*šu* *muq-qú-ta-át* gig-*su* gíd

10′ [diš gu.du.meš-*šú* *muq-qú-ta na-hi-id*: diš] ⸢gu.du 15-*šu*⸣ *šu-uh-hu-ṭa-át* gig-*su* man-*ni*

11′ [diš gu.du 150-*šú* *šu-uh-hu-ṭa-át* gig-*su* dugud: diš gu.du.meš-*š*]*u* ⸢*šu-uh-hu-ṭa* *na-hi-id*

12′ [diš gu.du 15-*šú* du$_8$-*át* gig-*su* man-*ni* : diš gu.d]u 150-*šu* du$_8$-*át* gig-*su* *na-hi-id*

13′ [diš gu.du.meš-*šú* du$_8$.meš gam : diš] gu.du.meš-*šu* *šal-ma* tin

14′ [diš gu.du.meš-*šú* ge$_6$.meš-*ma* ki.gub-*su* nu è]-⸢*a*⸣ *u* a nu *ú-še-rid* a.ga sìg-*iṣ* gam

---

15′ [diš uzu *šá-pu-la-šu*] *u* ⸢gu.du.meš-*šu*⸣ sì[g-*iṣ* šu ^{d}15]

16′ [diš uzu *šá-pu-la-šu*] *u* *kin-ṣi-šu* sìg-⸢*iṣ*⸣ šu ^{d}15

17′ [diš uzu *šá*]-⸢*pu-la-šu*⸣ bal.bal-*ut* gig-*su* ⸢man-*ni*⸣

18′ [diš uzu *šá*]-*pu-la-šu* bal.bal-*ut* hun.gá-*šú* tag$_4$-*šu* : uš$_4$ líl-*šú* kúr-*šú* šu 20 tin : aš gub-*az* [........]

19′ [diš uzu] *šá-pu-li-šu* *šá* 15 sìg-*iṣ* uš$_4$-*šú* nu dab *ina* nu zu *ú-rap-p*[*ad* .....]

20′ diš [uz]u *šá-pu-li-šu* *šá* 150 sìg-*iṣ-ma* gim dug$_4$.dug$_4$ x x [x]

21′ diš uzu *šá-pu-li-šu* *šá* 15 zi.meš *u* gi$_6$.meš *ana* ud.3.kám g[am]

22′ diš u[zu] *šá-pu-li-šu* *šá* 150 zi.meš *u* gi$_6$.meš *ár-hiš* g[am]

23′ diš dúr-*šú* gub-*iz* gam : diš dúr-*šú* gub-*iz* im.g[ú s]ig$_7$ ⸢si⸣ : x [...]

24′ diš dúr-*šú* bad-bad-*ir* tin : diš dúr-*šú* gub-*iz* x [..................]

25′ diš *ina* dúr-*šú* ⸢a.meš sa$_5$⸣.meš du-*ku* gig-*su* gíd : diš ⸢a⸣.meš ⸢sig$_7$⸣.meš du-*ku* na.b[i ...]

---

[1] My copy of this tablet was greatly facilitated by having to hand the edition of J. Scurlock, and editions of this tablet are being prepared by J. Scurlock and N. Heeßel independently. For this reason, the present edition is not based upon all the manuscripts but is restored after Labat, TDP. For the readings of the logograms in this tablet, cf. Heeßel, BAD.

TRANSLATION

col. i

1′ [If his buttocks are red, there is no attack (of disease); if] his [right buttock] is yellow, his disease will change.

2′ [If his left buttock is yellow, his disease is serious; if] his [buttocks] are (both) yellow, it is worrying.

3′ [If his right buttock is yellow, his disease is serious; if] his left [buttock] is black, it is worrying.

4′ [If (both) his buttocks are (both) black ....; if] his right buttock is bruised, he will linger and die.

5′ [If his right buttock is bruised .....; if (both)] his buttocks are bruised, he will die.

6′ [If his right buttock is dark ....; if] his left buttock is dark, his disease will change.

7′ [If (both) his buttocks are dark .....; if] his right buttock is swollen, his disease will change.

8′ [If his left buttock is swollen .....; if (both)] his buttocks have swelled up, his disease will change.

9′ [If his right buttock is caved in ....; if] his left buttock is caved in, his disease will be prolonged.

10′ [If (both) his buttocks are depressed, it is worrisome; if] his right buttock is raw, his disease will change.

11′ [If his left buttock is raw, his disease is serious; if (both) his buttocks] are raw, it is worrying.

12′ [If his right buttock is slack, his disease will change; if] his left buttock is slack, his disease is worrying.

13′ [If (both) his buttocks are slack, he will die; if] (both) his buttocks are well, he will recover.

14′ [If (both) his buttocks are black and his stools do not] appear nor has he passed water, his backside is affected; he will die.

15′ [If the flesh of his inner thighs] and buttocks is affected, [it is the Hand of Ishtar].

16′ [If the flesh of his inner thighs] and shins is affected, it is the Hand of Ishtar.

17′ [If the flesh of] his inner thighs was being displaced, his illness will change.

18′ [If the flesh] of his inner thighs was being displaced, his being free of disease (and it) has left him, the nature of his infection has changed him, it is the Hand of Šamaš, he will get better : if he stands up [.....].

19′ [If the flesh] of his inner left thigh bothers him (but) his mind is not affected, he wanders around without being aware of it, [..........].

20′ If the flesh of his inner left thigh bothers him and when he speaks .... [......]

21′ If the flesh of his inner right thigh keeps rising (pulsating) and is black, he will die within 3 days.

22′ If the flesh of his inner left thigh keeps rising and is black, he will die quickly.

23′ If his anus 'stood up', he will die; if his anus 'stood up', yellow pus (lit. mud) filled (it), ...

24′ If his anus is stopped up, he will recover; if his anus 'stood up' [.............]

25′ If reddish fluid flows from his anus, his illness will be prolonged; if yellow fluid (flows from his anus), that man [suffers from ....].

26′ diš *ina* dúr-*šú* zé sa$_5$ du-*ak* gíd-*ma* tin : ⸢diš⸣ [*ina*] ⸢dúr-*šú*⸣ *zu-ti* du-*ak* lù.lù sag.ba gam
27′ diš *ina* dúr-*šú* zé ge$_6$ [d]u-*ak* gam : diš *ina* dúr-*šú* ì šà-*šú* du-*ku* gam
28′ diš *ina* dúr-*šú* alan ad ti$^?$ di$^?$-*šú* šub.šub-*a* gam : diš *ina* dúr-*šú* uzu šub.šub-⸢*a*⸣ [..]
29′ diš *ina* dúr-*šú* múd mud šub.šub-*a* gam : diš *ina* dúr-*šú* uz[u] š[ub-.........]
30′ [diš *ina*] ⸢dúr-*šú* múd *i-te*⸣-*ez-zi*-⸢*ma* x⸣ [........]

obv. col. ii

1′ [diš še$_{10}$-*ú-šú* .... gam :] ⸢diš še$_{10}$-*ú*⸣ [sa$_5$.meš tin]
2′ [diš še$_{10}$-*ú-šú* sig$_7$.meš ....] : diš še$_{10}$-*ú-šú* *šal*-[*mu* .... (= TDP 134: 18)
3′ [diš še$_{10}$-*ú-šú* .... gig-*su*] gíd : diš še$_{10}$-*ú-šú* š[à ....
4′ [............] *i*[*t-te-n*]*ek-ki-ik* mur gig [.................

5′ [diš gìš-*šu* sa$_5$-*át* gig-*su*] gíd-*ma* tin : diš gìš-*šú* sig$_7$-*át* g[ig-*su* ....]
6′ [diš gìš-*šu* gi$_6$-*á*]*t* gam : diš gìš-*šú* *tar*-⸢*kát*⸣ *n*[*a-hi-id*]
7′ [diš gìš-*šu* *du-ʾ-mat*] gig-*su* *ú-šá-an-na-ah* : diš gìš-*šú* *nap-hat* *na*-[*hi-id*]
8′ [diš gìš-*šu* *muq-qu-t*]*a-át* tin : diš gìš-*šú* *šu-uh-hu-ṭ*[*a-at-ma* nu du$_8$-*ir* gam]
9′ [diš gìš-*šu* *šal-mat* tin] : diš gìš-*šú* *is-se-ker* gam : diš gìš-*šú* *maš*-[*da-at* ....]
10′ [diš gìš-*šu* *u* šà-*šú* kúm] úh *ú-kal* tùn-šà-*šú* gu$_7$-*šú* *u* šà-*šú* *ma-h*[*u* ....]
11′ [á^2-*šú* gìri^2-*šu* sag šà-*šú*] kúm na.bi gig *na-a-ki* gig-*su* šu din[gir-*šú* *u* ^{d}15-*šú*]
12′ [diš *ina* gìš-*š*]*u* múd sur šu ^{d}utu mu ki nu.gi [gam]
13′ [diš gìš-*š*]*u* *u* šir-*šú* *nap-hu* šu ^{d}*dil-bat* *ina* ki.[ná-*šú* kur-*su*]

14′ [diš kàš.meš-*š*]*u* sa$_5$.meš šu dingir-*šú* gíd : diš kàš.meš-*šu* sig$_7$.meš g[ig-*su* gíd ki.min ud.da tag-*it* gam]
15′ [diš kàš.meš]-*šu* ge$_6$.meš tag múd tag-*it* gam : diš kàš.meš-*šu* *ta*[*r-ka* gam]
16′ [diš kàš].meš-*šu* *it-te-né-es-ki-ru* gam : diš kàš.meš-*šu* d[u.meš gam]
17′ [diš kà]š.meš-*šu* *u* a.ri.a-*su* du.meš gam : diš [kà]š.meš-*šu* gi[m ..... gam]
18′ [diš k]àš.meš-*šu* gim a.meš gig-*su* gíd-*ma* tin : diš kàš.meš-*šu* gim esir [ki.min]
19′ [diš k]àš.meš-*šu* gim geštin gig-*su* dugud-*ma* tin : diš kàš.meš-*šu* gim ga [tin]
20′ [diš k]àš.meš-*šu* *taq-na* k[i.min]

26′ If red bile flows from his anus, (his illness) will be prolonged but he will live; if sweat flows [from] his anus, he is confused by (violation of) an oath, he will die.

27′ If black bile flows from his anus, he will die; if bowel fat flows from his anus, he will die.

28′ If he excretes a figurine of his ... from his anus, he will die; if he excretes flesh from his anus [.....].

29′ If he excretes dark-red blood from his anus, he will die; if he excretes flesh [............]

30′ If he voids blood from his anus and ... [...........................]

col. ii

1′ [If his stools are ...., he will die], if his stools are [red, he will recover].

2′ If his stools are yellow, ...], if his stools are healthy [.......

3′ [If his stools are ...., his disease] will be prolonged. If his stools among [........

4′ [If] he continually scratches [his ...], [he suffers from] a sick liver[1][.....

5′ [If his penis is red, his disease] will be prolonged and he will recover; if his penis is yellow, [his] disease [......]

6′ [If his penis is] black, he will die; his his penis is darkish, [it is] worrying.

7′ [If his penis is dark(-red), his illness *causes obstruction*; if his penis is swollen, [it is] worrying.

8′ [If his penis is] caved in, he will recover; if his penis is raw [and not loose, he will die].

9′ [If his penis is healthy he will recover]; if his penis is blocked up, he will die; if his penis has a welt [...]

10′ [If his penis and his epigastrium are hot], he retains phlegm, his *abdomen* hurts and his insides are spasmodic, [....],

11′ [his extremities and epigastrium are] hot, that man's illness is venereal, the hand of [his] god [and goddess].

12′ [If] blood drips [from] his [penis], it is the Hand of Šamaš; because of the Netherworld [he will die].

13′ [If] his [penis] and testicles are swollen, the Hand of Venus will [overwhelm him] in [his] bed.

14′ [If] his [urine] is red, it is the hand of his god, (his disease) will be prolonged; if his urine is yellow, [his] disease will be [prolonged; ditto, he is affected by sun-fever, he will die].

15′ [If] his [urine] is black, he is affected by the fatal disease, he will die; if his urine is dark, [he will die].

16′ [If] his urine is continually blocked up, he will die; if his urine keeps flowing, [he will die].

17′ [If] his urine and his sperm keep flowing, he will die; if his urine is [....] like [..., he will die].

18′ [If] his urine is like water, his illness will be protracted, but he will recover; if his urine is like pitch, [ditto].

19′ [If] his urine is like wine, his illness will be severe but he will get better; if his urine is like milk, [he will recover].

20′ [If] his urine is normal, ditto.

---

[1] Interpreting mur as *gabīdu* with Labat, TDP 134: 22 (reading ur_5), although 'lung' is also possible.

21′ [diš k]àš.meš-*šu* igi-*ma li-piš-tú* è.meš-*ni ina* edin t[ag-*it*]
22′ [diš k]àš.meš-*šu* igi-*ma* uzu.me-*šú* è.me-*ni ina* edin t[ag-*it*]

23′ [diš š]ir-*šu* sa$_5$.meš tin : diš šir-*šu* sig$_7$.[meš ....] (= TDP 136, 54)
24′ [diš š]ir-*šu* ge$_6$.meš tin : diš šir-*šu tar-ka* [...]
25′ [diš] šir-*šu du-ʾ-ú-ma* gig-*su* dugud : diš šir-*šu muq-qú-*[*ta$_5$* ....]
26′ [diš šir-*š*]*u šu-uh-hu-ṭa* gam : diš šir-*šu šal-*[*ma* tin]
27′ [diš šir-*š*]*u ze-ra* gam : *ana* nin.dingir.ra [dingir-*šú* te-*hi*]
28′ [diš šir-*šu*] ⸢*ze*⸣-*ra* eme-*šu i-te-nik-ki-ik* nundum.meš [*ú-na-aš-šak* ...]
29′ [diš] ⸢šir-*šu*⸣ [*na*]*p-hu na-hi-id* : *ana* nin.dingir.ra [dingir-*šu* te-*hi*]
30′ [diš] šir-*šu* ⸢mú⸣.meš-*hu* gìš-*šú sik-ka-ta$_5$* diri *ana* n[in.dingir.ra dingir-*šu* te-*hi*]
31′ [diš *ina*] šir-*šu* sìg-*iṣ ana* [n]in.dingir.ra dingir-*šú* te-*hi* : *ana* ⸢nin⸣.[dingir.ra dingir-*šú*....]
32′ [diš *ina*] šir-*šu* sìg-*iṣ u h*[*e-p*]*í eš-šú it-te-né-*[*es-ki-ra* ....]
33′ [diš é]llag *zi-kar-ti-šu* gaz-*át pa-pa-a*[*n* šà-*šú* .... kàš.meš-*šú* dab.dab ....]
34′ [diš] *šap-la-tu-šu nap-*[*ha* ....

35′ [di]š úr 15-*šu* sa$_5$-*át ú-*[*pa-su e-*...] (= TDP 138: 72)
36′ [diš] úr.meš-⸢*šu* sa$_5$⸣.[meš *na-hi-id* : diš úr-*šú* ....]
(broken)

rev. col. iii

1′ (broken)
2′ [diš *ina* úr-*šú* 15]0 sìg-*iṣ* [šà.meš-*šú eb-ṭu* sag.ki-*šú he-sa-at* gam]

3′ [diš *ri-bit-su šá* 15 g]u$_7$-*šú* šu dingir-*šú* tin : [diš *ri-bit-su šá* 150 gu$_7$-*šú* šu ^{d}15-*šú* tin] (= TDP 140: 43′)
4′ [diš *ri-bit-su šá* 15 *n*]*ap-hat-ma* gi$_6$-*át u ina* nu zu ⸢*ú*⸣-[*rap-pad* šu ^{d}im *ina* an.bar$_7$ sìg-*iṣ* gam]
5′ [diš *ri-bit-su šá*] 150 *nap-hat-ma* gi$_6$-*át u ina* nu zu *ú-*[*rap-pad* šu ^{d}*dil-bat ina šat ur-ri* sìg-*iṣ* gam]
6′ [diš *ri-biti r*]*i-biti* du$_{11}$.du$_{11}$-*si ina* dúr-*šú* zé *i-*[*te-eṣ-ṣi u* šir-*šú ze-ra* gam]
7′ [diš *ina ri-biti-š*]*u* sìg-*iṣ* š[u ^{d}im]
8′ [diš *ina ri-biti-š*]*u* sìg-*iṣ*-⸢*ma*⸣ *ina* kir$_4$-*šú* múd[1] mud šub.[šub-*a* šu ^{d}im gam]
9′ [diš *ina ri-biti-šu* sì]g-*iṣ-ma* dúr-*šú* kúr.kúr-*ir* [šu ^{d}nin-giš-zi-da]
10′ [diš *ina ri-biti-šu* sig-*iṣ-ma* múš-*šu uš*]-*qa-am-ma ina* e[din tag-*it* ki.min]
11′ [diš *ina ri-biti-šu* sig-*iṣ-ma*] m[úš-*šu*] ⸢*ih*⸣-*hi-su* suhuš.meš-[*šú i-tar-ru-ra* ....]
12′ [diš *ina ri-biti-šu* sig-*iṣ-ma ri-biti*] *ri-biti* du$_{11}$.du$_{11}$-*si* [*ina a-zi-ri-šú* zé *i-par*]-*ri* šu ding[ir-*šú* ...]

---

1 See Heeßel, BAD 179: 79′.

21′ [If] his urine is inspected and produces a fleshy-membrane, (the patient) was attacked from the steppe (i. e., by a demon).

22′ [If] his urine is inspected and produces his actual flesh, he was attacked in the steppe.

23′ [If] his testicles are red, he will recover; if his testicles [are] yellow [...].

24′ [If] his testicles are black, he will recover; if his testicles are darkish, [...].

25′ [If] his testicles are dark(-red), his disease is serious; if his testicles are caved in, [....].

26′ [If] his [testicles] are raw, he will die; if his testicles are whole, [he will recover].

27′ [If his testicles] are twisted, he will die; he [made sexual advances] towards the priestess of [his god].

28′ [If his testicles] are twisted, he continually scrapes his tongue, he [bites (his)] lips, [...].

29′ [If] his testicles are swollen, it is worrying; [he made sexual advances] towards the priestess [of his god].

30′ [If] his testicles are enflamed, his penis is full of pimples, [he made sexual advances] towards the priestess [of his god].

31′ [If] he is affected in his testicle, he made sexual advances towards the priestess of his god; he [....] to the priestess [of his god; if] he is affected [in] his testicle and <new break>, (his urine) is constantly stopped up [........].

33′ [If] the 'sack' of his masculinity is crushed, the ... of [his belly is ..., his urine is seized up...].

34′ [If] his nether regions are swollen [...

35′ If his right thigh is red, [his *mucous* is ....].

36′ [If] his thighs are red, [it is worrying; if his thigh ....].

rev. col. iii

2′ [If he] is affected [in his] left [thigh], [his bowels are cramped, his temple is puffed up, he will die].

3′ [If his perineum][1] hurts him [on the right], it is the Hand of his God, he will recover; [if his perimeum hurts him on the left, it is the Hand of his Goddess, he will recover].

4′ [If his perineum] is swollen on the right and dark plus he wanders [about] without knowing it, [it is the Hand of Adad, he is affected in the heat of the day, he will die].

5′ [If his perineum] is swollen [on the] left and dark, plus he wanders [about] without knowing it, [it is the Hand of Venus, he is affected at dawn, he will die].

6′ [If] he constantly cries, 'my street (i. e., perineum)! my street!', bile comes out from his anus [and his testicles are twisted, he will die].

7′ [If] he is affected [in] his [perineum], it is the Hand [of Adad].

8′ [If] he is affected in] his [perineum] and dark-red blood [constantly] protrudes from his nose, [it is the Hand of Adad, he will die].

9′ [If] he is affected [in his perineum] and his anus has an unhealthy appearance, [it is the Hand of Ningišzida].

10′ [If he is affected in his perineum and his face] is subdued, [he was attacked] in the steppe, [ditto].

11′ [If he is affected in his perineum and his] face has sunk, [his] lower extremities [shake ...].

12′ [If he is affected in his perineum and] he constantly cries, 'my street (i. e., perineum)! my street!', he throws up [bile in his sputum(?), it is the Hand of [his] God [...]

---

[1] lit. 'street'.

13′ [diš *ina ri-biti-šu ina su-ha*]-*ti* sìg-*iṣ* šu ding[ir-*šú*......]

14′ [diš] ⸢*bir*⸣-*ka*-[*šú*] g[u$_7$]-*šú* azag ding[ir-*šú*..........] (TDP 140 58′)

15′ [diš *bir*]-*ka-a* [*u* murub$_4$].⸢meš-*šu*⸣ *ina* ge$_6$ g[u$_7$.meš-*šú* su-*šú* kúm nu tuku azag ^{d}utu dab-*šú*]

16′ diš *pu-qa-a-š*[*u it-te-né-ep-ta-a* gam]

17′ diš *pu-qa-a*-[*š*]*u i*[*t-ta-n*]*a-a*[*z-qa*]-*pa* ti[n]

18′ diš *ki-i*[*n-ṣi-šú š*]*á* 15 [g]u$_7$-*šú* kúm-[*šú*] *mit-har* [šu ^{d}*eš*$_4$-*dar* mu ....]

19′ diš *k*[*i*]-*i*[*n-ṣi-šú š*]*á* 1[5]0 g[u$_7$-*šú* kú]m-*šú* nu *mit-har* g[ig-*su* gíd-*ma* tin$^?$]

20′ diš [*kin-ṣa-a-š*]*u* gu$_7$.[meš]-*šu* ⸢kúm⸣-*šú* nu *mit-har* [šu dingir-*šú* búr-*ru*]

21′ diš *k*[*in-ṣa-a-šu* gu$_7$.meš]-*šu* šu dingir uru-*šu* š[u dingir-*šú*]

22′ diš *kin-ṣa-a-š*[*u* gu$_7$.meš]-*šu* šu ^{d}utu mu k[ù.babbar zà.10.meš[1] tin]

23′ diš *kin-ṣa*-[*a-šu ki-is*]-*sa-tu*$_4$ *i-šá-a ina* du$_{11}$.du$_{11}$-*šú* [úh-*su* šub-*di-ma*] búr *ru-mi*-[*ka*]-*ti ik-bu-us*[2] [.............

24′ [d]iš *kin-ṣa-a*-⸢*šu*⸣ gi[g diri].meš-*šú* gu$_4$.ud.meš *u mim-ma* [*šá* gu$_7$ *i-ha-ru* ...]

25′ [d]iš *ina kin-ṣi-šu* [s]ìg-*iṣ* [šu ^{d}....] : diš *ina kin-ṣi-šu šá* 15 [sìg-*iṣ u ina* ka-*šú* múd buru$_8$ .....]

26′ [d]iš *ina kin-ṣi-šu šá* 150 *i*[*k*$^?$-*r*]*u u ina* ka-*šú* múd m[ud buru$_8$....]

27′ [d]iš gìri^2-⸢*šu*⸣ *šá* 15 gu$_7$-*šu* šu ^{d}⸢*eš*$_4$-*dar*⸣ diš gìri^2-[*š*]*u šá* 1[50 gu$_7$-*šu* šu ^{d}........]

28′ [d]iš gìri^2-*šu* gu$_7$.meš-*šu* šu ^{d}innin.na diš [gìri^2-*šu* gu$_7$.meš-*šu* šu ^{d}........ tin]

29′ [di]š gìri^2-*šu šá* 15 ⸢*i-maš-šar*⸣ [k]a-*šú ṣu-un-d*[*ur mi-šit-ti* maškim gíd-*ma* gam] (= BAD 154: 63′)

30′ [di]š [gìri]^2-*šu šá* 150 *i-maš-šar* [sìg]-*iṣ* [šu] ^{d}⸢ba.ba$_6$⸣ [sìg-*iṣ* gam] (= BAD 154: 64′)

31′ [diš gìri]^2-[*š*]*u šá* [1]5 ⸢*ik-te*⸣-*n*[*e*$^?$-*r*]*u*$^?$ šu ^{d}1[5] dab gu$_4$ [gam]

32′ [diš gìri]^2-⸢*šu šá* 150 *ik-te*⸣-*ner-ru* ⸢šu dingir-*šu*⸣ : diš gìri^2.meš *šá i*[*k-te-ner-ra* šu dingir hul dab-*su*]

33′ [diš gìri^2-*šu šá* 15]-⸢*šú*⸣ *ana šá* 1[50] lál-*at* [šu ^{d}.................]

34′ [diš gìri^2-*šu tur-r*]*a* [nu] zu-e én *i-la-at* [............ šid-*ma*.....]

35′ [diš gìri^2-*šu am-šá-ma* lál] nu zu-e *u* uš$_4$-*šú* nu dab [....] (= BAD 154: 64′ var.)

36′ [diš gìri^2-*šu it-t*]*e*-⸢*nen-gi*⸣-*ra* [šu ^{d}utu]

37′ [diš gìri^2-*šu it-te-nen-ṣi-la u it-t*]*a*-[*n*]*a-ak-na-an* š[u ^{d}.............]

1 See TDP 100: 5 and CAD A/2 439.

2 Cf. Labat, TDP 142: 16′, see AHw 994.

13′ [If] he is affected i[n his perineum, in his] cleft[1], it is the Hand of [his] God [...].

14′ [If his] knees hurt him, it is a sacrilege against [his] god [...].

15′ [If] his knees [and hips] hurt [him] in the night, (but) his body has no heat (fever), a sacrilege against Šamaš has seized him.

16′ If his (buttock)-cheeks [are always open, he will die].

17′ If his (buttock)-cheeks are always rising, he will recover.

18′ If [his] calf on the right hurts him (and) [his] temperature remains the same, [it is the Hand of Ištar, ...].

19′ If [his] calf on the left hurts [him] (and) his temperature does not remain the same, [his] illness [will be prolonged and he will recover[?]].

20′ If his [calves] hurt him (and) his temperature does not remain the same, [it is the Hand of his God, resolved].

21′ If [his] calves hurt] him, it is the Hand of the God of his city / Hand [of his God].

22′ If his calves [hurt] him, it is the Hand of Šamaš because of an (unpaid) [tithe, he will get better].

23′ If [his] calves have *k.*-disease (and) when he speaks [his spittle comes out], resolved; he stepped in dirty bath water, [...........

24′ If his calves are full of illness (and) jump about, and whatever [he eats he vomits, ...].

25′ If he is affected in his calf [it is the Hand of ...]: if [he is affected] in his right calf, and he throws up blood from his mouth [....].

26′ If his calf on the left *is short* and [throws up] dark-red blood from his mouth [...].

27′ If his foot on the right hurts him, it is the Hand of Ištar; if his left foot [hurts him, it is the Hand of ...].

28′ If (both) his feet hurt him, it is the Hand of Inanna; if his feet hurt him, it is the Hand of ..., he will recover].

29′ If he drags his foot on the right (and) his mouth twitches, [it is a stroke (caused by) the Snatcher(-demon), it will be prolonged and he will die].

30′ If he drags his foot on the left, [he has been struck a] blow by the [Hand] of Baba, [he will die].

31′ [If] his foot on the right keeps shrinking, it is the Hand of Ištar; it is seizure by a ghost, [he will die].

32′ [If] his foot on the left keeps shrinking, it is the Hand of his God; if (both) his feet keep shrinking, [the Hand of a God; evil has seized him].

33′ [If] his [foot on the right] stretches out towards his left, [it is the Hand of ....].

34′ [If] he is [not] able to [turn his foot], [let him recite] the incantation *ilat* [and ....].

35′ [If his feet are cataleptic and] he cannot [stretch them out], and his mind is not affected, [...]

36′ [If his feet] keep crossing, [it is the Hand of Šamaš].

37′ [If his feet become paralysed and become] contorted, it is the Hand [of ....]
(remainder of column broken)

---

1 See Labat, 206 n. 14, arguing for 'pubis', which is supported by J.-M. Durand, *Florilegium Marianum* VII (Paris, 2002), 136–137, 139–140, in which he demonstrates that *suhatu* refers to the pubic region.

col. iv.
[gap of c. 5 lines]

1′ [diš gìri^{2}-*šu*] x ....

2′ [diš] ⸢gìri^{2}-*šu*⸣ ta *tuḫ-ri* ⸢gig šub⸣-[*ma* ....

3′ [diš gìri]^{2}-*šu ú-ḫúl-a*[1] ⸢gig-*su*⸣ man-*ni* : diš ⸢gìri^{2}-*šu*⸣ [...]

4′ [diš gìri]^{2}-[*š*]*u* diri kuš *šá* ki.ta[2] *t*[*e-b*]*a* diš *ina* gìri^{2}-*šu* sìg-⸢*iṣ* x x šu⸣ ^{d}maš.tab.ba

5′ [diš *ina* gìri^{2}-*š*]*u šá* 15 sìg-*iṣ* šu ^{d}utu *ana* [ud..kám gam] : diš gìri^{2}-*šu šá* 150 sìg-*iṣ* šu ^{d}⸢15 gíd⸣-*ma* gam[3]

6′ [diš *ina* gìri^{2}-*š*]*u šá* 15 sìg-*iṣ u* du$_{11}$.d[u$_{11}$-*si pu-qud-de*]-*e* ^{d}utu ⸢ta⸣ ^{d}maš.tab.ba

7′ [diš *ina* gìri^{2}-*š*]*u* ⸢*šá*⸣ 150 sìg-⸢*iṣ*⸣ *u* d[u$_{11}$-*si pu-qud-de*]-⸢*e*⸣ ^{d}15 *ana* ^{d}maš.tab.ba[4]

8′ [diš *ina* gìri^{2}-*š*]*u* sìg-⸢*iṣ*⸣ *u* d[u$_{11}$-*s*]*i* [*pu*]-*q*[*ud-de-e*] ^{d}15 *ana* ^{d}maš.tab.ba (TDP 144: 37′)

9′ [diš *ina* gìri]^{2}-*šu* murub$_{4}$ [sì]g-[*i*]*ṣ* murub$_{4}$.me[š]-*šú* gig ud.[x].meš x [...*ana*] ud.41.kam šu ^{d}15

10′ diš u.meš gì[ri^{2}-*š*]*ú* [*tar-k*]*u* gíd-*ma* gam : diš u.meš gìri^{2}-*šú u*[*ṣ-ṣi-l*]*a-šú-ma* šu ^{d}*iš-ḫa-ra*

11′ [diš u].meš gìri^{2}-[*š*]*ú* ⸢dar$^{?}$⸣.[meš] x *ina* ka-*šú* ⸢gur⸣ mu kù.[babbar zà.10].⸢meš$^{?}$-*ma*$^{?}$ šu⸣ ^{d}[u.gu]r$^{?}$ gam (TDP 144: 43′ and CAD Š/2 194)

12′ [diš u.m]eš gìri^{2}-*šú* múd sa$_{5}$.meš-*ma* gu$_{7}$.meš-*šú ana la-ba-ṣu* gur-[*šum-ma*] gam (TDP 144: 45′–46′)

13′ (traces)

14′–16′ ....

17′ [diš ....] gìr[i^{2}-*šú* ....]

18′ [diš kuš *šá* ki.ta gì]ri^{2}-*šú* [zi] ⸢sag.du dab⸣-*s*[*u u* šà-*šú tur-ru-ur* gam]

19′ [diš *ka-bit-ma* gìri^{2}-*šú šá* 1]50 : *i*-⸢*ka*⸣-*na-an u* [*i-tar-ra-aṣ* gam] (TDP 144 56′)

20′ [diš sa gìri^{2}-*šú* du-*ku-ma šá* šu^{2}-*šú n*]*e*-⸢*e-ḫu ár*⸣-*ḫiš* úš [al.ti]

21′ [diš sa gìri^{2}-*šú* du-*ku-ma šá* šu^{2}-*šú* gar-*nu* ki].ta gig ku$_{4}$-*šú* níg.⸢gig⸣ [igi-*ma* tin]

22′ [diš sa gìri^{2}-*šú* zi.meš-*ú* igi^{2}-*šú ana* í]l dugud sag.du-*su u* sag š[à-*šú e-em* šu ^{d}....]

23′ [diš *ta-kap* ir zi.in.gi]-*šu* [kúm nu tuku] tin

24′ [diš *ta-kap* ir zi.in.gi-*šu* kúm] tuku *ki-iṣ*-[*ṣa*]-*ta* diri ug[u-*šú i-ša*]g-g[*ú-um* ti-*uṭ šum*$_{4}$-*ma* gig-*su*] ⸢tag$_{4}$-*šum*⸣-*ma* tin

[1] CAD E 41 s.v. *e'ēlu*, D = coagulate.

[2] see Labat, TDP 144: 54 *mašku ša šaplānu* gìri^{2}-*šú te-bi*.

[3] cf. Heeßel, BAD 154: 61′–62′

[4] Cf. Heeßel, BAD 155: 92.

col. iv

1′ [If his foot] ....

2′ [If] his foot *drops* from an aching tendon [and ....

3′ [If] his foot is *coagulated*, his illness will change; if his foot [..................

4′ [If] his [foot] drifts[1] (and) the sole of the foot rises; if he is affected in his foot, ..., it is the Hand of the Twins.

5′ [If] he is affected [in] his [foot] on the right, it is the Hand of Šamaš, towards the [... day he will die]; if he is affected in his left foot, it is the Hand of Ištar, (the illness) will be prolonged and he will die.

6′ [If] he is affected [in] his [foot] on the right and he always cries out, it is Šamaš' order from the Twins.

7′ [If] he is affected [in] his [foot] on the left and he [cries, it is] Ištar's order to the Twins.

8′ [If] he is affected [in] his [foot] and cries, [it is] Ištar's order to the Twins.

9′ [If in] his [foot] the middle is affected (and) his hips ache, ... days ..[..up to] the 41st day, it is the Hand of Ištar.

10′ If the toes of his foot [are] dark, (his illness) will be prolonged and he will die; if the toes of his foot make him lame, it is the hand of Išhara.

11′ [If] the toes of his foot are full of cuts, ... *returned* from his mouth, because of an (unpaid) tithe, it is the Hand of Nergal?, he will die.

12′ [If the] toes of his foot are full of blood and hurt him (and) turns into a *labāṣu*-demon, he will die.

13′–17′ ....

18′ [If the sole of] his foot [rises], he is seized in the head, [and his bowel is quaking, he will die].

19′ [If he is troubled and his foot] on the left: twists and [stretches out, he will die].

20′ [If the sinews of his foot 'go' while the ones of his hands] are still, he will die quickly; [he will live].

21′ [If the sinews of his foot 'go' while of his hands are stationary], illness has entered him from below, he has [witnessed] a sacrilege [and he will recover].

22′ [If the sinews of his foot rise up], it is difficult [to] raise [his eyes, he is hot in] his head and [his] epigastrium, [it is the Hand of .....].

23′ [If there is a prickling from sweat,] his ankles [have no heat], he will recover.

24′ [If there is a prickling from sweat, his ankles] have [heat], it is full of *k*.-disease and [his] head buzzes [(but) he will live. If his illness] leaves him, he will recover.

---

[1] cf. CAD N/2, ***neqelpû***, 'to drift, sail downstream', and MSL 9 78 f., gìri-gá ba-an-gur$_4$ (var. du) = (*še-pí*) *i-te-eq-lip-an-ni*. Heeßel, BAD, 416, translates this word as 'schwindlig werden', which fits the contexts he cites but is not appropriate for our passage.

No. 50 AMT 22,2

AC = K3550 = AMT 22,2 (collated)[1]
AN = VAT 8269 (BAM 253) = ll. 11–28
AO = K 5834 + (BAM 579 iii 20–24, *suālu*) = rev. 22–24

cf. also BAM 95 1–4[2], AMT 21,2 and for both texts, PRSM 19, 55 f. and 56 f.

1 AC [diš na g]ú *u* sag-*šú ú-zaq-qata-su* igi.meš-*šú* nigin.meš-*du*
2 AC [^{na4}ki]šib gú-*su* sìg.sìg-*su* sa gú-*šú* gu$_7$.meš-*šú*
3 AC [*i-d*]*a-a-šú* gaba-*su šá-šal-la-šú u* maš.sìla.meš-*šú* gu$_7$.meš-*šú*
4 AC [im *i*]-*kal-la* šà.meš-*šú* mú.mú.meš-*hu ir-ru-šú i-ár-ru-ru*
5 AC [x] ⌜x⌝ šu^2-*šú* gìr-*šú ù kin-ṣa-šú i-kaṣ-ṣa-ṣa-šú*
6 AC [*šim*]-*mat* tuk-*ú lu* murub$_4$.meš-*šú* gig *lu* éllag.meš-*šú* tag.meš-*šú*
7 AC [*l*]*u hi-níq-tu* gig *lu hi-niq* dúr gig *lu hi-niq* bún
8 AC [g]ig *lu sa-hi*[3] éllag gig *lu* zé gig *lu a-mur-ri-qa-nu* gig
9 AC [lu] nam.érim gig *lu maš-ka-du lu* sa.gal *lu* šu.gedim.ma
10 AC [lu *šu-k*]*ul u šá-qi lu* sag.hul.ha.zu gig *ana maš-tak-ti-šú*[4] *bul-lu-ṭi*
11 AC [^{ú}]úkuš.hab ^{na4}úkuš.hab ^{ú}*si-hu* ^{ú}*ár-gan-ni* ^{ú}*ba-ri-rat*
AN ^{ú}úkuš.hab $^{na4.ú}$min ^{ú}*si-hu* ^{ú}*ár-gán-nu* ^{ú}za.hum[5] ^{ú}*ar-man-nu*
12 AC [x x ^{giš}*š*]*u-šum* suhuš ^{giš}*šu-šum* ^{giš}nam.tar níta
AN ^{ú}*ak-tam* ^{ú}*šu-šum* suhuš ^{ú}*šu-šum* ^{ú}nam.tar níta
13 AC [x x x *kam-k*]*a-du* ^{ú}áb.duh ^{ú}*áp-ru-šú* ^{giš}naga.si
AN suhuš ^{ú}min ^{ú}*kam-ka-du* ^{ú}áb.duh ^{ú}*áp-ru-šú* ^{ú}naga.si
14 AC [x x x ^{ú}]ku$_6$ suhuš ^{ú}ku$_6$ ^{ú}*ṣa-ṣu-*[*un-t*]*u*$_4$ ^{ú}eme.ur.gir$_7$
AN ^{giš}še.ná.a numun ^{giš}min ^{ú}*ṣa-ṣu-un-tú* ^{ú}eme.ur.gir$_7$ ^{ú}ku$_6$ suhuš ^{ú}ku$_6$
15 AC [.......................................] ⌜x ^{ú}*a-la*⌝*-mu-u* ^{ú}⌜geštin⌝.ka$_5$.a
AN ^{ú}a.zal.lá numun ^{ú}min ^{ú}*ṣa-da-nu* ^{ú}*a-la-mu-u* ^{ú}geštin.ka$_5$.a
16 AC [.......................................] ⌜ x x x ti x x ⌝
AN ^{ú}lag.gán ^{šim}gúr.gúr ^{šim}li gazi^{sar} *ši-te-e* gazi^{sar}
17 AN ^{ú}kur.kur numun ^{ú}kur.kur ^{šim}gír ^{šim}sal
18 AN $^{šim.d}$maš ^{šim}gam.ma ^{ú}nu.luh.ha $^{ú.zè}$min
19–20 AN broken
21 AN ^{ú}sikil ⌜^{ú}⌝[.................] x ^{ú}ki.^{d}iškur [...] x x -na
22 AN ^{ú}*a-nu-nu-tú* ^{ú}⌜*ši*⌝-[*im*$^?$]-*ra* ^{ú}*tara-muš* ^{ú}igi-*lim*
23 AN ^{ú}igi-*ešra* ^{ú}*kur-ka-nam* ^{ú}kur.ra ^{ú}*ur-nu-*[*ú* ^{giš}gišim]mar.tur
24 AN ^{giš}šul.hi ⌜^{ú}⌝[*a*]-*ri-bu*[6] ^{ú}[..] x a peš$_{10}$.^{d}íd úh.^{d}íd
25 AN ^{ú}*še-ma-ha* ^{ú}*tuš-ru* hénbur ^{giš}dìh hénbur ^{giš}kiši$_{16}$ ^{giš}eren

---

[1] The ductus of this tablet is similar to that of text No. 32 (AMT 56,1) and may have been written by the same scribe.

[2] See text No. 21.

[3] passage cited in CAD S 67a, but see also ibid. 56b, *sahhu* and also *sihhu* < zah, (scar). These are all likely to be the same word, referring to *sāhu*-disease of the kidneys and bladder. Cf. BAM 78: 17 (reference courtesy M. Stol) for a text against a spleen ailment (l. 1: diš na *tu-lim-šú* gu$_7$-*šú* ud *u* ge$_6$ *la i-ṣal-lal* [*ana* ti]-*šú* ...). Line 17 (at the end of the recipe) has: *sa-hi* bir x [....], probably referring to *sāhu*-disease in the kidney.

[4] Cf. CAD M/1 171, *maltaktu*, 'water clock', perhaps related to *latāku*, CAD L 111, given there as 'meaning uncertain', associated with oil (*šaman latāki*). We would suggest a bi-form of *natāku*, 'to drip', which would fit well with the water clock. The metaphor here is that the body functions like a water clock, for which there is a parallel in Aristotle, citing Empedocles, comparing breathing with the workings of a water clock (see Aristotle *On Respiration* 7 473b, Loeb edition vol. viii, 445 f.).

[5] For *sīhu*, although one might expect lum.ha for *barīrātu* in this sequence.

[6] Usually *šēp aribi*, if this is the same plant.

TRANSLATION

1 [If a man's] neck and head cause him pain and he has vertigo,
2 [and] his neck vertebrae constantly cause him pain and the veins of his neck hurt,
3 his arms, chest, back and shoulders hurt,
4 he retains [wind], his bowels are bloated, his intestines discharge (a putrid liquid),
5 ... his hands, feet, and shins gnaw (at him),
6 he has paralysis, either his hips are ailing or his kidneys constantly afflict him
7 or he suffers from a stricture, or stricture of the anus, or stricture of the bladder,
8 or he suffers from a 'scar' of the kidney or suffers from bile or from jaundice
9 [or] suffers from a curse or suffers from *maškadu*-disease or *sagallu*-disease or the 'Hand of a Ghost'(-disease)
10 [or] being given (bewitched) food and drink or is suffering from the 'evil-attendant-demon'; to heal his 'clock-works' (i. e., body functions),
11 cucumber and ditto-stone, *sīhu*, *argānu*, *barīrātu*,
12 *aktam*, *šūšu*-tree and root, male mandrake,
13 male mandrake-root, *kamkadu*, *kamantu*, *aprušu*, horned alkali,
14 *šunû*, *urânu*, seed of *urânu* (var. seed of *šunû*), *ṣaṣumtu*, 'dog's-tongue'-plant,
15 *azallû*, *azallû* seed, *ṣadānu*, *alamû*, fox-vine-plant,
16′ field-clod'-plant, *kukru*, juniper, *kasû*, shoots[?] of *kasû*,
17 *ata'išu*, *ata'išu* seed, myrtle, *šimeššalû*,
18 *nikiptu*, *ṣumlalû*, *nuhurtu*, flour of *nuhurtu*
19–20 ....
21 *sikillu*, [...........] *qudru* [...]...
22 *anunūtu*, fennel[?], *taramuš*, *imhur-līm*,
23 *imhur-ešra*, *kurkānû*, *nīnû*, *urnû*, young date palm (*suhuššu*),
24 *šalālu*(-reed), *aribu*[?], *rutītu*(-mineral),
25 boxthorn, *tušru*, sprout of *baltu*-thorn, sprout of acacia-thorn, cedar,

26 AN ⸢ì.giš$^{!}$⸣ ^{giš}*dap-r*[*a*]*-nu* gi.du$_{10}$.ga ^{šim}man.du pap 75 ú.meš šeš

---

27 AN *mal-ma-liš ta-ka-sim* [*ana*$^{?}$] *lìb-bi* kàš.meš *ru-še-te-e šá* lú.meš
28 AN ⸢a⸣.meš gazi^{sar}*u* kaš šub-*di* [*ina* š]à ra.meš-*su* gig dù.a.bi su.na du$_{8}$

---

gap
rev.

1′ AC [..............................] súd x x [..................
2′ AC [....................................] *lap-*⸢*pu lat*⸣-[*ku*[1] ...

3′ AC [...................... l]i$^{?}$ *lap-pu* [..................]
4′ AC [....................] x illu ^{šim}bulug ^{ú}kur.⸢gi.rín.na x x ⸣ [....]
5′ AC [................] x tar ì.giš ka.ka.sa$_{5}$[2] *ana na-hir-šú* [gar-*an*]

6′ AC [............] x ⸢suhuš$^{?}$⸣ ^{giš}gúr.gúr ^{šim}li ^{ú}kur.kur ^{ú}*a-ši-*⸢*i*⸣ [.....]
7′ AC [............] x ša$^{?}$ sig$_{5}$ diš-*niš* gaz ki dída ⸢sig$_{5}$⸣[3] hi.hi x [.......
8′ AC [.........*ina*] ⸢a gazi^{sar}⸣ *i-ra-muk* ì.giš ^{šim}gúr.gúr šéš-[*su* din]

9′ AC [....] x ^{ú}kur.ra ⸢^{giš}li⸣ ^{giš}šinig suhuš ^{ú}kur.kur ⸢$^{\text{šim.d}}$maš ^{šim}gúr.gúr⸣
10′ AC [....] hi.hi *te-sér-šú*$^{!}$*-ma*[4] *ina-eš*

11′ AC [......] ⸢x *ana*$^{?}$ lú$^{?}$⸣ *bul-*⸢*lu-ṭu*$^{?}$⸣ ^{šim}gúr.gúr ^{šim}li ^{ú}har.har numun ^{ú}*qut-ri*
12′ AC [........] ⸢ú.meš⸣ šeš.meš gaz sim zà.hi.li *qa-lu-*⸢*ti*⸣
13′ AC [ina ^{urudu}]šen.tur *tara-bak ina* kuš šur lá-*su-ma* din

---

14′ AC [.....................] ⸢*ga*⸣*-bu-u* ^{ú}nu.luh.ha ú bábbar ^{šim}li ^{šim}gúr.gúr
15′ AC [....................] diš-*niš* ⸢gaz⸣ sim *ina* ì.udu éllag udu níta gaba.làl
16′ AC [.............*al*]*la-nu* dù *ana* dúr-*šú* gar-*an alla-nu kal-la* ti
17′ AC [.......... ^{ú}a.zal].lá ^{ú}kur.kur ^{ú}kur.ra ^{ú}⸢*úr-né*⸣*-e* ^{ú}nu.luh.ha
18′ AC [..............^{gi}]^{š}man.du ⸢mun x ì$^{?}$.udu$^{?}$⸣ udu *lu-u* máš.gal
19′ AC [................] x meš lú [..............] x x *qí-lip* zú.lum.ma x x
20′ AC [................] ì.giš [...................] ⸢*ú*$^{?}$⸣*-na-šar*$^{?}$
21′ AC [..............] lum ⸢è.a x x x x x a

---

lower edge

22′ AC [..................... gi]š.⸢šà$^{?}$⸣.gi$^{?}$ ^{šim}gúr.gúr ^{šim}li gázi^{sar} *sah*$^{?}$*-lu-u*
AO diš na sa x [..] gázi^{sar} *sa*[*h*.....
23′ AC [....................] har.har[5] ^{ú}*ur-né-e* ^{ú}kur.ra ^{ú}hur.sag
AO [.............................]^{ú}*ur-nu-*[*u* ....
24′ AC [............................] x 15 ú.meš *ina* kaš a níg.àr.ra [hi.hi *ina* dúr-*šú*] dub-*ak*
AO ^{ú}maš.tab.ba [..........................] *ina* kaš a níg.àr.[ra ....]

---

1 See CAD L 200, BAM 3 iv 22
2 Might this be a pseudo-logogram for the plant/stone name *kakkassu/kakkussu* (CAD K 60)?
3 *našpu*.
4 Cf. CAD S 228–9.
5 from AMT: these signs are no longer visible on the tablet (coll.)

26 oil of *daprānu*, sweet reed, *suādu*, total of these 75 drugs,

27 you cut (them) up equally and add it to red human urine,
28 juice of *kasû* and beer, you bathe him [in] the ingredients, and all the illness in his body will be dissolved.

gap

rev. (on A)

1′ Crush [..................................] .... [............
2′ [..], a tested tampon.

3′ [..................] tampon [................
4′ [...................] resin of *baluhhu*, *kurkānû* ...[..........
5′ [.............]... oil of .... [you put it] into his nostril.

6′ [.........] root?of *kukru*, juniper, *ata'išu*, *ašû*, [.....
7′ [........] .... crush together and mix with *frothy*[1] *billatu*-beer ....
8′ he will wash [his ..... in] *kasû*-juice and anoint [himself with] *kukru*-oil [and he will improve].

9′ [......] *nīnû*, juniper, tamarisk, root of *ata'išu*, *nikiptu*, *kukru*
10′ mix [...], you rub him and he will get better.

11′ [.....] in order to heal the man, *kukru*, juniper, *hašû*, *qutru* seed,
12′ crush and sieve these [...] drugs, you decoct (them) in roasted *sahlû* in
13′ a small vessel, spread it on leather and bind him (with it) and he will improve.

14′ [...............] alum, *nuhurtu*, 'white'-plant, juniper, *kukru*,
15′ [....................] crush and sieve together, in fat of a kidney of a male sheep and wax
16′ [................], make a suppository and insert it into his anus. Take a suppository (and) *bowl*,
17′ [...........] *azallû*, *ata'išu*, *nīnû*, *urnû*, *nuhurtu*,
18′ [............] *suādu*, salt, .. fat(?) of a sheep or goat,
19′ [.........] ..... [...........], date-peel ...,
20′ [.....................] oil of [...........] ....
21′ [..............] ....

22′ If a man ... [..............................]... *kukru*, juniper, *kasû*, *sahlû*,
23′ [.....................] *hašû*, *urnû*, *nīnû*, *azupīru*,
24′ *māštu*, [......... mix] 15 drugs in beer and groats-water, pour it [into his anus].

[1] See above, text No. 9 iv 13.

No. 51 Lexical tablet which includes many disease names. Bab. Excav. No. 47097 (Photo2940/2941) (plates 36–37)

obv.

[a]-⸢gar⸣- r[a]	[x x x]	
[a]-gar-ra	x [x x]	
[a]-gar-ra	*bi*- x – [x]	
[a-ga]r-gar-ra	*qú-lì*[*p-tu*]	'scaly skin'
[x] x gar-ra	*es-l*[u_4]	'constipated'
a-gal-la-ti-la	*ka-ši im-*tu_4	'helps against poison'
a-gal-la-ti-la	*ma-li-a me-e*	'dropsy' lit. 'full of fluid'
a íd-gál	MIN	
a hul-a	MIN[1]	
a-bar-ra	*sim-*tu_4	'red'?[2]
a-bar-ra	*te-qú-ú-*tu_4	'*Augenblitzen*'[3]
a-bar-ra	*haṣ-bi-*tu_4	'splinter/greenness'[4]
a-bar-ra	*re-hu-*tu_4 *a-hi-*tu_4	'strange emission'
a-bar-ra	MIN *na-kar-*tu_4	'foreign emission'
a-bar-ra	MIN *pa-ra-su*	'to stop the emission'
a-bar-bar-ra	*nam-šu*	'dew'[5]
a-bar-bar-ra[6]	zu_x(*su*)-tu_4 *i-bàr-ru-ur* in_6	'sweat blurs the eye'[7]
a-hal-hal	MIN	
a-kaš$_4$-kaš$_4$	MIN[8]	
a-bar-dug$_4$	*bi-hu-ú* = *bī'u*	'Durchlass'[9]
a-bar-dug$_4$	*iz-bu-um*	'malformed foetus'[10]
a-bar-dug$_4$	*ku-bu-um*	'miscarriage'
a-bar-⸢dug$_4$⸣	⸢*a*⸣*-hu-um*	'strange (birth)'
a-bar-[dug$_4$]	[*zu-*tu_4 *i-bàr-ru*]-*ur* in_6	'[sweat] blurs the eye'[11]
a-bar-[dug$_4$]	[x x] -tu_4	
a-bar-kúr-x	[x x] -tu_4	
a-bar-kúr-x	[x x x]	
⸢a⸣-bar-kár-kúr	[x x x]	

rev.

a-ra-ah	ŠU	
a-ra-ah	*na-hal-*lu_4	'wadi'[12]

---

[1] The tablet shows the number 3 rather than MIN.

[2] > *siāmu*, describing the eye, as in the following two lines.

[3] cf. AHw 1361 s. v. *tiqqûtu*.

[4] Cf. AHw 348 s. v. *hiṣibtu*, or < *haṣābu*, 'grün sein', *ibid.* 331.

[5] *nalšu*, 'dew', another possible metaphor for a medical problem.

[6] See PSD A/1 50.

[7] See CT 18 49 ii 17, for a similar expression.

[8] The tablet shows the number 3 rather than MIN.

[9] AHw 134, CAD B 297, referring to a drainage opening in a wall, which we interpret here as a metaphor for diarrhoea.

[10] see PSD A/1 49 and 50, also for the following entry, and cf. MSL IX 29. For the translations of *izbu*, *kūbu*, and *ahû*, cf. CT 18 49 ii 8–11 and CT 19 33 (80-7-19, 307): 10–13.

[11] see l. 17 above.

[12] Cf. CAD N/1 124, giving Sum. as uh.ru.um, har, hur.ru.um, one of which might reflect our text.

a-ra-ah	*šu-um-qú-*tu_4	'struck with pestilence'
a-ra-ah	IZI *te-eb-*tu_4	'high (lit. risen) fever'
⸢a⸣-ra-ab	ŠU	
[a]-ra-ab	IZI *te-eb-*tu_4	'high fever'
[a]-ra-ab	*ra-ab-bu-ú*	'soft'
[a-r]a-zu	*su-up-pu-ú*	'to pray'
[a-ra]-zu	*te-ès-li-*tu_4	'prayer'
[a-ra-z]u	*te-me-qu*	'prayer'
[x x x]	[*a*]-⸢*a*?⸣ *it-tu-ur* x	
[x x x]	[*m*]*á-an-gu*	'paralysis'
[x x x]	[x]-*a-an-nu*	
[x x x]	[*la*]-*a-b*[*u*](?)	'skin disease'
(traces)		

(rest broken)

Notes: cf. MSL 13 p. 74 s.v. a-bar-ra, with a gloss *sà-ah-sà-ha-t*[*um*], see also MSL 15 p. 43: 322–323.

School texts

No. 52 BM 42576 + 43546 + 43589 (81-7-1, 336 + 1310 + 1353); (Babylon)

publication: I. L. Finkel, FsWGL 159 f.
recipe for a sore anus (dúr.gig)

obv.

2 gar gúr.gúr 1 gar ⸢li⸣
[1 g]ín ^{šim}gig 1 gín *ka-mu-nu*
1 g[ín] *a-zu-pi-ri* 1/2 gín *ha-*⸢*še-e*⸣
1 gín *uh-hu-lu* 1 gín *si-i-hu*
1 gín *ár-gan-nu*
1 ⸢gín⸣ *ba-ri-ra-tu*$_4$
1 [gín] *ir-ru-ú u* 1 <gín> *tara-muš*
⸢*ina*⸣ x + [.... sìla ka]š še.bar šeg$_6$-*šal*
⸢*a*⸣-[*di-i a-na*] ⸢1/2⸣ sìla gur.re
[*mar-ha-ṣ*]*u šá* dúr gig

---

rev.

[......] ^{šim}li
[....] x *ka-mu-nu*
x x *si-im-bi-ri*
⸢ú⸣ babbar ⸢ukuš⸣.hab$^{!}$
m[*á*]*l-ma-liš ta-sa-qu*
ina làl hi.hi ⸢*alla*⸣*-nu šá*
dúr gig du$_{10}$.ga

1/2 ⸢gín⸣ *ka-mu-nu* 4-*ut ak-tam*
[1 g]ín *mur-ri* 4-*ut* ^{šim}hab
[*i-n*]*a* kaš sumun hi.hi
[....] *šá* ⸢uh⸣ *u ri-šu-tú*

TRANSLATION (cf. I. L. Finkel)

You boil (l. 8) 2 gar of *kukru* 1 gar of juniper,
[1] shekel of *kanaktu*, 1 shekel of *cumin*,
1 shekel of *azupiru*, half shekel of *hašû*,
1 shekel of horned alkali, 1 shekel of *sīhu*
1 shekel of *argannu*
1 shekel of *barīrātu*
1 [shekel] of *irrû* and 1 (shekel) of *taramuš*
in x litres of barley beer
until it is reduced to half litre.
A lotion for a 'sick rectum'.

You crush (l. 15) [....] of juniper,
[....].. of *kamūnu*,
... of *šibbiru*[1]
'white' plant, cucumber,
in equal amounts
and mix in honey; a suppository for
improving rectal disease.

Mix (l. 20) one half shekel of *kamūnu*, a 4th (measure) of *aktam*,
[1] shekel of *murru*, a 4th (measure) of *ṭūru*
in old beer,
[a lotion?] for lice and itching.

---

[1] = *šibburatu*? / šimbirida?

No. 53 BM 42342 (81-7-1, 102); (Babylon)

publication: I. L. Finkel, FsWGL 163 f.
recipe for 'stricture' (*hiniqtu*)

1 gar gu$_4$.gal
1 gar gu$_4$.tur
1 gar numun ⸢gada⸣
1 gar ^{šim}li
1 gar *mu-un-du ka-si-ia*
1 gar *si-in-du* gig.ba
1/2 gar ^{ú}kur.ra
1/2 ⸢gar⸣ ^{ú}*úr-né-e*
1/2 gar ^{ú}*ha-še-*⸢*e*⸣
1/2 gar ^{ú}*e-la-lim*
šal-šú gar ^{ú}nu.luh.ha
1/2 gar *ka-mu-nu*
1 gar ^{šim}gúr.gúr
1/2 gar ^{ú}*ak-tam*
1/2 gar ^{ú}maš.tab.ba
1/2 gar *kar-šú*
1/2 gar numun ^{ú}*ši-mit-tu*$_4$
1/2 gar numun ^{ú}numun.hur.sag
1/2 gar *si-in-du* x
1/2 gín ^{ú}kur.ku[r]

rev.

2 gín ^{šim}gig
1/2 gín ^{giš}eren
1/2 gín ^{giš}šur.mìn
1/2 gín ^{šim}gír
1/2 gín ^{šim}sal
2 gín ^{šim}mug *sa-pan*
2 gín gi.du$_{10}$.ga
1/2 gín ^{šim}šeš
2 gín *kur-ban-ni* a.šà
3 gín ^{šim}mìn.du
1/2 gín *si-i-hu*
1/2 gín *ar-ga-nu*
⸢1/2 gín⸣ *ba-ri-rat*
2 gín úkuš.hab
pap 34 ú.hi.a *i-na*
1 bán 1 sìla kaš še.[b]ar šeg$_6$-*šal*
a-di 1 bán 1 sìla gur *ta-šah-hal*
1 gar ì.giš *hal-ṣu*
1 gar ì.[nu]n.na
1 gar ⸢ì.udu⸣ udu.nita
1 gín ⸢*in-za*⸣*-ru-ú*
1/2 [g]ín *hi* x *-a-na*
ši-[*i*]*m*$^?$*-ru*$^?$ x x x ru
[..] x x [...] ku

left edge

a.meš ì.giš *ina* igi dù-*uš mar-*[*ha*]-*ṣu šá hi-*⸢*niq*⸣-*tú*

No. 54 BAM 89 (Assur)

AB	=	Ass. 13955bu = BAM 89
Y	=	K 2433+ [text no. 24 iv 6′–7′]

1	AB	diš na *k*[*i-is* šà gig ....]
2	AB	ninda *u* a *tur-ra* šà-*šú* x [......]
3	AB	tùn.šà-*šú ub-*⸢*bu*⸣-*ṭa-at* [.......]
4	AB	^{ú}*tara-muš ina* kaš.sag na[g-*ma*]
5	AB	^{šim}li ^{šim}gúr.gúr ^{giš}[................]
6	AB	súd *ina* ì.udu hi.hi šu.si [dù-*uš*]
		ana dúr-*šú* gar-*an-ma* t[i]

rev.

8	AB	diš na *a-ha-šú kìn-ṣa-šú ki-ṣil-la-šú* [gig]
	Y	[diš.na] ⸢á$^{?}$⸣-*šú* [................................gi]g
9	AB	na.bi *qé-reb* dúr.gig ^{šim}[....]
	Y	na.bi *qé-reb* dúr gi[g]
10	AB	ì.udu ^{šim}gig súd *ina* ì.ud[u hi.hi]
	Y	[..]
11	AB	šu.si dù-*uš ana* dúr-*šú* gar-*an-m*[*a* ti]
	Y	⸢šu.si⸣ dù-*uš ana* dúr-*šú* gar-*a*[*n*]

TRANSLATION

If a man [suffers from] colic [...........]
(and) food and drink are regurgitated, his bowel .....
his *abdomen* is cramped ....
he drinks *taramuš* in premium beer,
crush juniper, *kukru*, ...
and mix (them) in fat, [make] a pessary
and insert it into his anus and he will improve.

rev.

If a man's arms, shins, and ankles [are sore],
that man is sore in the rectum.
Crush ..[...], fat, *kanaktu*, [mix them] in fat,
make a pessary and and insert it into his anus and [he will improve].

No. 55 BAM 258 (Assur)

A 216 (BAM 258)

[.............] babbar
[...................]-*ra*
x x [....] a
gú.gal
gú.tur
ú numun *la-di-ri*
numun gada
ina kaš.sag
šeg_6-*šal*
làl *u* ì
ana igi šub
ana dúr-*šú* dub

TRANSLATION

Boil [.............................] pea, lentil, *ladiru*-seed (herb) (and) flax seed in premium beer, put honey and oil into it, and pour it into his anus.

No. 56 BAM 117 (Assur, kidney disease text)

VAT 13910 (BAM 117)

[diš.na ....] *mu-ṣa* gig *ana* ti-*šú*
[......................................] *úr-né-e* ^{ú}*ak-tam*
[....................................^{ú}h]ar.har ^{ú}*kar-kar-te*
[............................ ^{ú}nam.t]i.la ^{šim}gúr.gúr
[.........................^{ú}*hal-ta-p*]*a-an-nu* ^{giš}šùr.mín
[....................................] gazi^{sar} ^{giš}man.du
[................................^{š}]^{im}buluh
(traces)
[.......................................].meš
[.............................. ^{urudu}]šen.⸢tur⸣
[.............................*ina*] ⸢mul_4⸣ *tuš-bat*
[.................................] x -*šú* ⸢nag⸣-*ma* ti

No. 57 BAM 118 (Assur, kidney disease text)

VAT 13908 (BAM 118)

1′ [............................] x an.zah.ge$_{6}$: :

2′ [..........................] ⸢u$_{5}$⸣.gar.ib^{mušen} : :

3′ [..................................... ^{ši}]^{m}šeš : :

4′ [..................................^{ši}]^{m}šeš ^{šim}še.li babbar a.geštin.na diš-*niš*
5′ [..................................*tu*]*š-bat ina* ^{urudu}šen.tur šeg$_{6}$-*šal u$_{4}$-ma* šeg$_{6}$.gá
6′ [.................................^{ši}]^{m}buluh ì *hal-ṣa ana* šà šub *ana* gìš-*šú* dub-*ak*

7′ [..........................] $^{⸢ú⸣}$*úr-ni-i ina* ì *hal-ṣa ana* gìš-*šú* dub
8′ [..] súd : :

Indices

Catalogue of incipits in BAM VII

Medical texts tend to duplicate individual recipes rather than entire compositions, and it is therefore useful to record incipits of medical recipes, i. e., passages beginning with diš na (= *šumma amīlu*) or incantations beginning with én.

Renal Disease Texts

No. 1 CBS 19801 BAM 396

10′ diš na *ta-at-ti-kam šá šīnāti maruṣ*

14′ diš na *ša-a-ši-tu-nam un-nu-ut ù ma-gal ittenebbi*

23′ diš na *kalīt-su ikkalšu qablā-šú iltanappatā-šú ù šīnāti-šú kīma šināt imēri peṣâ arki šīnāti-šu dama ú-kal-la-ma amīlu šû mu-ṣa-am maruṣ*

col. ii

25′ diš na *abna maruṣ*

col. iv

3 [diš n]a *ina ušari-šú dama ú-tab-ba-kám kīma aššāti kakka ma-hi-*[*i*]*ṣ*

6 [d]iš na *i-na-aṭ-ma i-na alāki-šu re-hu-us-su illak-ma la īdi kīma ša ūri-šu illak-ma ma-as-ra-ah ušari-šu bubu'ti ma-li*

13 diš na *iška-šú maruṣ*

15 diš na *iška ēda* <*maruṣ*> *zuqaqīpa balṭa urrubba šamni tumalli*

No. 2 K 2405 = + AMT 31,1 +

1 [diš na] *mi-na-tu-šú ittanašpakā idā-šú kim-ṣa-a-šú ù bir-ka-šú* [*ikkalā-šú*]

3 [diš] na *naglabā-šú ikkalā-šú i-ta-an-na-ah im-ta-na-aš-ši ramānu ṭe*$_4$*-en-šú i*[*š-ta-na-an-ni*]

16 diš na *hi-niq-ti ellibuhhi maruṣ*

18 diš na *ana šīnāti-šú aš-ṭu-ú-tì* x [*hi-ni*]*q-ti ellibuhhi maruṣ*

33 diš na *hi-niq ellibuhhi maruṣ*

35 diš na gig *hi-niq ellibuhhi maruṣ*

col. ii

3 [diš na *hi*]*-niq-ti maruṣ*

22 diš na *qablā-šú lu ina alāki-šú lu ina ṣalāli-šú lupputu-šú u*[*šar-šú* ....] *uzaqqat-su ú-ha-ma-at-su i-tar-rak-šú arki šīnāti-šú iš-t*[*i-nu* ....]

No. 2a

Text B_1 = K 7230

5′ [d]iš na *i-na-aṭ-ma ina alāki-šu re-hu-us-su illak-ma la īdê [kīma š]a ūri-šu illak-ma ma-as-ra-ah ušari-šu bubu'ti ma-li*

9′ [diš na *ina alāki-šú r*]*e-hu-su illak-ma la īdi ka-la ú-ri-šú* [..............] *bubu'āti ṣehherēti mali*

12′ [diš na *ištu*] *ušari-šú damu šarku uṣṣū-šú kīma ṣi-bit barbari lu* x [.....]

14′ [diš na ...... *t*]*as-li-a-te-šú ilappatū-šú šīnāti-šú ṣubbutā*$^{t[a}$ ....]

Text B_2 =AMT 40,3 = K 13403

9′ [diš na...*nup*]*puh-ma libbi-šú ṣa-bit-m*[*a* ....

Text B_4 = S 467 (AMT 58,5)

3′ diš na sa tùm [............

6′ diš na *ina šināti-šú da*[*ma ú-tab-ba-kam* ....

9′ diš na *kis libbi-šú mahiṣ* [............................

B_5 = K 5864

2′ [diš.na *uš*]*ar-šú uzaqqat-su u_4-ma šināti-šú i-šá-ti-nu re-*[*hu-su iddâ*[a] *ina libbi-šú ṣa-bit-ma*]

No. 3 VAT 9871 + 10397 BAM 111

16 [diš.n]a *ušar-šú ú-zaq-qa-su u_4-ma šināti-šú i-šá-ti-nu re-hu-su iddâ*[a]

col. ii

15′ diš na *ša-a-ši-ta-na un-nu-un-ta*

21′ diš na *šināti-šú ut-ta-na-tak ka-la-a la i-la-a' ellibuhha-šu he-sa-at*

Ms. YY = A 239 (BAM 161 v 15–20)

15 diš na *ana šināti-šú ma-gal ittenebbi*

No. 4 VAT 9870 + 10095 BAM 112

17′ [diš.n]a *ušar-šú ú-zaq-qa-su u_4-ma šināti-šú i-šá-ti-nu re-hu-su iddâ*[a]

34′ [diš.na *ušar-šú*] *uzaqqat-su u_4-ma šināti-šú i-šá-ti-nu re-hu-su iddâ*[a]

col. ii

6′ diš na *ušar-šú īmim* [....................] *ṣēta kašid* x [................

8′ diš na [*uša*]*ri-šú šāru iš-biṭ* [..

11′ diš na *ušari-šú šāru iš-biṭ* [.............................] *bubu'ti malû*

15′ diš na *qablā*^{2}*-šú maruṣ-m*[*a* ....

17′ diš na *ina ušari-šú dama ú-tab-ba-ka kīma sinništi kakka ma-hi-iṣ*

No. 6 VAT 8693 BAM 115

14′ [diš.n]a *ina ṣalāli-šú šināti-šú iš-tin-ma*

rev.

4′ [diš.na *ina ṣal*]*āli-šú šināti-šú* ⌜*iš-tin*⌝-[*ma* ....

No. 7 A 267 BAM 116

1 diš na *mu-ṣa maruṣ*

rev.

8′ diš na *ana šināti-šú ma-gal ittenebbi*^{bi}

No. 8 AMT 66,7 = S 261

7 diš na *mu-ṣa maruṣ*

18 [diš na *kalīt-su ikkalšu qablā-šú iltanappatā*]*-šú ù šināti-šú kīma šināt imēri peṣâ arki šināti-šu dama ú-kal-la-ma amīlu šû mu-ṣa-am maruṣ*

No. 9 AMT 82,1 + = K 4957+ kidneys tablet 3

1 diš na da[b *kalīt-su*................................

39 én ⸢^{d}⸣[gu.la.................] ⸢x *at-ti-ma*⸣ dingir.mah *at-ti-ma mu-bal-li-ṭa-at pagra*

44 én ^{d}gu.la nin an.ta gal [an.ú]r.ta n[am.t]a.[è]

col. ii

1′ ⸢én⸣ *a-ta-mar* [*pa*]-⸢*né-e*⸣-*k*[*i* ^{d}*gu-la a-s*]*u-gal-la-tú ṣir-tú*

9′ [én *a*]-*na* ^{d}*gu-la lik-tar-ra-ba ka-liš tubqāti*

39′ diš na *lu abna mu-ṣa maruṣ* [...................................

col. iii

9′ diš na *libbi ušari-šú maruṣ-ma šināti-šú uttanatak*

col. iv

19′ [diš n]a *išik-šú mun-ga ṣabit*

20′ diš na *išik-šú šarka ú-kal*

21′ diš na *mi-qit ir-ri irtaši*

31′ (catchline): diš na *ina la si-ma-ni-šú qablā*[*-šú ikkalā-šú*] (see text No. 22)

Addendum: VAT 9024 (= KAR 73) obv.

1 [*e-nu-m*]*a* diš na *lu-u pàr-dan-nu lu-u š*[*a*]*h-hi-h*[*u*]

No. 11 K 6493 +

39′ én [^{d}g]*u*-[*l*]*a* nin an.⸢ta⸣.gal an.ú[r.ta nam.ta.è] (see No. 9: 44)

No. 13 AMT 39, 6 = Rm II, 375

6′ [dub.x.kam] diš na *kalīt-su* [*aklat-su*]

7′ [diš na .... *i-te-ni*]*k-ki-ik amīlu šû abna šá-hi-ih-ta* [*maruṣ*....

No. 14 K13405 + S 804 + 926 (all AMT 89,4) + 2160 (AMT 53,8)

4′ diš na *hi-niq-ti q*[*ablī* ....

6′ [diš n]a *abna maruṣ* x [.................

8′ diš na *abnu š*[*a*]*h-hi-hu* x [..................

No. 15 AMT 2,7 (K 1847)

3′ [diš na .... *mar*]*ṣā*^{a} *abna maruṣ-ma* ⸢*la ṣa-a*⸣-[*du* ....

8′ [diš na ....] x *itaddâ*^{a} *embūb hašê-šú ú-na-qar-šú* [.............

No. 16 = AMT 66,11 + = K 11230 + 11280 + 16437 + S. 126

6′ [diš na.............] x *ù šināti-šú it-ta-na-aṣ-ba-ta*

17′ [diš na ... *m*]*aruṣ*

18′ [diš na ... *m*]*aruṣ*

No. 17 BAM 113 VAT 10818

3′ [diš na ......] x *-dir-šú qilip šīrī-šú ši-ši-t*[*u ma-li*]

6′ [diš na ....] *ú-ta-na-har amīlu šû hi-niq-*[*ti* ....

Rectal Disease Texts

No. 21 BAM 95 = VAT 13752+ 13791 + 14190 + 14373

10 diš na *ur-šu dan-nu bāb šuburri-šú ṣabit-ma bāb šuburri pehi*^{hi}

14 diš na *šuburra-šú ha-niq-ma šuburra-šú ur-še u um-ṣa-a-ti mali*

19 diš na *kim-ṣa-a-*[*šú*] *itebbâ e-sil ši-hat šīri irtaši*^{ši}*dama utabbaka amīlu šû šuburra maruṣ qāt* ^{d}*māmīti*

21 diš na *šuburra maruṣ-ma šuburra-šú e-sil*

23 [diš na] *n*[*ik*]<*kim*>*-ti šuburri maruṣ qerbū-šú nuppuhū*^{hu}

27 diš na *šuburra marṣa maruṣ dama i-te-ez-zi qé-reb šuburri-šú i-ha-áš*

29 diš na *dama ina šuburri-šú ú-tab-ba-ka amīlu šû qer-bé-ni šuburri maruṣ*

36 diš na *šuburra maruṣ*

colophon: gaba.ri *šum-ma qāt* [*eṭimmi* ....

No. 22 S. 36 + AMT 43,1 + 57,6 *ina lā simānišu*:

1 diš na *ina la si-ma-ni-šú qablā-šú ikkalā-šú kim-ṣa-a-šú i-za-qata-šú bur-ka-šu i-kaṣ-ṣa-ṣa-šú amīlu šû ina meṣ-hi-ru-ti-šú šuburra maruṣ*

19 diš na *ina meṣ-hi-ru-ti-šú šuburra maruṣ amīlu šû* z[i$^{?}$.................

23 diš na *ina meṣ-he-ru-ti-šú šu*[*burra maruṣ* ....

col. ii

12 diš na *takāltu ikkal-šú*

col. iii

14′ diš na *damu ina šuburri-šú kīma sinništi ša na-ah-šá-te imtanaqquta*^{a} *ta-hi-su-ma muruṣ šuburri la iraššī ter-di-it ir-ri maruṣ*

col. iv

1 diš na *qab*[*lā-šú* ....-*s*]*u*

3 diš na *akala ikkal-ma i-*[*p*]*àr-ru šikara išatti-ma* [............] *amīlu šû šuburra marṣa* [*maruṣ*]

19′ [diš na *l*]*i-kis muruṣ šuburri qerbu* [.......................... (catchline)

20′ [dub x kam] diš na *ina la si-ma-ni-šú qab*[*lā-šú ikkalā-šú kim-ṣa-a-šú*](catchline)

No. 23 AMT 40,5 = K 6545 +

rev. col. iii

9′ diš na *qerbū-šú nuppuhū akalu u šikaru muṭṭû it-te-né-es-sil amīlu šû hi-ni*[*q-ti* ....

14′ diš na *mi-na-tu-šú ittanašpakā irat-su u šašalla-šú ikkalu-šú idā-šú k*[*im-ṣa-a-šú u bir-ka-šú*]

col. iv

29′ [diš.na *ṣalil-ma šit*]-⌜*ta-šú*⌝ *eli-šú iṭāb itebbi-ma i-ka-*⌜*šu-uš*⌝ (catchline)

30′ [diš na *ina la si-ma-n*]*i-šú qablā-šú ikkalā-šú* (catchline)

No. 24 AMT 47,1 = K 2433 +, *ina lā simānišu* Tablet 4

1 diš na *ṣalil-ma šit-ta-šu eli-šú iṭāb itebbi-ma i-ka-šu-uš īta[r-ma....]*

3 diš na *ṣalil-ma itebbi-ma pa-nu-šú nu-pu-hu amīlu šû šuburra marṣa [maruṣ]*

5 diš na *ṣalil-ma ši[t-ta-šu eli-šú iṭāb itebbi-ma i]-ka-šu-uš īta[r-ma. ....]*

col. ii

1 [diš] n[a *in-n]im-me-er i-te-ni[k-ki-ik] šāra ina šuburri-šú ú-kal akala u mê tur-ra i-sil-ti šuburri maruṣ*

8 diš na *šuburra marṣa maruṣ-ma i-te-nik-ki-ik šāra ina šuburri-šú ú-kal*

21 diš na *akala ikkal šikara išatti qerbū-šu nuppuhū ú-na-paq amīlu šû* ....

24 diš na *šuburra marṣa mar[uṣ-ma* ....

col. iii

1 diš na *šer'ān šuburri-šú iltanapp[at* .... *amīlu šû šuburra maruṣ]*

4' diš na *ki-ṣil-la-šú ikkalā* ....

6' diš na *ki-ṣil-la-šú ikkalā* ....

18' [diš na *šuburra mar]ṣa maruṣ-ma šuburra-šú e-sil*

20' diš na *akala ikkal šikara išatti-ma e-si-il ru'āti i-šal-la qerbū-šú [it-tan-n]a-bi-ṭu ir-ru-˹ú-šu i-ár-ru-ru amīlu šû šuburra marṣa maruṣ*

col. iv

1' [diš na *bāb šuburri-šú nuppuh ú-na-paq qer]-bé-nu maruṣ um-ṣa-tu*$_4$

6' [diš na] *idā-šú [kìn-ṣa-šú ki-ṣil-la-šú mar]uṣ amīlu šû qé-reb šuburri maruṣ*

13' diš na *šuburra marṣa mar[uṣ-ma di-ik-š]á irtaši* (= catchline)

14' dub-4-kam diš na *ina la si-ma-[ni-šú qablā] ikkalā-šú*(= catchline)

No. 25 = AMT 58,2, *ina lā simānišu* Tablet 5 (see YBC 7123+ 13');

1 diš na *šuburra marṣa maruṣ-ma di-ik-šá ir[taši*^{ši} *u mê libbi-šú la i-ma-har ru'ta ina šuburri-šú ú-tab-ba-ka]*

8 diš na *šuburra marṣa maruṣ-ma di-ik-ša irtaši aka[la u mê libbi-šú la i-ma-har ru'ta ina šuburri-šú ú-tab-ba-ka]*

12 diš na *libba-šú man-*g[*u*.........................

No. 26 BAM 96 EHE 331 + VAT 8694 + 14118

5' [diš na *akala ikkal šikara išatti qerbū-šu nuppu]hū ú-na-paq*

12' [diš na.............................]*-šú naši qablū-šú iltanappatū-šú akala u šikara ip-ru*

23' [diš na ....*m]a-le-e si-ka-tim*

col. ii

1 diš na *qerbū-šú ilap[patū-šu] mi-na-tu-šu puṭṭurā amīlu š[û* ....]

9 diš na *muruṣ šuburri maruṣ*

14 diš na *qablā-šú ikkalā-šú iš-dú*$^{?}$*-šú puṭṭurū [amīlu š]û muruṣ šuburri [maruṣ]*

18 diš na *šuburra marṣa maruṣ u šināti-[šú...]* x a x [............ *amīlu šû*] *šuburra marṣa maruṣ*

20 diš na *šuburra marṣa maruṣ-ma hašê-[šú* ....

col. iii

2' diš na *pīt*(?) *šu[burri-šú nuppuhu*^{hu} *ú-na-paq qer-bé-nu muruṣ] um-ṣa-tu*$_4$

8' diš na *šināti-šú ina šuburri e-te-rim [šuburra] marṣa [maruṣ]*

10' diš na *qer-bé-na* gig

No. 27 BAM 88 = VAT 10723

–1′ [diš na diš na *mi-na-tu-šú ittanašpakā irat-su u šašalla-šú ikkalū-šú*]
10′ [diš na *šuburra marṣa mar*]*uṣ-ma šuburra-šú uzaqqat-su*
13′ [diš na *šuburra marṣa mar*]*uṣ-ma di-ik-ša irtaši*^{ši} [*akala u mê libbi-šú la i*]*-ma-har ru'ta ina šuburri-šú ú-*[*tab-bak*]
17′ [diš na] *qerbū-šú nuppuhū*^{hu} *ir-ru-šú* [*kīma*] *šá išqippi ma-gal iqabbû*^{ú} *amīlu šû ni-kim-ti šāri u ṣēta maruṣ*

No. 28 BAM 104

42 diš na *pīt*(?) *šu*[*burri*]*-šú nuppuhu*^{hu} *ú-na-paq i qer-bé-nu muruṣ um-ṣa-tu*$_4$

No. 29 AMT 44,5 (S 1587)

2′ [diš na ....] x *-a ši-hat šīri* [*maruṣ* ...
6′ [diš.na *šuburra maruṣ-ma šit-t*]*a -šú ina libbi-šú i-ta-na-bal*

No. 30 AMT 40,4 + 57,5 = S 1283 + 1947

4′ diš na *dama ina šu*[*burri-šú ú-tab-ba-ka* ....
9′ diš na *šuburra marṣa maruṣ-ma lìb-ba-šu ṣabit-su it-te-nen-sil*
12′ diš na *šuburra maruṣ-ma šuburra-šú e-sil*
30′ diš na *akala ikkal šikara išatti-ma*

No. 31 BAM 182 (O. 194)

2′ diš na *ušaru-šú ú-zaq-qa-ta-šú*
3′ diš na *ušaru-šú ú-kas-sa*<*as-su*> *hi-níq-ti ka*[*līti* ....
5′ [d]iš na gìš*-šú ú-zaq-qat-su*
6′ diš na *ina ušari-šú dama ú-tab-ba-ka kīma sinništi kakka ma-hi-iṣ*
7′ [diš n]a *maš-ka*$_{15}$*-dù ṣabit-su*
11′ diš na *maš-ka*$_{15}$*-dù maruṣ*
14′ én *maš-ka*$_{15}$*-dù iš-tu ṣe-er-*<*ret*> *šá-ma-me ur-dam*
18′ [én] *a-re-eh-hi ra-ma-ni a-ra-ah-hi zu-u*[*m-ri* ....
25′ [én ......] x *bu-uh-ru bu-ha-ru šu-ú maš-*[*ka-du*

rev.

4′ [diš na *dama*] *šuburri-šú i-te-ez-zi ur-ši ina* x [...
7′ [diš na *šu*]*burra maruṣ-ma um-ṣa-ti šu-ti*
9′ [diš n]a *šuburra maruṣ-ma šuburra-šú e-sil*
11′ diš na *šuburra maruṣ šuburra-šú ú-zaq-qat*^{2}*-su qerbū-šú in-n*[*i-bi-ṭu*] *ú-ta-sal*
13′ diš na *šuburra marṣa maruṣ-ma e-sil*
17′ [diš na *šubu*]*rra maruṣ* [.................] ....
21′ [diš n]a *šuburra maruṣ* [...
23′ diš na *šuburra marṣa maruṣ-*[*ma* ....

No. 32 AMT 56,1 = K 8248

1 [diš na *mi-na-tu-šú ittanašpakā ir*]*at-su u šašalla-*[*šú*] *ikkalū-*[*šú*] [*idā-šú kim-ṣa-a-šú u bir-ka-šú*] *ikkalā-šú kalâti itti-šú lu sû 15 lu šá* 150 [*mahiṣ-su-ma ina mùš-tin-ni*]*-šú dama ú-kal-lam amīlu šû hi-níq-ti šuburri maruṣ*
8 [diš na *šuburra mar*]*ṣa maruṣ-ma šuburra-šú ú-zaq-qat-su qerbū-šú it-ta-nin-b*[*i-ṭ*]*u ú-ta-as-sal*

10 [diš na *šubur*]*ra marṣa maruṣ-ma šuburra-šú ú-zaq-qat-su*

12 [diš na *akala ik*]*kal šikara išatti-ma e-si-il ru'āti i-šal-la qerbū-*[*šú it*]*-tan-na-bi-ṭu* [*ir-ru-*⌜*ú-šu*] *i-ár-ru-ru amīlu šû šuburra marṣa maruṣ*

No. 33 AMT 43,5 K 9441

5 diš na *šuburra marṣa maruṣ-ma e-*[*sil....*

7 *akala ikkal šikara išatti-ma e-si-il ru'āti* [*i-šal-la qerbū-šú it-tan-na-bi-ṭu*] *ir-ru-šu i-ár-ru-ru amīlu šû šuburra marṣa maruṣ*

11 [diš] na *šuburra marṣa maruṣ-ma libba-šú ṣabit-su it-te-nin-s*[*il* ....

13 [diš na] *šuburra marṣa maruṣ-ma e-sil ù ú-nap-paq i-* ..[.........................

No. 34 BAM 168 = VAT 9138

1 diš na] *qerbū-šú nuppuhū*^{bu} *ir-ru-šú* [*kīma*] *šá išqippi ma-gal iqabbû*^{u} *amīlu šû ni-kim-ti šāri u ṣēti maruṣ šikin-šú ilabbir-ma qāt eṭemmi*

18 diš na *ši-biṭ šāri hi-miṭ ṣēti ši-biṭ šāri šim-ma-tú ri-mu-tú šá-áš-šá-ṭu qāt eṭimmi qāt māmīti šuburra maruṣ kala murṣi*

45 diš na *hi-niq-ti ellibuhhi maruṣ*

62 diš na *libba-šú umma iraššī*^{ši} *ummi libbi šá-ha-ṭi*

66 diš na *e-sil-ti libbi-šú šu-šu-ri u ur-še huppî um-ṣa-a-te qut-tu-pi*

70 diš na *ina la si-ma-ni-šú qablā-šú ikkalā-šú kim-ṣa-a-šú i-za-qata-šú pēmī-šú i-tan-na-ah bur-ka-šu i-kaṣ-ṣa-a-šú amīlu šû*(!) *ina meṣ-hi-ru-ti-šú šuburra maruṣ*

No. 35 BAM 99 = VAT 13726 *ina lā simānišu*

1 [diš na *ina*] *šuburri-šú dama ú-tab-ba-ka amīlu šû qer-bé-nu maruṣ*

17 diš na *dama i-te-zi qé-reb šuburri-šú i-za-qat-su kī*[*ma* ....

19 diš na *damu ina šuburri-šú kīma sinništi ša na-ah-ša-te imtanaqquta*^{a} *t*[*a-hi-is-su-ma*]

25 diš na *šuburra marṣa maruṣ dama i-te-ez-zi qé-reb šuburri-šú i-ha-áš*

27 diš na *ina šuburri-šú dama ú-*[*tab*]*-ba-ka kīma sinništi kakka ma-hi-iṣ*

30 [diš na *ina šuburri-šú dama ú-ta*]*b-ba-ka amīlu šû qer-bé-nu maruṣ*

rev.

42 diš na *ina šuburri-šú kīma sinništi ša na-ah-ša-te imtanaqquta*^{a} *ta-hi-su-ma*

56 (colophon): 7 *nis-hu* gaba.ri é.sa.bad *šá* bal.ti^{ki}

No. 36

2 diš na *damu ina šuburri-šú kīma sinništi ša na-ah-ša-te imaqquta ta-hi-is-su-ma*

No. 37 AMT 95,3 + = K 8182

11′ [diš na *šināti-šú ut-ta-na-tak*] *ka-la-a lā ilē'i*

18′ [diš na ....] *i-šah-hu-uh qerbū-šú em-ru*

col. ii

3′ diš na *i-kab-bat* sa [.......................

No. 38 AMT 100,3 = K 8369

4′ [diš na ..... *u*]*r-ši sāmi ana ur-eš huppî*

21′ [diš na *ina šuburri-šú dama ú-tab-ba-ka am*]*ilu šû qer-be-ni šuburri maruṣ*

No. 43 Text No. 23 STT 100

3′ [diš na *šāru ina libbi-šú issanahhur-ma ú*]*-na-pih ma-la i-kal-la amīlu šû šuburra maruṣ*

11′ diš na *šāru ina libbi-šú issanahhur-*[*m*]*a*$^{?}$ *ú-*⸢*na-pih*⸣ [..............

No. 45 K 2428 + 2548 + 6728

8′ diš na *maš-k*[*a-dù ṣabit-su*

12′ A diš na *maš-ka-da ṣab*[*it-su* ....

col. ii

7′ A diš na *naglabu ṣab*[*it-s*]*u*

11′ A én *maš-ka-du maš-ka-d*[*u man-za-a*]*s-su nar-ba-as-su*

19′ A én *lib-li* ^{d}girra *li-*[*nu-uh qab-l*]*i*

21′ A én *bēl šipri u balāṭi* ^{d}é.a [......................

24′ A diš na *maš-ka-du maruṣ*

No. 46 AMT 69,8 = K 6056

rev.

1 diš na *šēpā-šú* gar x [......................

5 diš na *šer'ān* [*qabli lu-ub-bu-ki* ....

No. 47 AMT 57,1 = 81-7-27, 72

rev.

4 [diš n]a *šuburra marṣa ma*[*ruṣ-ma* ....

No. 48 (Assur catalogue of incipits)

No. 50 AMT 22,2 = K3350

1 [diš na *kiš*]*adu u rēšu-šú ú-zaq-qata-su pānū-šú iṣṣanundū*^{du}

Sumerograms

a	*mû*
á	*idu*
a.ab.ba	*tâmtu*
a.gar.gar	*piqqannu*
a.geštin.na	*ṭābātu*
á.gú.zi.ga	*šēru*
a.rá	*adi*
a.ri.a	*rebûtu*
a.šà	*eqlu*
ad$_6$	*pagru*
al.la.na	*allānu*
al.ús.sa	*šiqqu*
al.šeg$_6$.gá	*bašlu*
alan	*ṣalmu*
am.si	*pīru*
an.dah.šum	*andahšu*
an.záh / na$_4$.an.zah	*anzahhu*
an.záh.ge$_6$	*kutpû*
anše	*imēru*
àr	*ṭênu* (*teṭên*)
az	*asu*
azag	*asakku*
àš.šár	*šumma*
ba.ba.za.^{d}íd	*pappasītu*
babbar	*peṣû*
bal	*naqû* (*tanaqqi*)
bal / bal.bal	*nabalkutu*
bar	*muššuru* / *uššuru* (*tumaššar*)
bar	*qilpu*
bára.ga	*halṣu*
bi.iz.bi.iz	*natāku*
bún	*napāhu*
bún / bun / see uzu.bun	*ellibuhhu*
búr	*pašāru*
buru$_5$	*erbu*
buru$_5$ íd.da	*ereb nāri*
buru$_5$.en.me.li	*šā'iltu*
buru$_5$.úš.ku$_6$	*erbu*? see PSD B 216
buru$_8$	*arû*
dab / dab$_5$	*ṣabātu* (*ṣubbutu*, *ṣabit*)
dabin(zì.da.še)	*tapinnu*
dam	*aššatu*

dara$_4$.maš	*ajjalu*
dè	*dikmennu pēmtu*
día(kaš.ús.sa)	*billatu*
dida(kaš.ú.sa)	*billatu*
dílim.a.bár	*itqūru*
diri	*mahāhu* (*tamahhah*)
diri	*malû* (*mali*)
diš-*niš*	*ištēniš*
dù	*epēšu* (*teppuš*)
dù.a.bi	*kalama*
du.du	*alāku* (*ittanallak*)
dù.dù.bi	*epištašu*
du$_{10}$.ga	*ṭiābu* (*iṭib*) / *ṭābu*
du$_{10}$.gam	*kimṣu* / *kamāṣu*
du$_{11}$.ga	*qabû* (*iqabbi*)
du$_8$.du$_8$ / du$_8$.meš	*paṭāru*
dub	*šapāku* (*tašappak*)
dub	*sarāqu* (*tasarraq*)
dub.dub / dub.meš	*šapāku* (*ittanašpakā*)
dug.a.da.gur$_5$	*adagurru*
dug.bur.zi	*pursītu*
dug.kal	*urruppu*
dug.kam	*diqaru*
dug.utul$_7$	*rabīku*
dugud	*kabtu*
dúr	*šuburru*
dúr	*ašābu*
è	*aṣû*
é.gar$_8$	*igāru*
é.gi$_4$.a-^{d}utu	*kallat Šamaš*
e$_{11}$	*elû* (*tušellâ*)
egir	*arka*
éllag	*kalītu*, see also uzu.éllag
eme.šid / eme.dir	*ṣurāru*
én	*šiptu*
ésir	*ittû*
eš	*pašāšu*
ga	*šizbu*
gá / ga.nu$_{11}$.mušen	*lurmu*
gaba	*irtu*
gaba.làl	*iškūru*
gada	*kitû*
gal	*rabû* (*rubbû*)

gal$_4$.la	*ūru*
gar (verb)	*šakānu*
gar.ib.u$_5$.mušen	*rikibti arkabi*
gar (noun)	*šiknu*
gaz / gaz.meš	*hašālu, hepû, huppû*
ge$_6$	*ṣalāmu* (*ṣalmu*)
ge$_6$	*mūšu*
gen / du	*alāku*
geštin	*karānu*
geštin.kala.ga	*karānu dannu*
geštin.šur.ra	*karānu ṣahtu*
gi.du$_{10}$.ga	*qanû ṭābu*
gi.dub.ba	*qanṭuppu*
gi.gíd / giš.gi.gíd	*embūbu*
gi.guhšu (sig$_4$+sig$_4$.šú)	*guhšû*
gi.sag.kud	*takkussu*
gi.zú.lum.ma	*kūru*
gi.šeš (*tâmti*)	*misis tâmti* (variant)
gi.šul.hi	*qan šalāli*
gibil	*edēšu*
gíd	*šadādu* (*išaddad*); *arāku* (*urruku*)
gig	*marāṣu marṣu*
gig	*murṣu*
gim	*kīma*
gin	*alāku*
gín	*šiqlu*
gír.gír	*zaqātu* (*uzaqqat*)
gìr.pad.du	*eṣemtu*
gír.tab	*zuqaqīpu*
gír.šu.i	*naglabu*
gìri	*šēpu*
gissu	*ṣillu*
gìš	*ušaru*
gìš nu zu	*lā petītu*
giš.apin	*epinnu*
giš.az	*asu*
giš.dìh	*baltu*
giš.eren	*erēnu*
giš.erin.úš	*šupuhru*
giš.esi	*ušû*
giš.geštin.ka$_5$.a	*karān šēlibi*
giš.gi.zú.lum.ma	*kūru*
giš.gi$_6$.pàr	*lipāru*
giš.gišimmar.tur	*suhuššu*
giš.ha.lu.úb	*haluppû*
giš.hab	*hūratu*
giš.hašhur	*hašhuru*
giš.kiri$_6$	*kirû*
giš.kiši$_{16}$	*ašāgu*
giš.kiši$_{16}$(ú.gír).hab / ${}^{\text{ú}}$gír.hab	*dadānu*
giš.kun	*rapaštu*
giš.lagab.munu$_4$	*buqlu*
giš.lam.gal	*buṭuttu*
giš.lum.ha (ú.lum.ha, lum.ha)	*barīrātu*
giš.ma.nu	*e'ru*
giš.maš.huš	*kalbānu*
giš.nàga	*esittu*
giš.nam.tar / tal(.nita)	*pillû*
giš.nim	*baltu*
giš.nu.úr.ma	*nurmû*
giš.tara.muš	*taramuš*
giš.tukul	*kakku*
giš.kiši$_{16}$.hab	*dadānu*
giš.úr.tál.tál	*uzun lalî*
giš.zú.lum.ma	*suluppu*
giš.še.ná.a	*šunû*
giš.šinig	*bīnu*
giš.šú.a giš / ú.sila$_{11}$.gá	*littu*
giš.zú.gišimmar	*zû*
gú.bí.ku$_6$	*kuppû*
gu.du	*qinnatu*
gú.gal	*hallūru*
gú.níg.àr.ra	*kiššēnu*
gu$_7$	*akālu*
gub	*kânu* (*tukân*)
gùb	*šumēlu*
gub.gub	*izuzzu* (*ittanazzaz*)
gur	*tūrtu*
gur	*târu*
gurun	*inbu*
hád.du / hád.a	*abālu urruru*
hénbur(še.kak)	*habburu*
hi.hi	*balālu*
hur.meš	*hašû*
ì / ì.giš	*šamnu*
ì.nun.na	*himētu*
ì.udu	*lipû*
íb.tag$_4$	*rēhtu*
íd	*nāru*
igi	*īnu / pānū*
igi	*amāru*

igi.4.gál	*rebūtu*
igi.bar	*naplusu*
igi.du$_8$	*amāru*
íl	*našû* (*našāku*)
illu	*hīlu*
im	*šāru*
im.gá.li	*kalû*
im.gú	*qadūtu*
im.gú.en.na	*qadūt šikani*
im.gú.gar.rin.na	*adattu?*
im.kal.la	*kalû*
im.sahar.babbar.kur.ra	*alluharu*
im.sahar.ge$_6$.kur.ra	*qitmu*
im.sahar.na$_4$.kur.ra	*gabû*
im.si.sá	*iltānu*
ir	*zu'tu*
iti.zíz.àm	*šabāṭu*
izi	*išātu*
ka	*pû*
ká .bar	*bābu kamû*
ka.a.ab.ba	*imbū tâmti*
ka.inim.ma	*šiptu*
ká.mud	*bāb šuburri*
kaš	*šikaru*
kàš	*šinātu*
kaš.lú.tin.na / kaš.sag.lú.tin.na	*šikar sābî*
kaš.sag	*šikaru rēštû*
kašbir(KAŠ.A.SÙ)	*hīqu*
kéš	*rakāsu*
kéš.da	*riksu*
ki	*ašru*
ki	*erṣetu*
ki	*itti*
ki nu.gi	*erṣetu lā târi*
ki.ná	*ṣalālu* (*ṣalil*); *eršu*
ki.ta	*šaplītu*
kin	*šipru*
kir$_4$	*appu*
kisal (var. of gín)	*šiqlu*
kù	*ellu*
kù.babbar	*kaspu*
kù.gi	*qutāru*
ku.ku	see CAD Q 208
ku$_6$	*nūnu*
ku$_7$.ku$_7$	*matqu*
kud	*parāsu*
kúm / kúm.kúm	*bahrūtu; buhhuru; emēmu, ummumu, ummu*
kur	*kašādu* (*kašid*)
kur	*šadû*
kuš	*mašku*
kuš.edin	
lá	*ṣamādu* (*taṣammid*)
lá	*maṭû* (*muṭṭû*)
lá	*naṣmadu / naṣmattu*
lag.a.šà	*kirbān eqli*
lagab.munu$_4$	*šibirti buqli*
lál	*ṣamādu* (*taṣammid*)
làl	*dišpu*
li.dur	*abukkatu*
lú.a.zu	*asû*
lú.aš.gab	*aškāpu*
lù.lù	*dalāhu*; *adāru* (*adir*)
lugud	*šarku*
luh	*mesû*
luh.mar.tu	*šibburratu*
MA	(measure = gín)
mah	*ṣīru*
man	*šanītu*
mar / (mar.meš)	*eqû*
mar.gal	*išqippu*
maš.dà	*ṣabītu*
máš.gal	*urīṣu*
maš.sìla (maš.sìla^2)	*naglabu* (*naglabā*)
maškim	*rābiṣu*
mí.aš.gàr	*unīqu*
mí.ur	*kalbatu*
mí.šah	*šahītu*
mú / mú.meš / mú.mú	*napāhu* (*tanappah*)
mu.ni	*šumšu*
mu.ùr.ra.ku$_6$	*girītu*
mud	*da'mu*
múd	*damu*
mud (see also ká.mud)	*uppu*
mul / múl / mul$_4$	*kakkabu*
mul.ug$_5$	*kakkab āribi* (CAD A/2 266)
mul.ud$_5$ / mul.ùz	*kakkab enzi*
mun	*ṭābtu*
mun.kù.pad	*šibirti ṭābti*
munu$_4$	*buqlu*

munus	*sinništu*
murub$_4$	*qablu*
muš	*ṣerru*
mušen	*iṣṣuru*
na.bi	*amīlu šû*
na$_4$	*abnu*
na$_4$.bur	*pūru*
na$_4$.duh.ši.a	*dušû*
na$_4$.gi.dub-*tamti*	*qanṭup tâmti*
na$_4$.ka.gi.na(dib.ba)	*šadânu*
na$_4$.kišib	*kunukku*
na$_4$.kur-*nu* (dib)	*šadānu*
na$_4$.na.zà.hi.li	*urṣu*
na$_4$.ni.bu	*janibu*
na$_4$.pa	*ajartu*
na$_4$.peš$_4$.a.ab.ba	*išqillat tamtim*
na$_4$.peš$_4$.anše	*biṣṣur atāni*
na$_4$.ú.níg.bùr.bùr	*pallišu*
na$_4$.zálag	*zalāqu*
na$_4$.zú	*ṣurru*
na$_4$.šà.giš.ge$_6$na$_4$.šuba	*šubû*
nag	*šatû (išatti)*; *šaqû*
nag.nag / nag.meš	*šatû* (Gtn); *šaqû*
naga.si	*uhūlu qarnānû*
nagar	*allānu*
nam.érim / nam.rim / ^{d}nam.érim	*māmītu*
nam.lú.u$_{18}$.lu	*amīlūtu*
níg.àr.ra	*mundu*
níg.lá	*naṣmattu*
níg.na$_4$	*lipāru*
nigin	*lamû (talammi)*
nigin	*sihru / sahāru* (Gtn)
nigin	*ṣâdu* (Gtn)
ninda	*akalu*
ninda.ì.dé.a	*mirsu*
nindu	*tinūru*
níta / nita	*zikaru*
nu.nu	*ṭamû*
numun	*zēru*
nundum	*šaptu*
nunuz	*pēlu*
pa	*aru*
pap	*napharu*
pú	*būrtu*
peš$_{10}$-^{d}íd	*kibrītu*

ra (ra.meš)	*rahāṣu* (*tarahhaṣ*)
sa	*šer'ānu*
sa.gal	*sagallu*
sa.sal.(meš)	*šašallu*
sá.sá	*kašādu* (*kašid*)
sa$_5$	*sāmu*
sa$_5$	*sīmutu*
sag šà	*rēš libbi*
sag.ki	*pūtu*
sahar	*eperu*
sar see mú	*napāhu* (*tanappah*)
si.sá	*ešēru* (*šūšuru*)
sig	*qatnu*
síg	*šipātu*
sìg	*mahāṣu* (*mahiṣ*)
síg.àka	*itqu*
síg.hé.me.da	*tabarru*
sig$_4$.al.ur$_5$.ra	*agurru*
sig$_5$	*našpu / damqu*
sig$_7$	*arqu*
sikil	*ellu*
sìla	*qû*
sim	*napû*
siskur	*nīqu*
sù / sù.sù	*salāhu*
súd	*sâku*
suhuš	*šuršu*
sumun	*labāru* (*labiru*)
sur	*ṭerû* (*teṭerri*)
šà	*libbu*
šà / šà.meš	*qerbu / qerbū*
šáh	*šahû*
še	*še'u*
šè	*ana*
še$_{10}$	*zû*
še$_{10}$.^{d}iškur še.gín	*šimtu*
še.sa.a	*laptu*
šed$_7$	*kaṣû*
šeg$_6$	*bašālu* (*tušabšal*)
šen.tur	*tamgussu*
šeš(.meš)	*annûti*
šéš	*pašāšu* (*tapaššaš*)
šid	*manû*
šid	*lâšu* (*talâš*)
šika	*haṣbu*
šim / šim.hi.a	*riqqu / riqqū*
šim.bal	*ballukku*
šim.buluh	*baluhhu*
šim.^{d}maš	*nikiptu*

šim.^{d}nin.urta	*nikiptu*
šim.gam.ma	*ṣumlalû*
šim.gig	*kanaktu*
šim.gír	*asu*
šim.gúr.gúr	*kukru*
šim.hab	*ṭūru*
šim.im.di	*suādu*
šim.li	*burāšu*
šim.man.du	*suādu*
šim.mug	*ballukku*
šim.sal	*šimeššalû*
šim.še.li / še.li	*kikkirânu*
šim.šeš	*murru*
šim/ú.^{d}maš	*nikiptu*
šir	*išku*
šu	*qātu*
šu.gedim.ma (var. šu.gud)	*qāt eṭemmi*
šu.si	*ubānu*
šub	*nadû* (*iddâ*)
šub.šub	*maqātu* (*imaqqut*)
šum.šir.dil	*turû*
šur	*ṣahtu*
šur.min / giš.šur.min / šur.mìn	*šurmēnu*
tab	*himṭu* (*himiṭ*)
táb.táb	*ṣurrupu*
tag / tag.tag	*lapātu* (*tulappat*)
tag$_4$	*ezēbu*
tar	*nakāsu* (*nakis*)
te	*ṭehû*
téš.bi	*ištēniš*
ti / tin	*balāṭu*(*bulluṭu*)
ti.la	*balṭu*
túg	*ṣubātu*
tuh.še.giš.ì	*kupsu*
tuk / tuku	*išû; rašû* (*irtaši*)
tùn / tùn.šà	*tākaltu*
tur.meš	*ṣehhērūti*
tuš	*ašābu*
u	*ubānu*
ú / ú.hi.a	*šammu*
ú.a.zal.lá	*azallû*
ú.áb.duh	*kamantu*
ú.an.ki.an.di / an.ki.nu.di	*ankinutu*
ú.an.nu.ha.ra	*annuharu*
ú.aš.tál	*ardadillu*
ú.babbar	*šammu peṣû*
ù.bu.bu.ul	*bubu'tu*
ú.^{d}maš	*nikiptu*
ú.^{d}utu	*šam Šamaš*
ú.dili	*ēdu*(?)
ú.eme.ur.gi$_7$	*lišān kalbi*
ú.esi	*ušû*
ú.gamun	*kamūnu*
ú.gamun [= tin.tir]. (ge$_6$.ki)	*zibû*
ú.gazi.sar	*kasû*
ú.geštin.hád.du.a	*munzīqu*
ú.geštin.ka$_5$.a	*karān šēlibi*
ú.gír	*ṣadānu*
ú.gír.hab (var.ú.gur$_4$.hab?)	*dadānu* var.
ú.gír	*uh-ha-ah*
ú.hab	*hūratu*
ú.har.har	*hašû*
ú.har.lum.ba.šir	*harmunu*
ú.hur.sag	*azupīru*
ú.igi-*ešra*	*imhur-ešrâ*
ú.igi-*lim*	*imhur-līm*
ú.in.úš (in$_6$.úš)	*maštakal*
ú.ki.^{d}iškur	*qudru*
ú.ki.kal	*sassatu*
ú.gír	*ašāgu*
ú.kù.babbar	*ajarkaspi*
ú.ku$_6$	*urânu*
ú.kur.gi.rín.na	*kurkānû*
ú.kur.kur	*ata'išu*
ú.kur.ra	*nīnû*
ú.kur.zi	*samīdu*
ú.lag.a.šà	*kirbān eqli*
ú.lag.gán	*kirbān eqli*
ú.maš.tab.ba	*māštu*
ú.nam.tal / tar	*pillû*
ú.níg.bùr.bùr	*pallišu*
ú.níg.kud.da ú.níg.sù.sù / sì.sì	*sāpinu*
ú.níndu edin	*illūri ṣēri*
ú.nu.bal	*tullal*
ú.nu.luh.ha	*nuhurtu*
ú.peš$_4$.anše	*bişşur atāni*
ú.si.sá	*šurdunû*
ú.sikil	*sikillu*
ú.sum.sikil	*šamaškilu*
ú.sumun.dar	*šumuttu*
ú.šiš.ba.na	*šizbānu*

ú.tál.tál	*urânu*
ú.tara.muš	*taramuš*
ú.tur.ra	*haltappānu*
ú.úkuš.hab(sar)	*irrû*
ú.ukuš.ti.gi.la / lu	*tigilû*
ú.úkuš.ti.gil.kur.ra	*tigilat šadî*
ú.zì.nu.luh.ha	*tiātu*
u_4.bú.bú.ul	*bubu'tu*
u_5.gar.ib.mušen	*rikibti arkabi*
ud(ud.meš)	*ūmu*
ud.da	*ṣētu*
ud.sa_9	*mišlam?*
udu.níta	*immēru*
ugu	*muhhi eli*
ugu.súh.ha	
úh	*ru'tu*
umbin	*ṣupru*
úr	*išdu / sūnu / pēmu*
ùr	*ūru*
ur.bar.ra	*barbaru*
ur.gi_7	*kalbu*
úr.kun / uzu.úr.kun	*rapaštu*
ur.mah	*nēšu*
ur_5.gim	*kīam*
urudu	*erû*
urudu.šen.tur	*tamgussu*
útul (see dug.útul)	*diqāru*
usduha[u_8.udu.hi.a]	*ṣēnu*
úš	*pehû (pehi)*
úš	*sekēru (tesekker)*
$uš_4$	*ṭēmu*
ùz	*enzu*
uzu	*šīru*
uzu ka.izi	*šumû*
uzu.bun	*ellibuhhu*
uzu.éllag	*kalītu*
uzu.me.hé	*himṣu*
uzu.zag	*imittu*
zà.10.meš	*ešrētu*
zà.hi.li(sar)	*sahlû*
zabar	*siparru*
zé	*martu*
zi	*nasāhu*
zi	*tebû (ittenebbi)*
zi	*nasāhu*
zì(.da)	*qēmu*
zì.gig	*qēm kibti*
zì.gú	*qēm kakki*
zì.gú.gal	*qēm hallūri*
zi.in.gi	*kiṣallu*
zì.kum	*isqūqu*
zì.$munu_4$	*qēm buqli*
zi.zi / zi.meš	*tebû (ittenebbi)*
zì.zíz.àm	*qēm kunāši*
zu	*idû*
zu	*le'u (ila'e)*
zú	*šinnu*
zú.lum	*suluppû*
zú.lum.ma dilmun^{ki}	*asnû*

PLATES

No. 2 Ms. B

K 2405 + 2449 + 8757 + S 32b + 150 + 1983

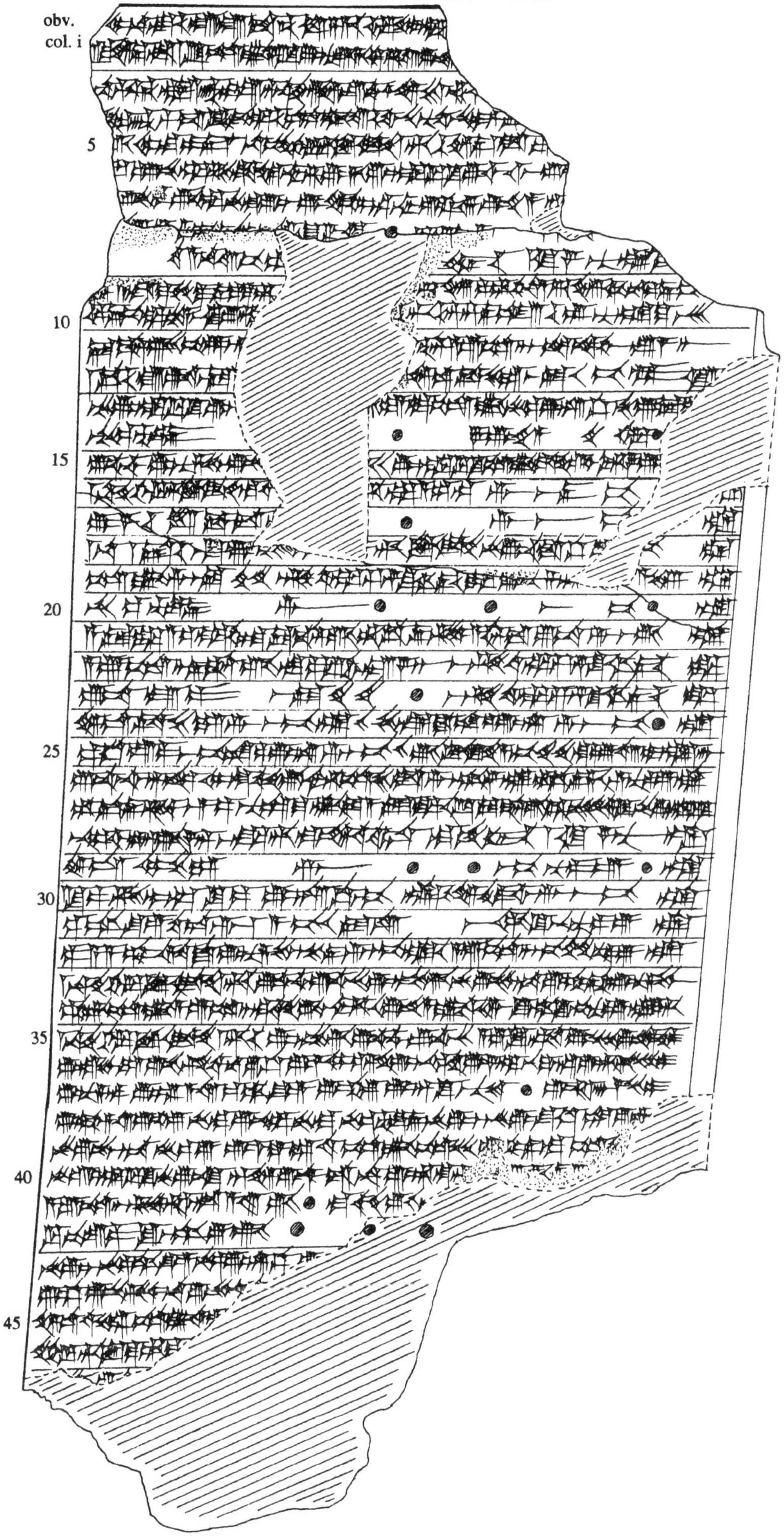

K 2405 + 2449 + 8757 + S 32b + 150 + 1983

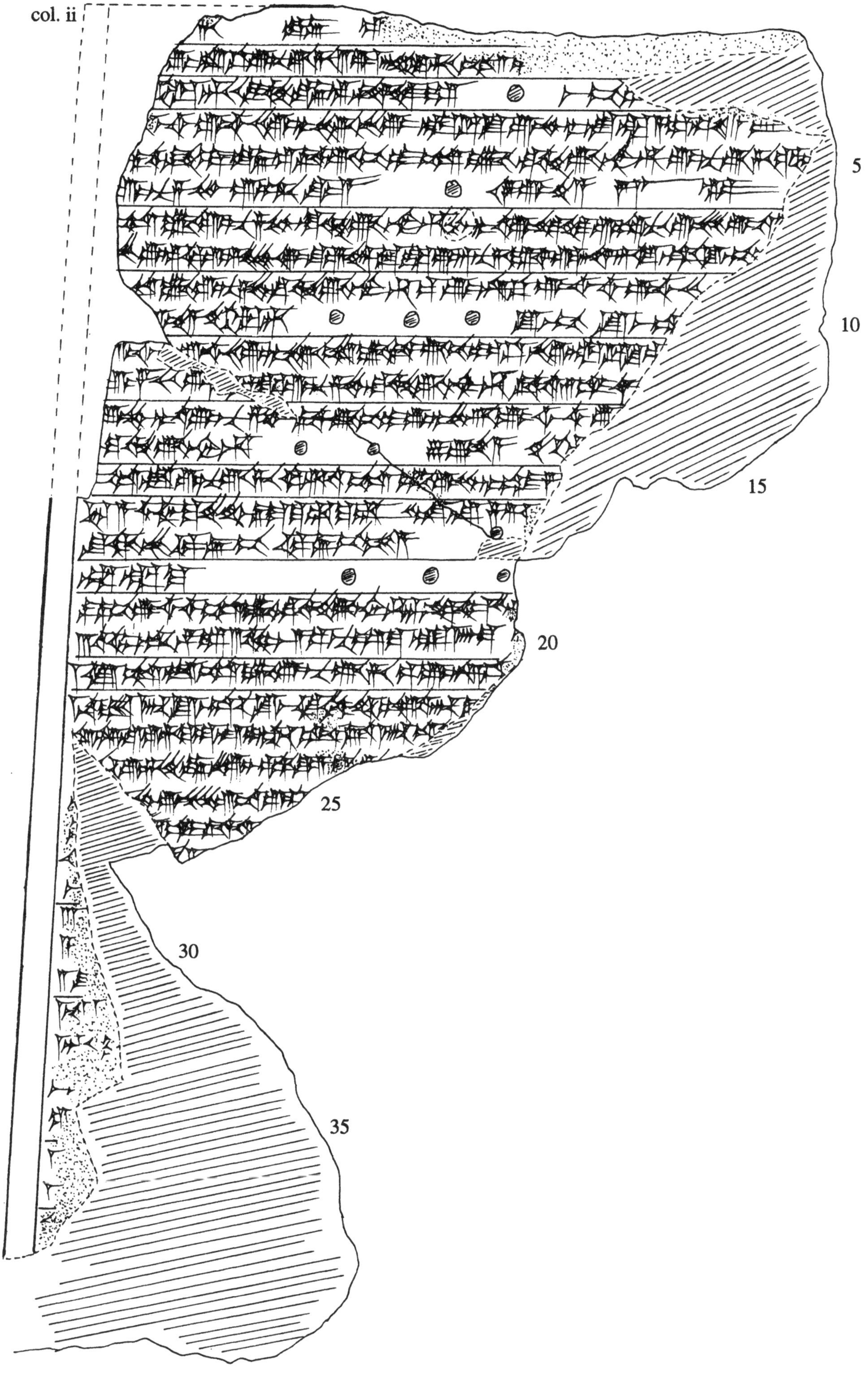

K 2405 + 2449 + 8757 + S 32b + 150 + 1983

rev.

Ms. B1 K 7230

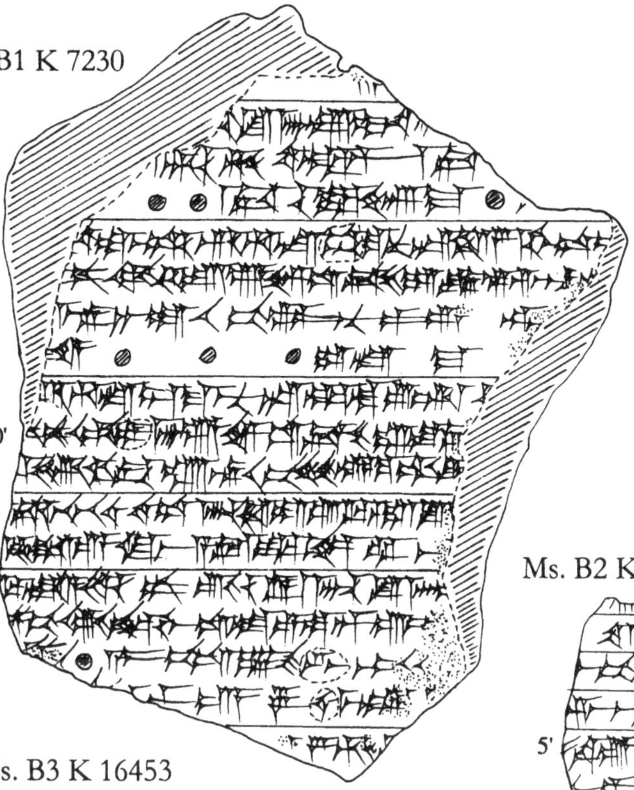

Ms. B2 K 13403

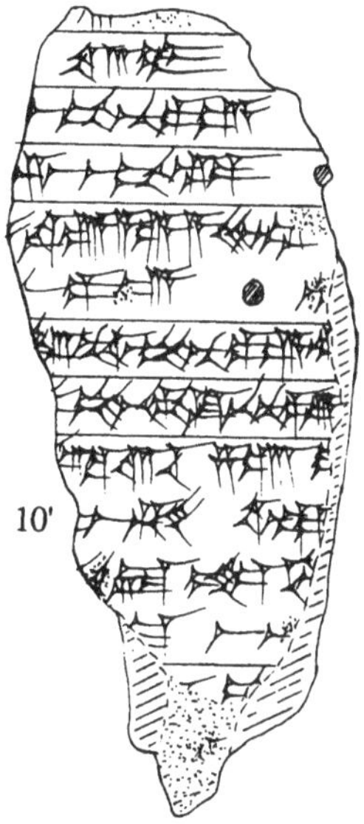

Ms. B3 K 16453

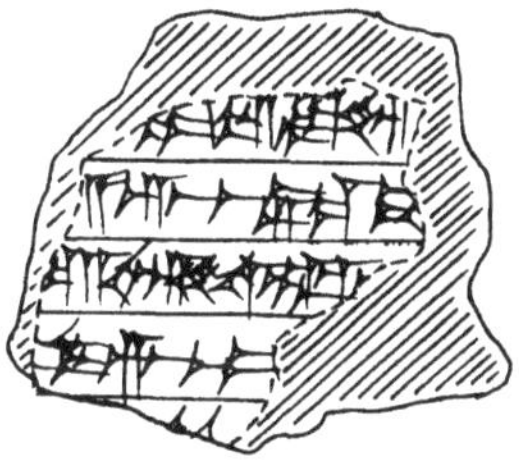

Ms. B4 S 467

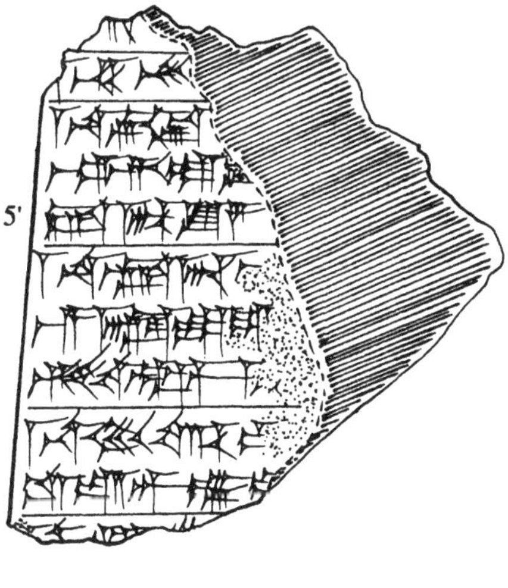

Ms. B5 K 5864

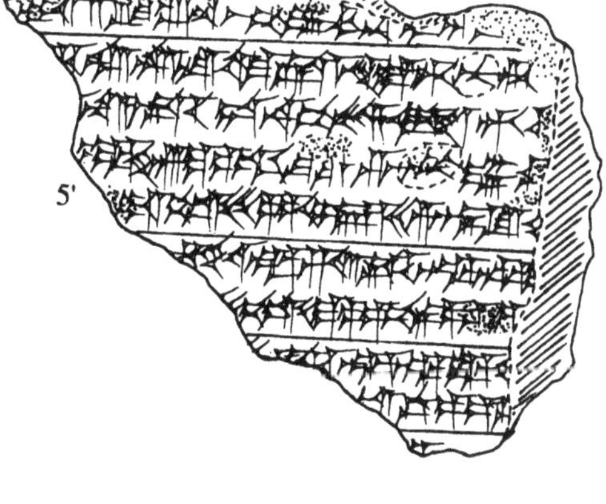

K 4957 + 11742 + S 110 + 516 + 679 + 761 + 2058

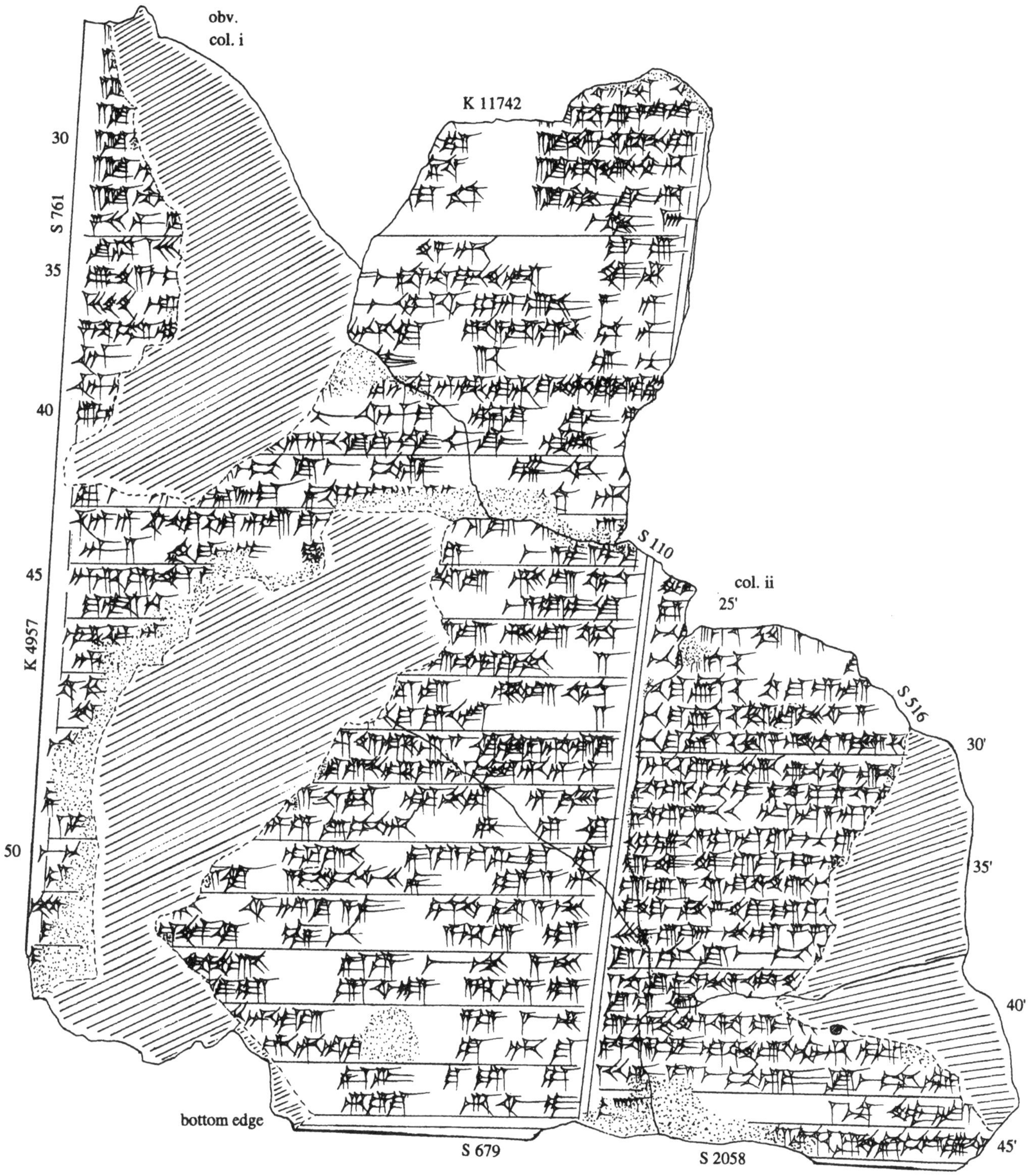

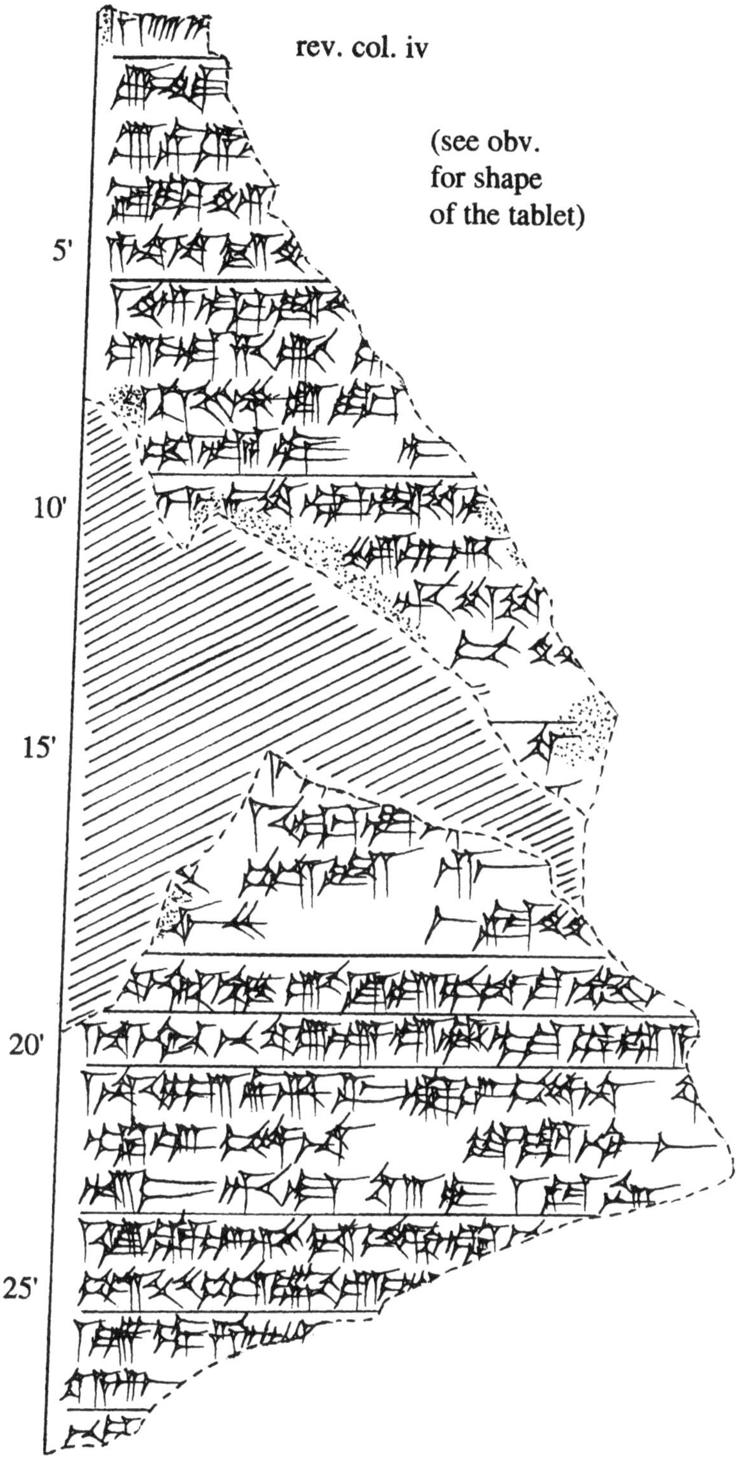
rev. col. iv
(see obv. for shape of the tablet)
5'
10'
15'
20'
25'

No. 9b Ms. J
K 2960 + 10268 + 14977 + Rm II, 315

obv.
col. i

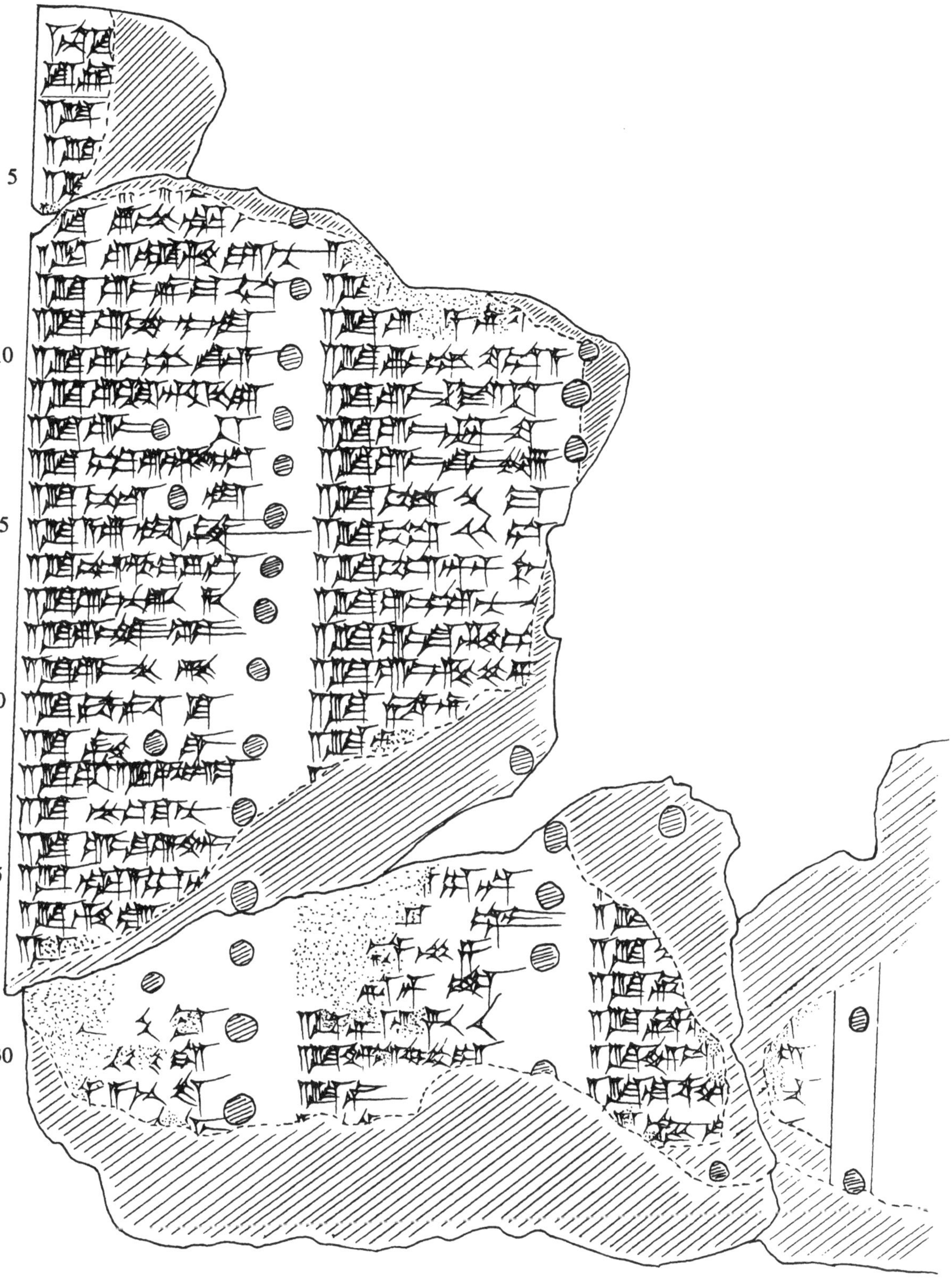

col. ii

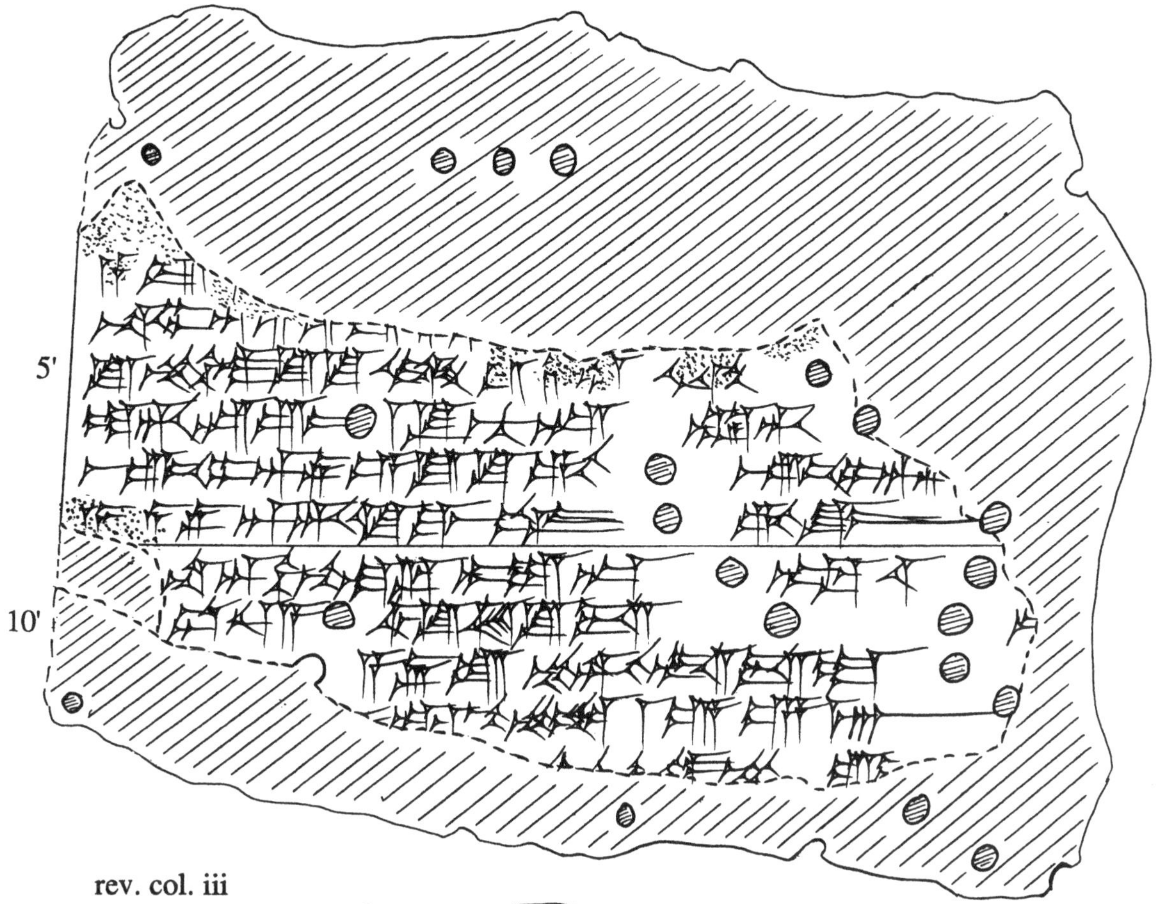

rev. col. iii

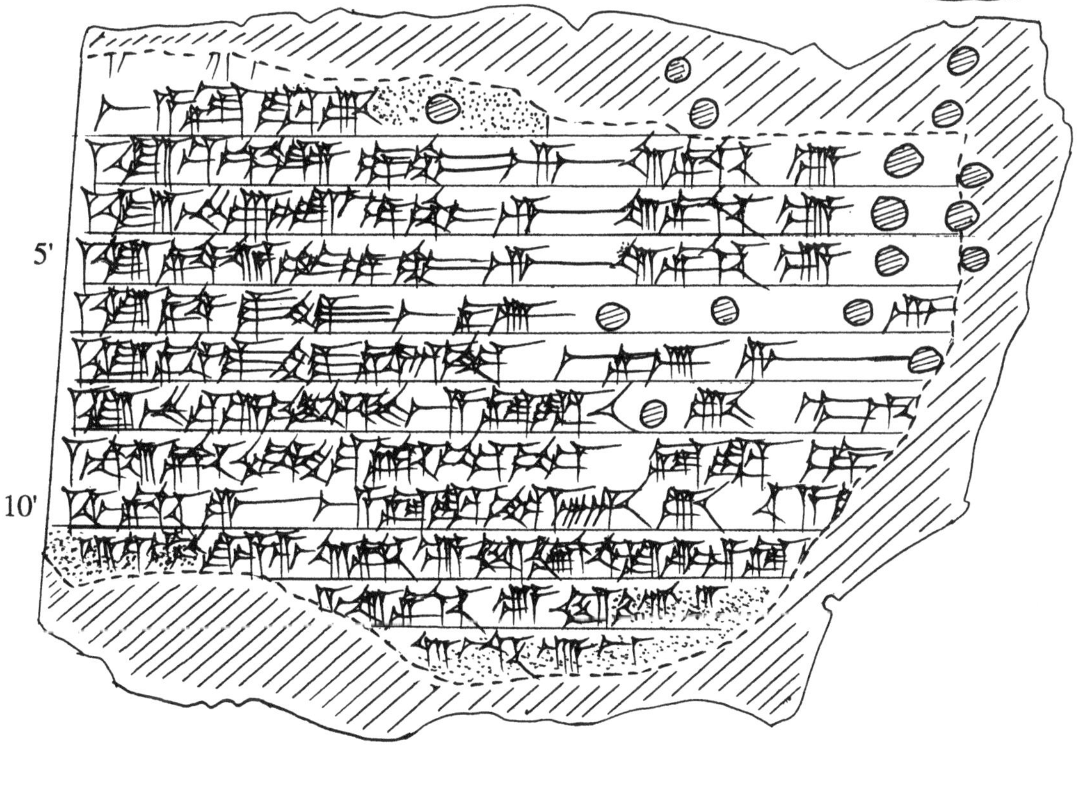

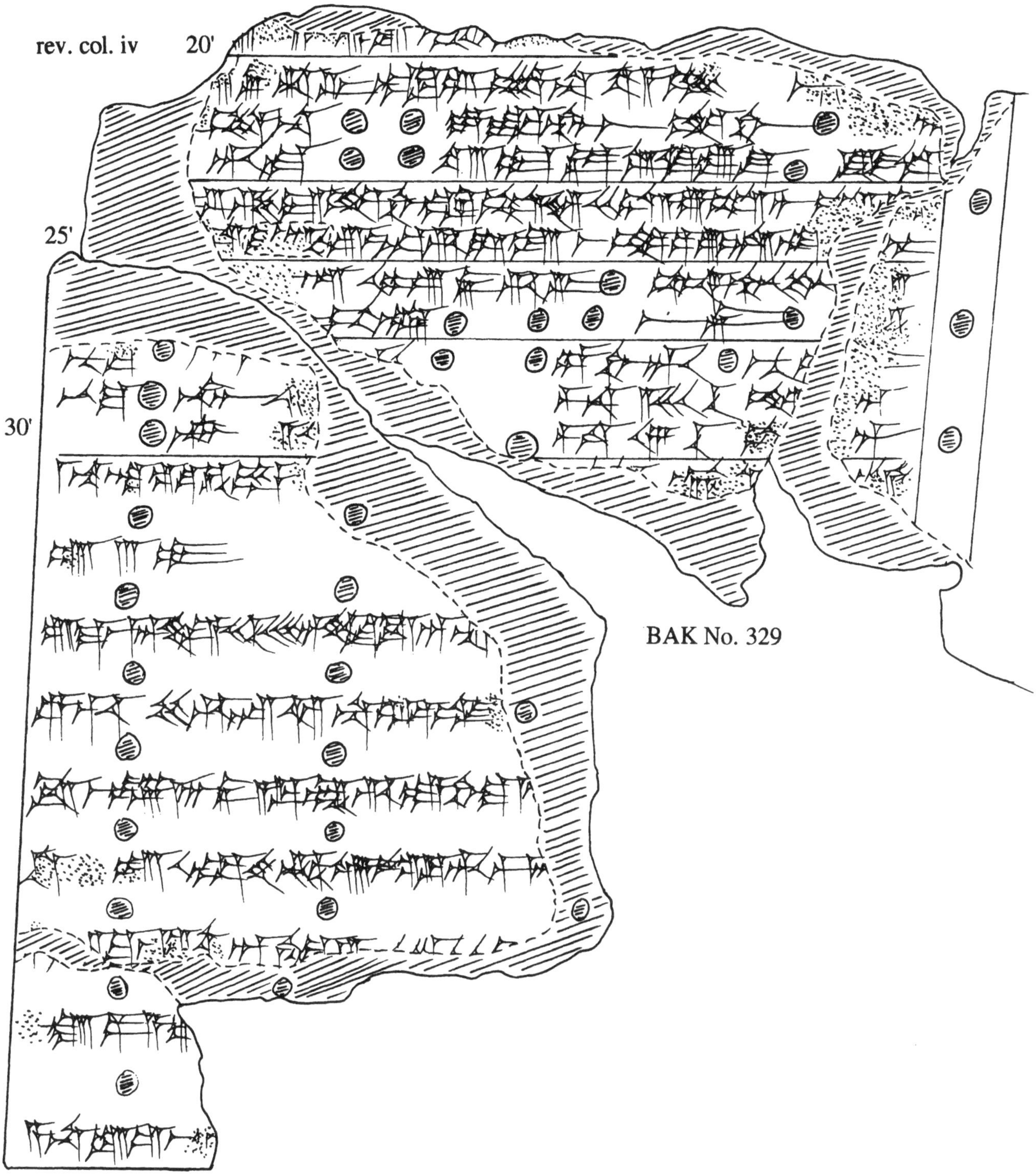

BAK No. 329

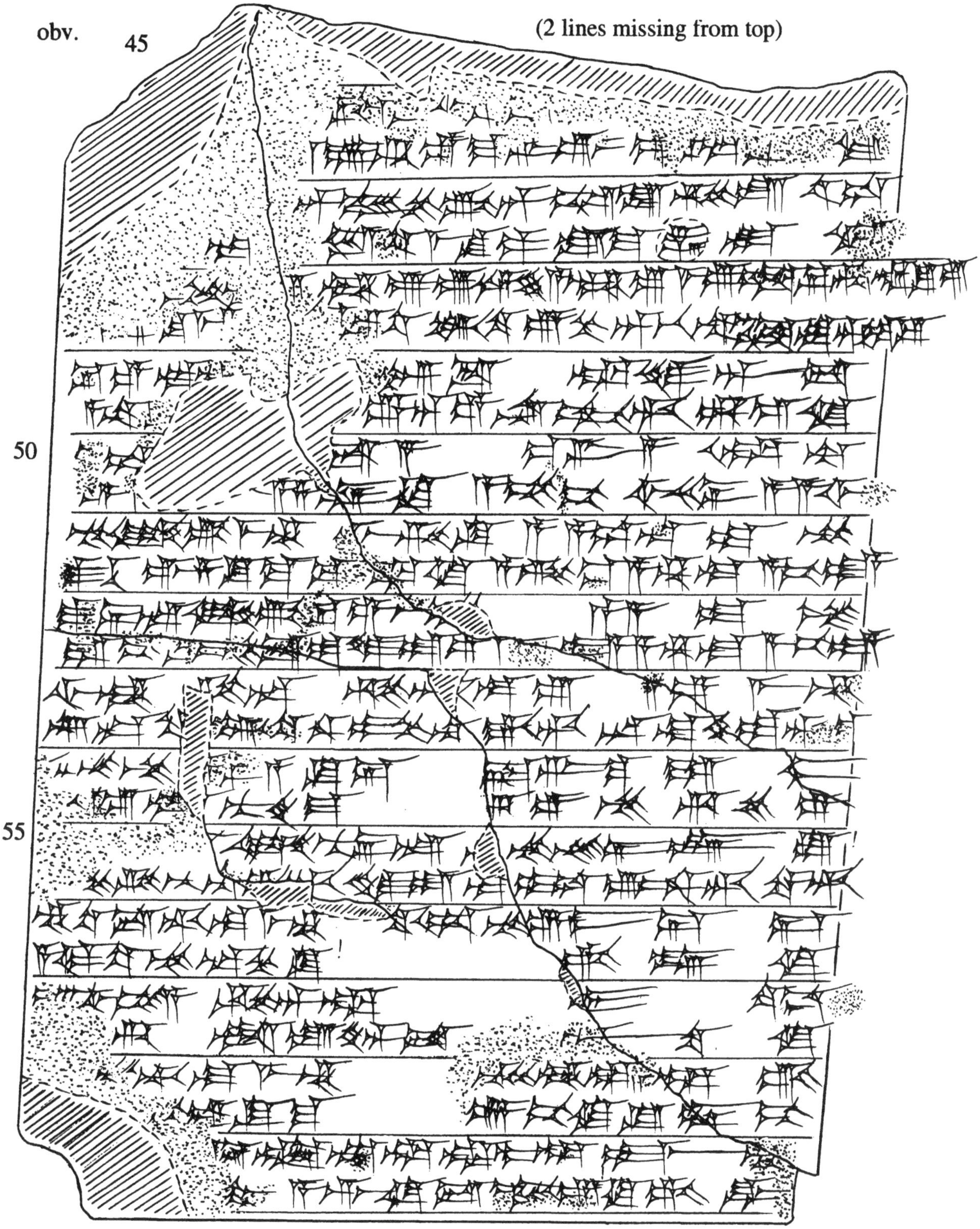

(poor scribe - text full of errors!)

rev.

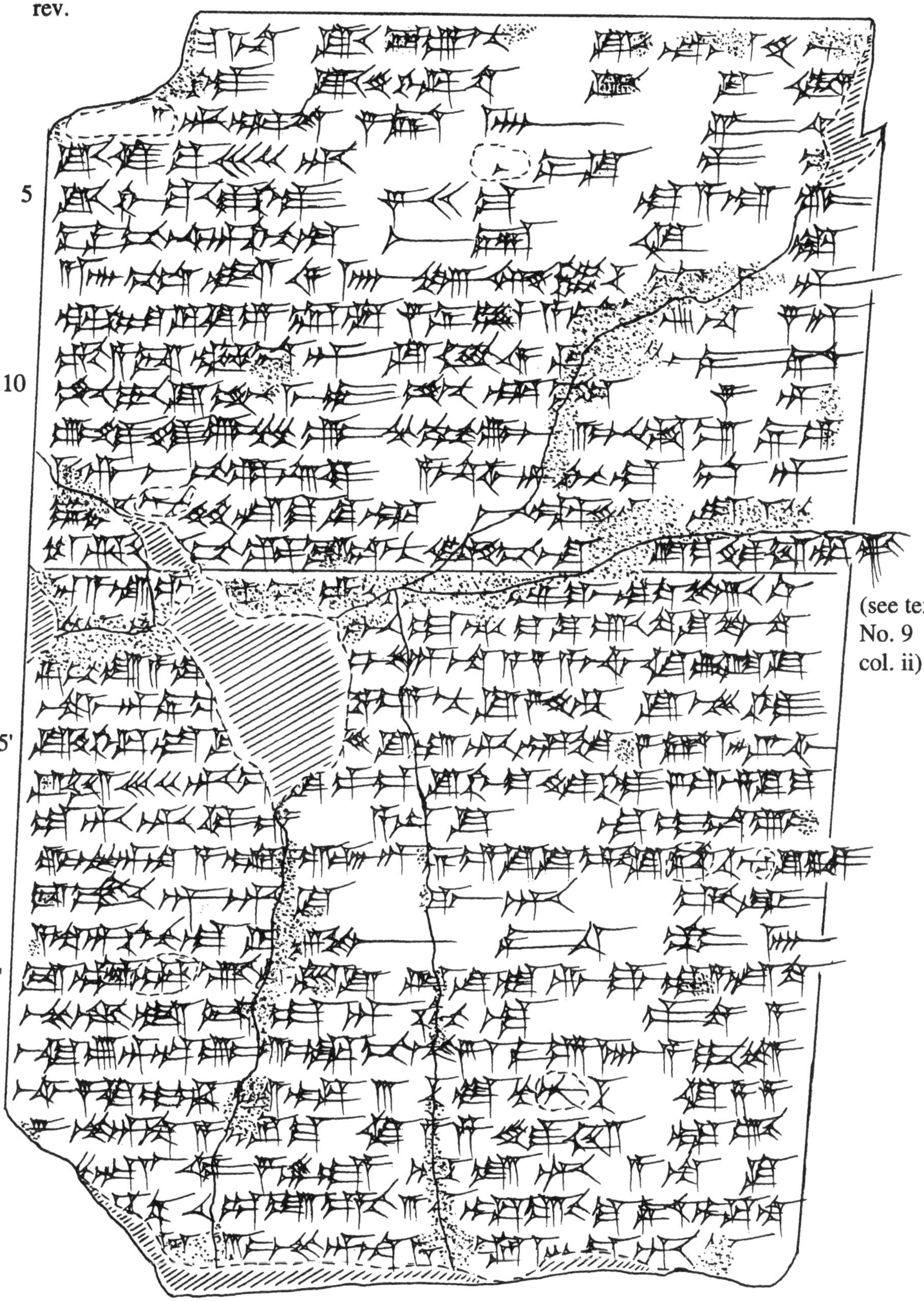

(see text No. 9 col. ii)

No. 12 Ms. M
K 11829

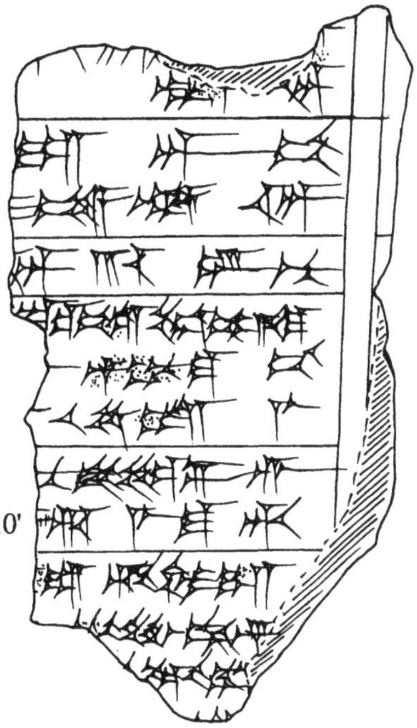

No. 11 Ms. L
K 6493 + 6811 + Bu 91-5-9,52 (+) K 10676

obv.

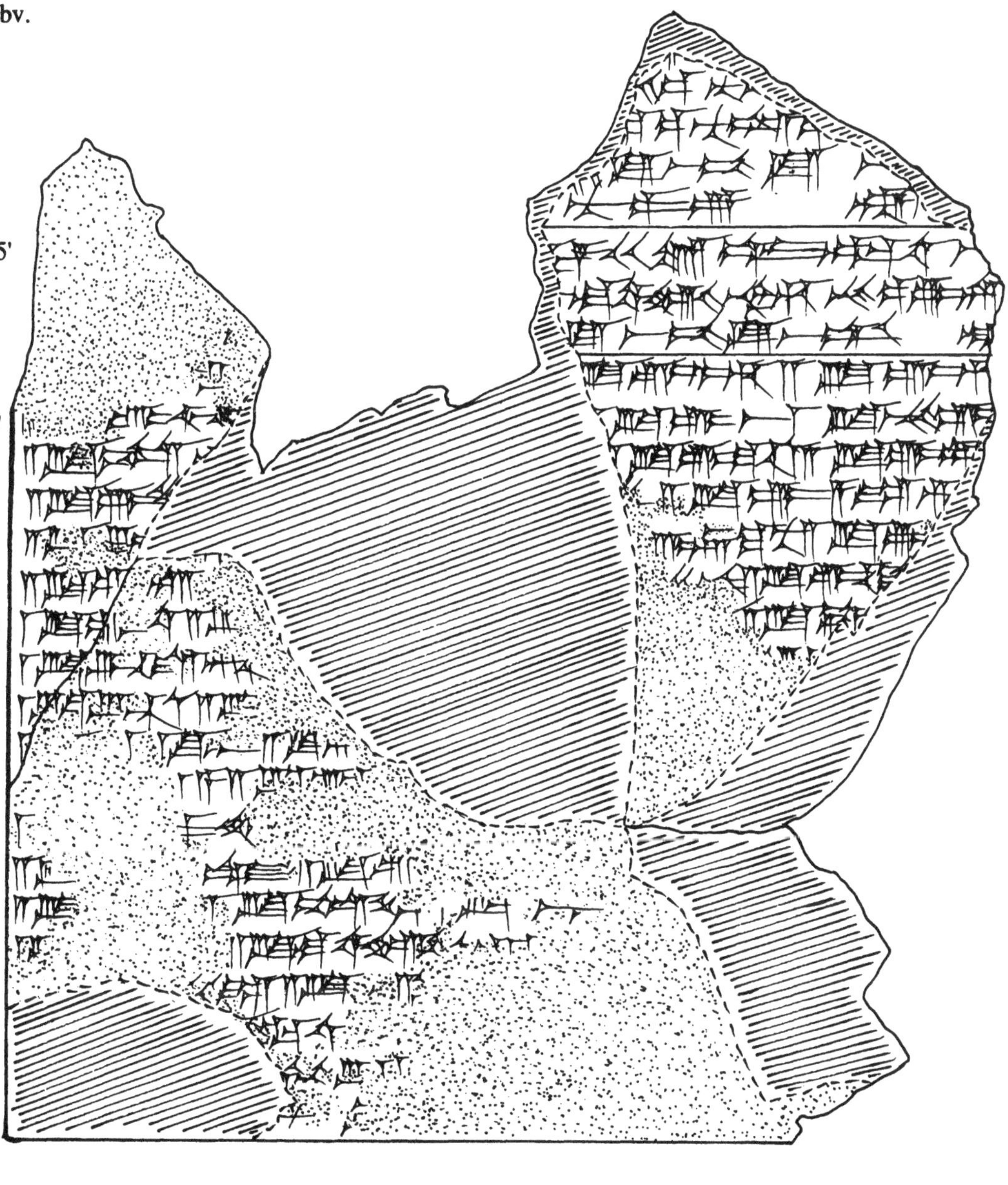

rev.

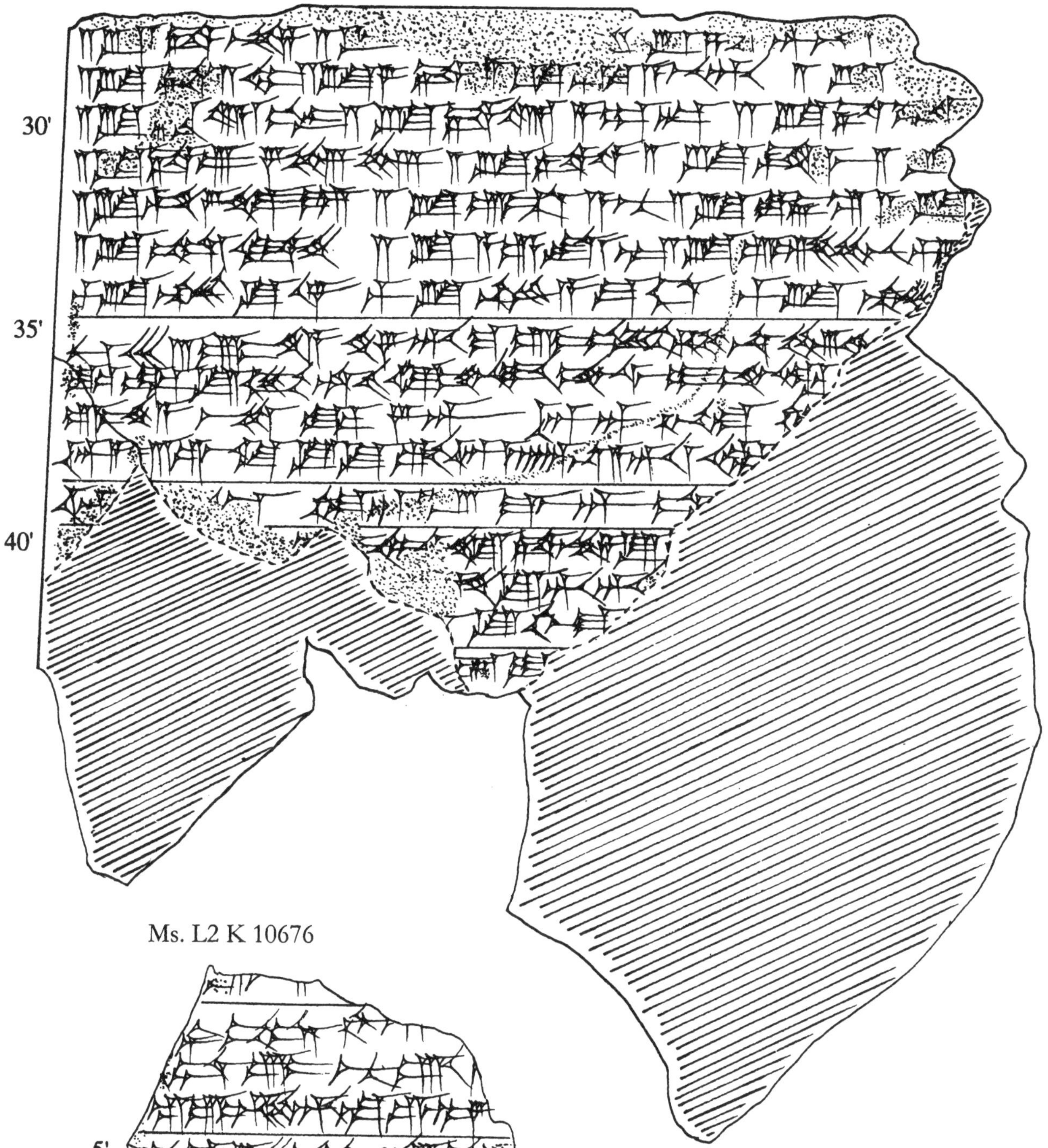

Ms. L2 K 10676

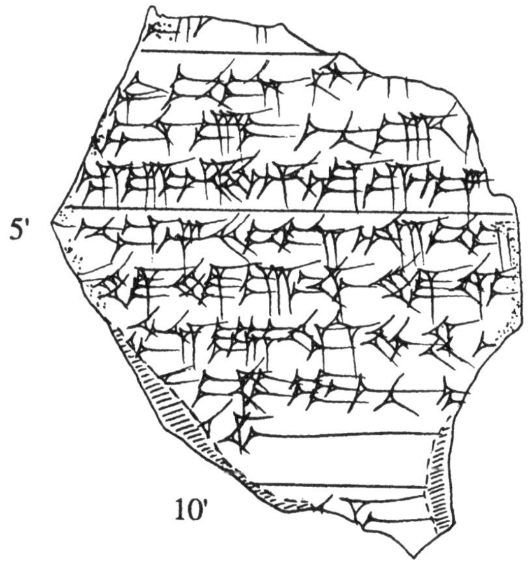

No. 14 Ms. o
K 13405 + S 804 + 926 + 2160

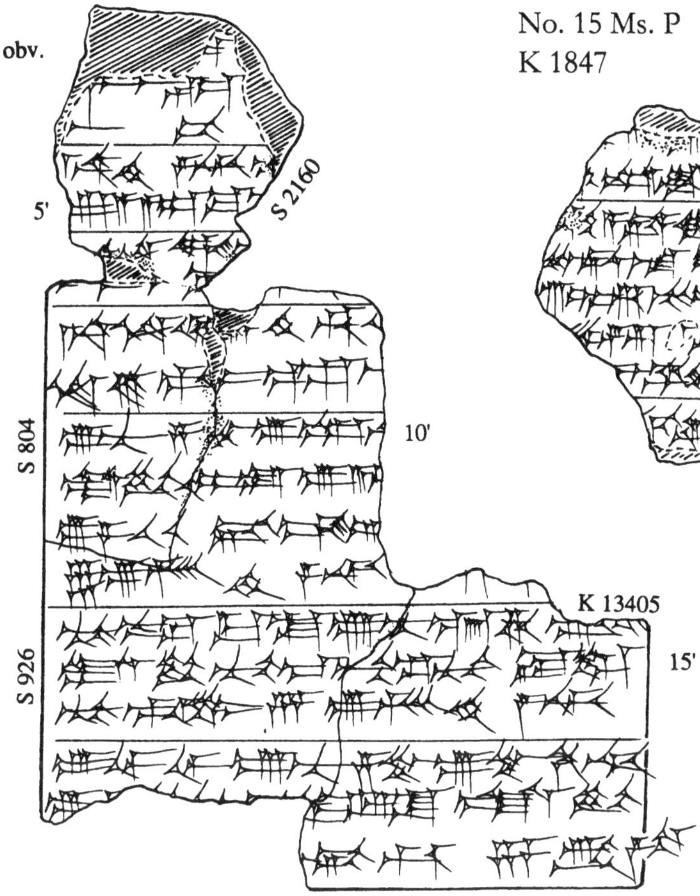

No. 15 Ms. P
K 1847

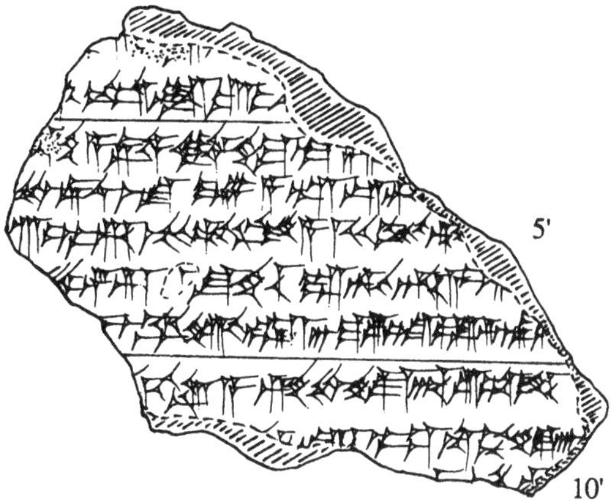

K 13405 + S 804 + 926 + 2160

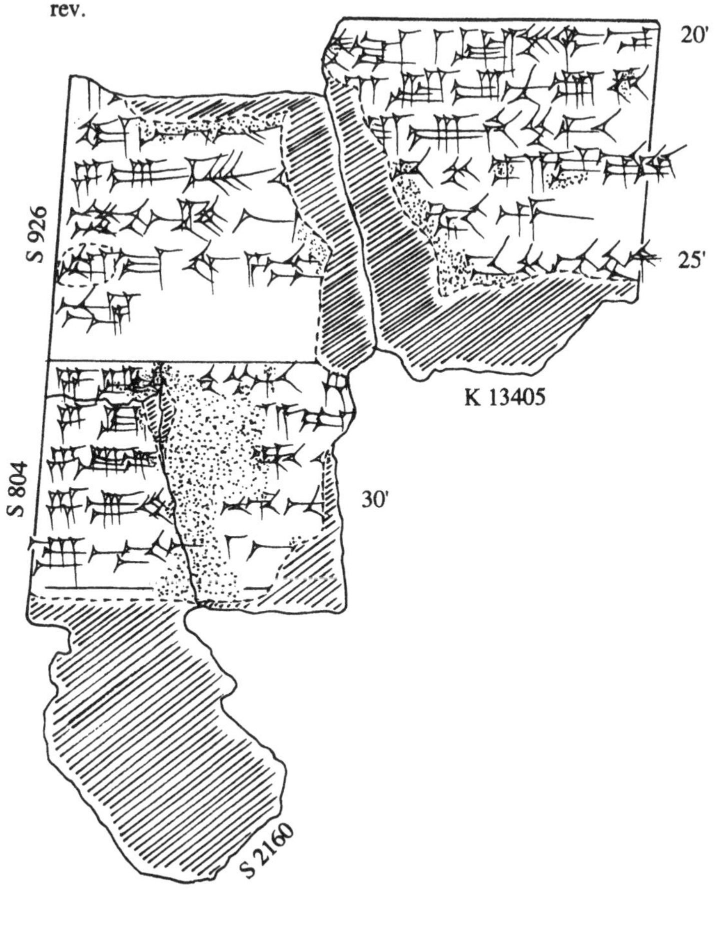

No. 16 Ms. Q
K 11230 + 11280 + 16437 + S 126

col. i

col. ii

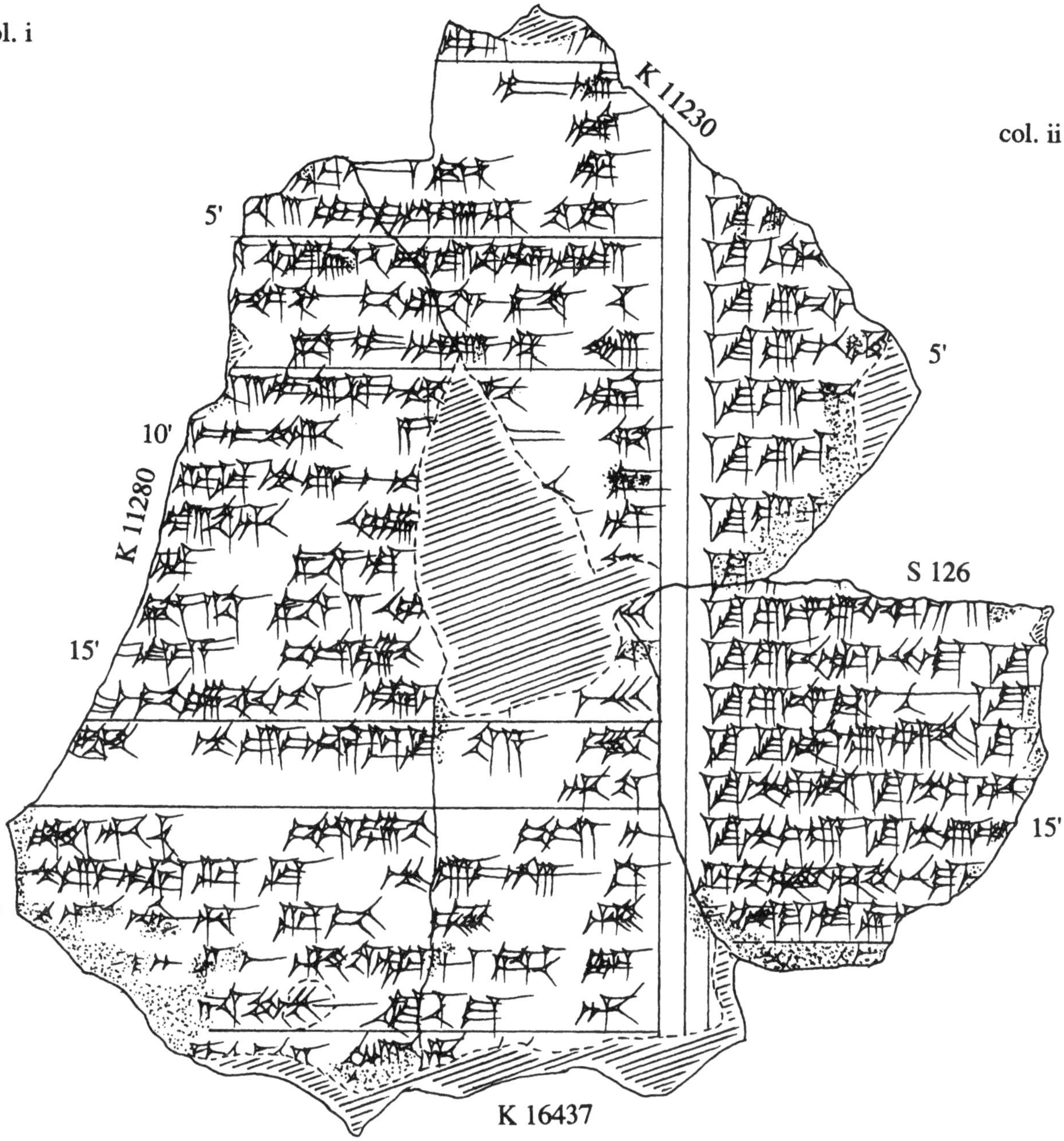

No. 22 Ms. WS 36+ 215 + 449 + 1245 + 1372 + 1452 + 1628 + 1646 + K 7925 + K 9091 (+) K 3453 (+) K 5955 + 14453

obv.
col. i

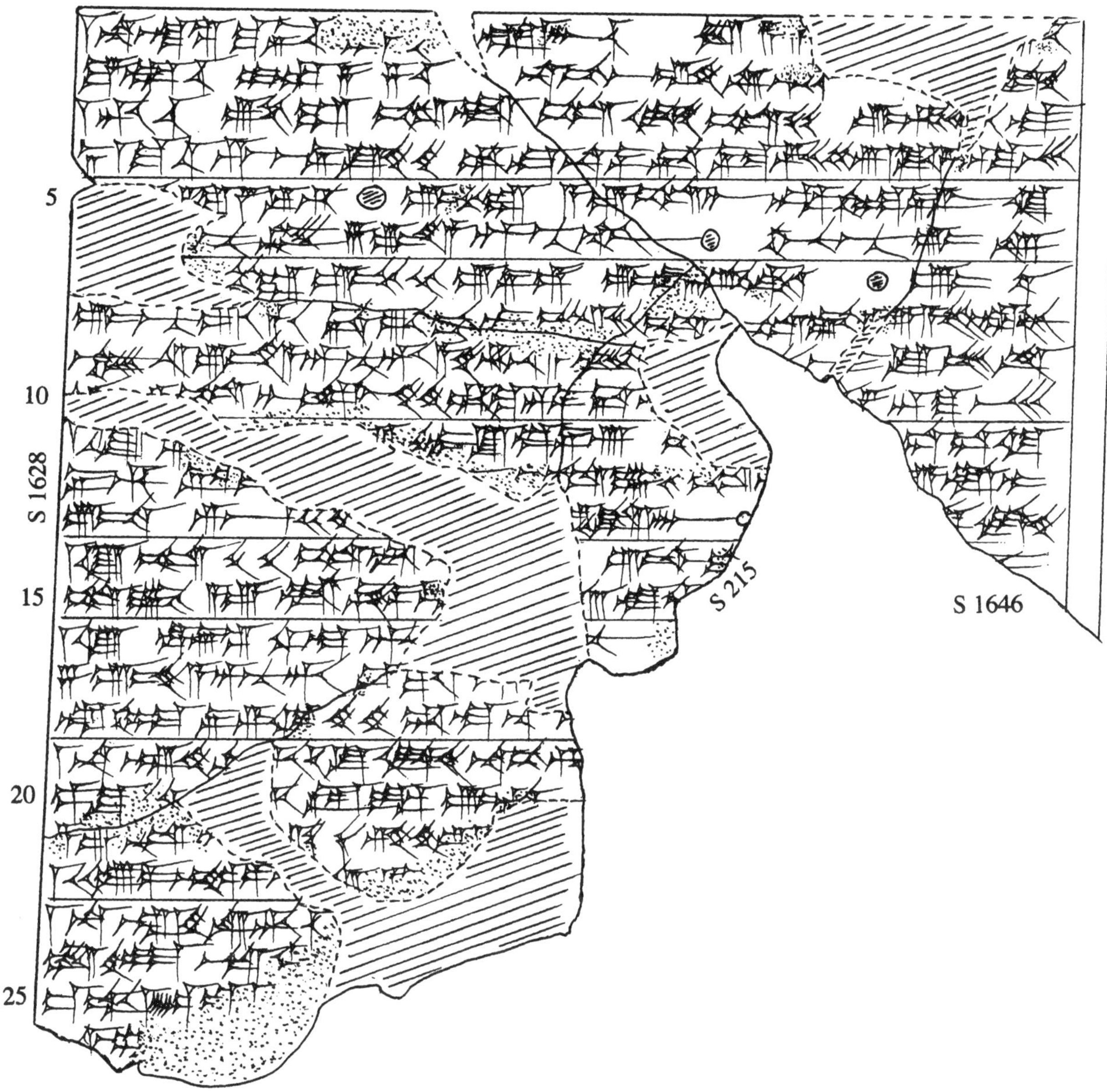

S 36+ 215 + 449 + 1245 + 1372 + 1452 + 1628 + 1646
+ K 7925 + K 9091 (+) K 3453 (+) K 5955 + 14453

obv.
col. ii

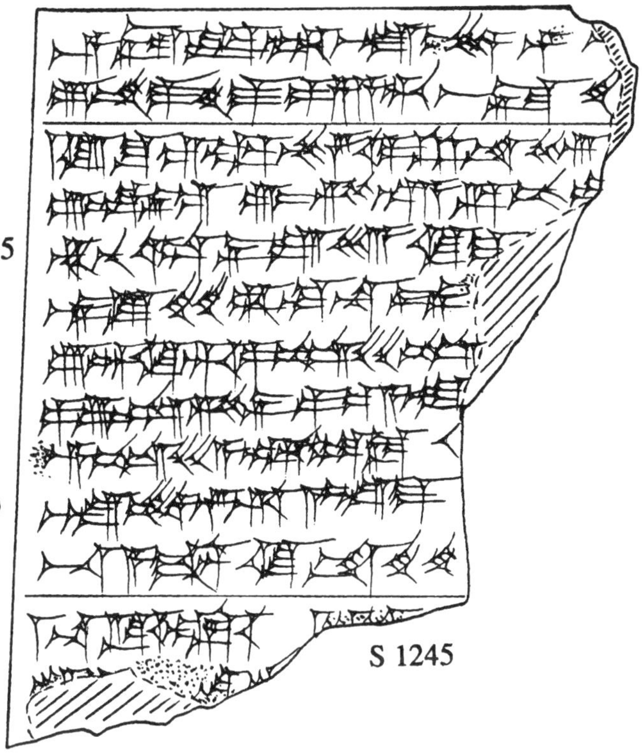

S 1245

K 3453

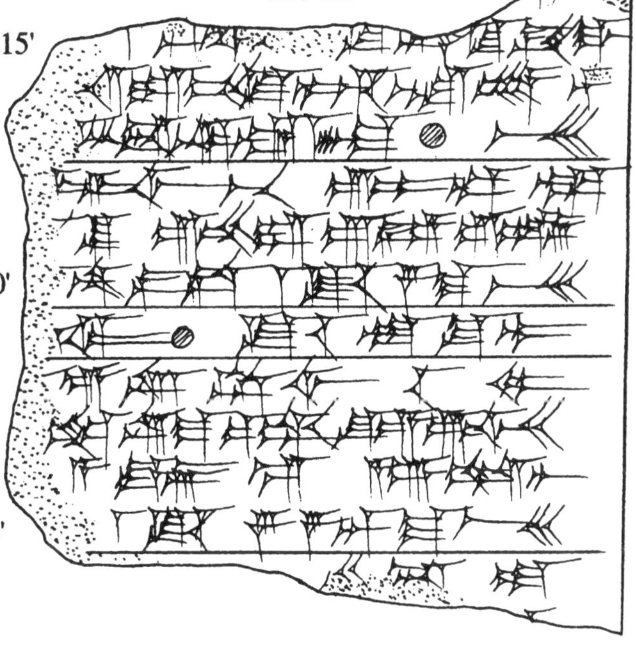

S 36+ 215 + 449 + 1245 + 1372 + 1452 + 1628 + 1646
+ K 7925 + K 9091 (+) K 3453 (+) K 5955 + 14453

rev. col. iii

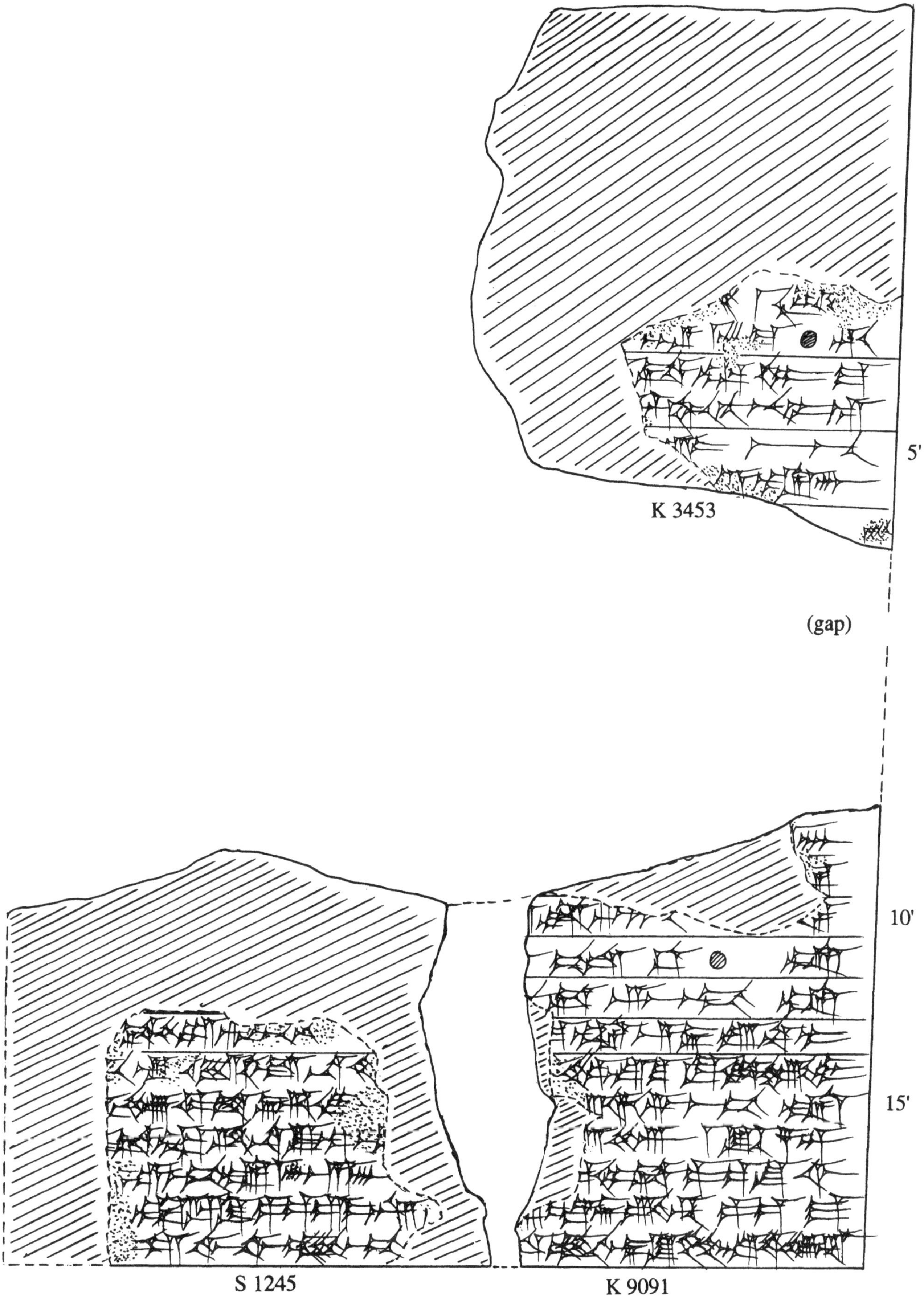

S 36+ 215 + 449 + 1245 + 1372 + 1452 + 1628 + 1646 + K 7925 + K 9091 (+) K 3453 (+) K 5955 + 14453

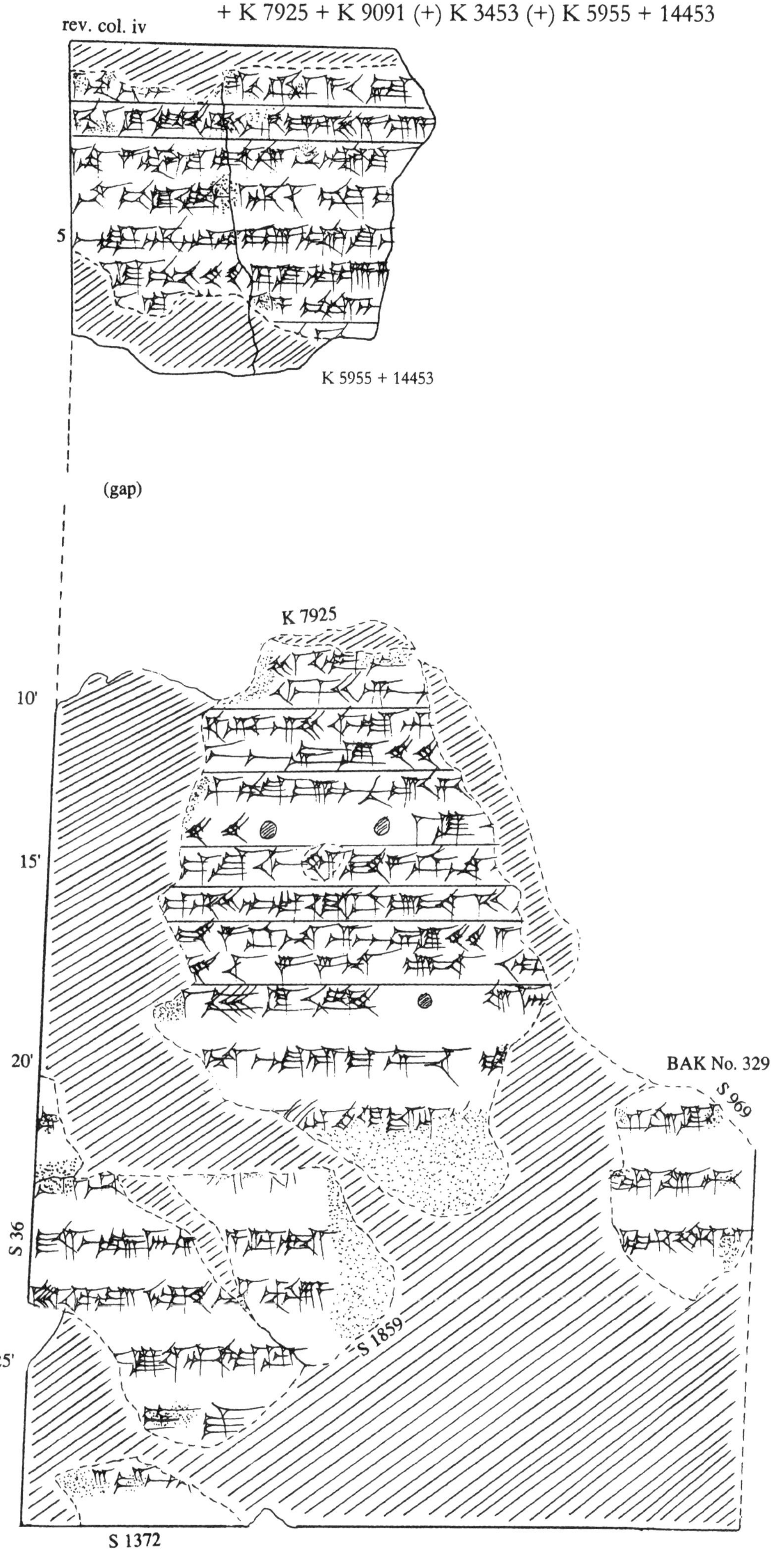

rev. col. iii

No. 23 Ms.X

K 6545 + 8355 + 9030

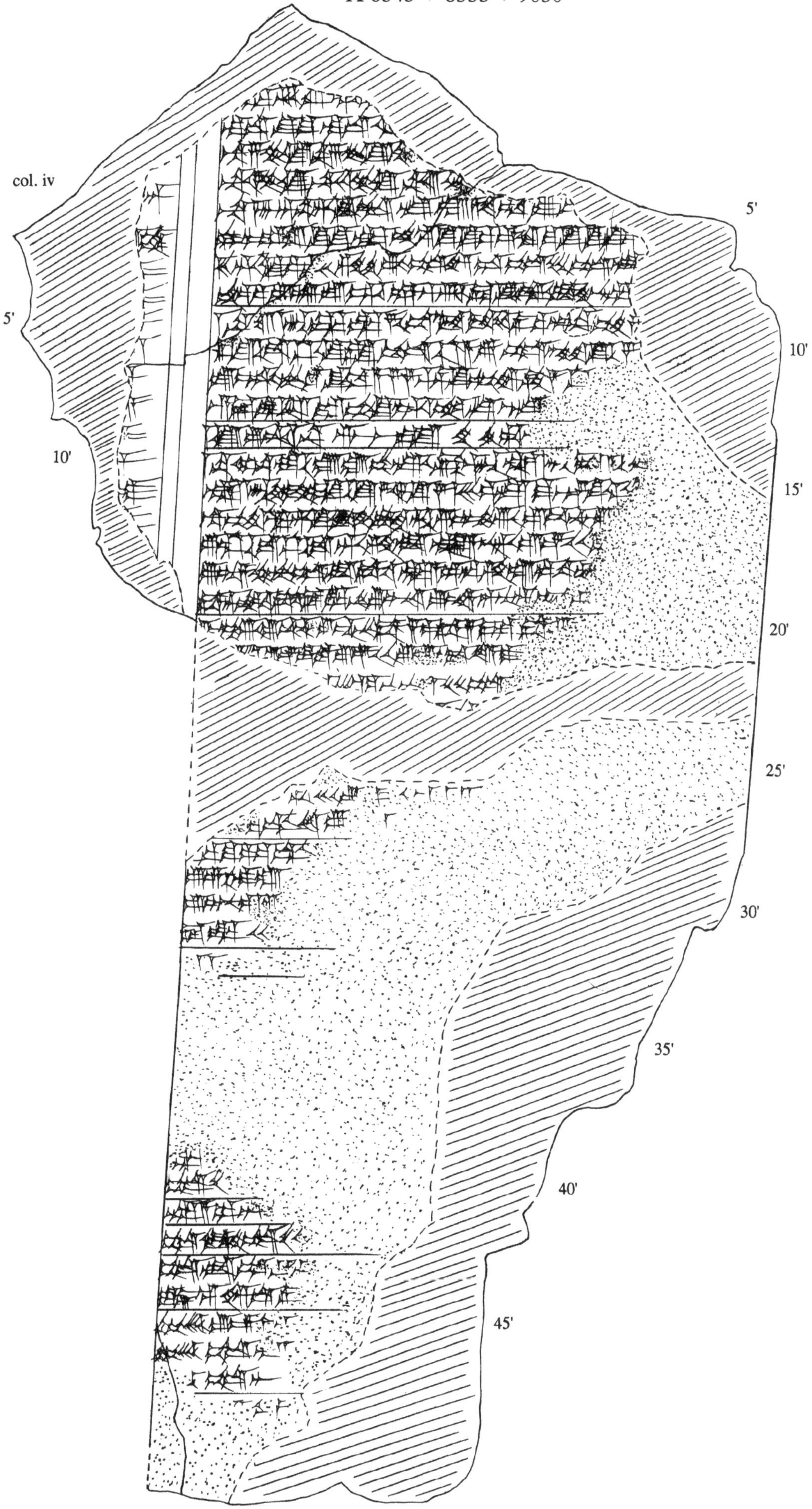

K 6545 + 8355 + 9030

rev. col. iv

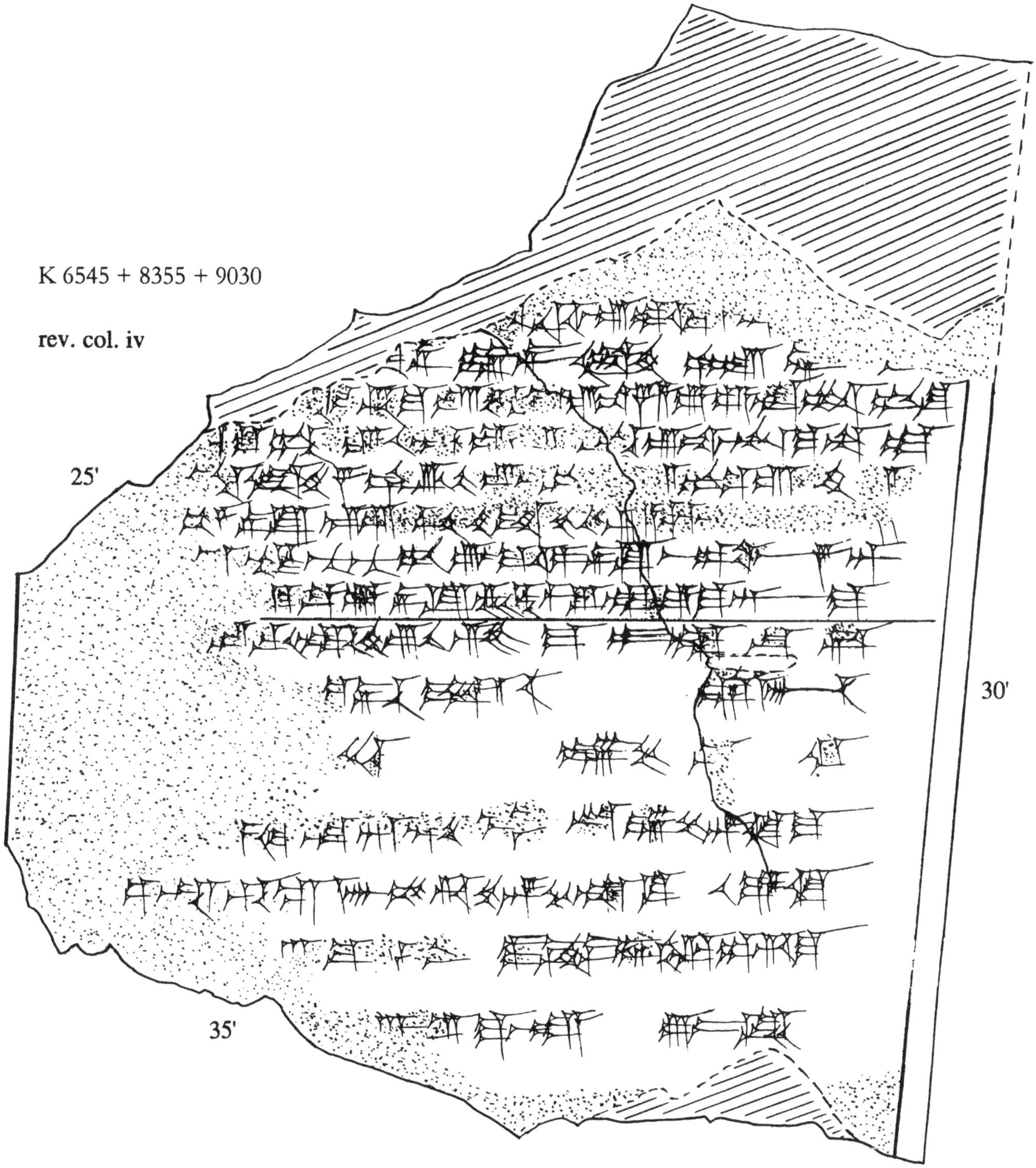

No. 24 Ms. Y
K 2433 + 3989 + 4019 + 7818 + 8172 + 14216 + 14772 + 15762 + 16409 + S 357

obv.

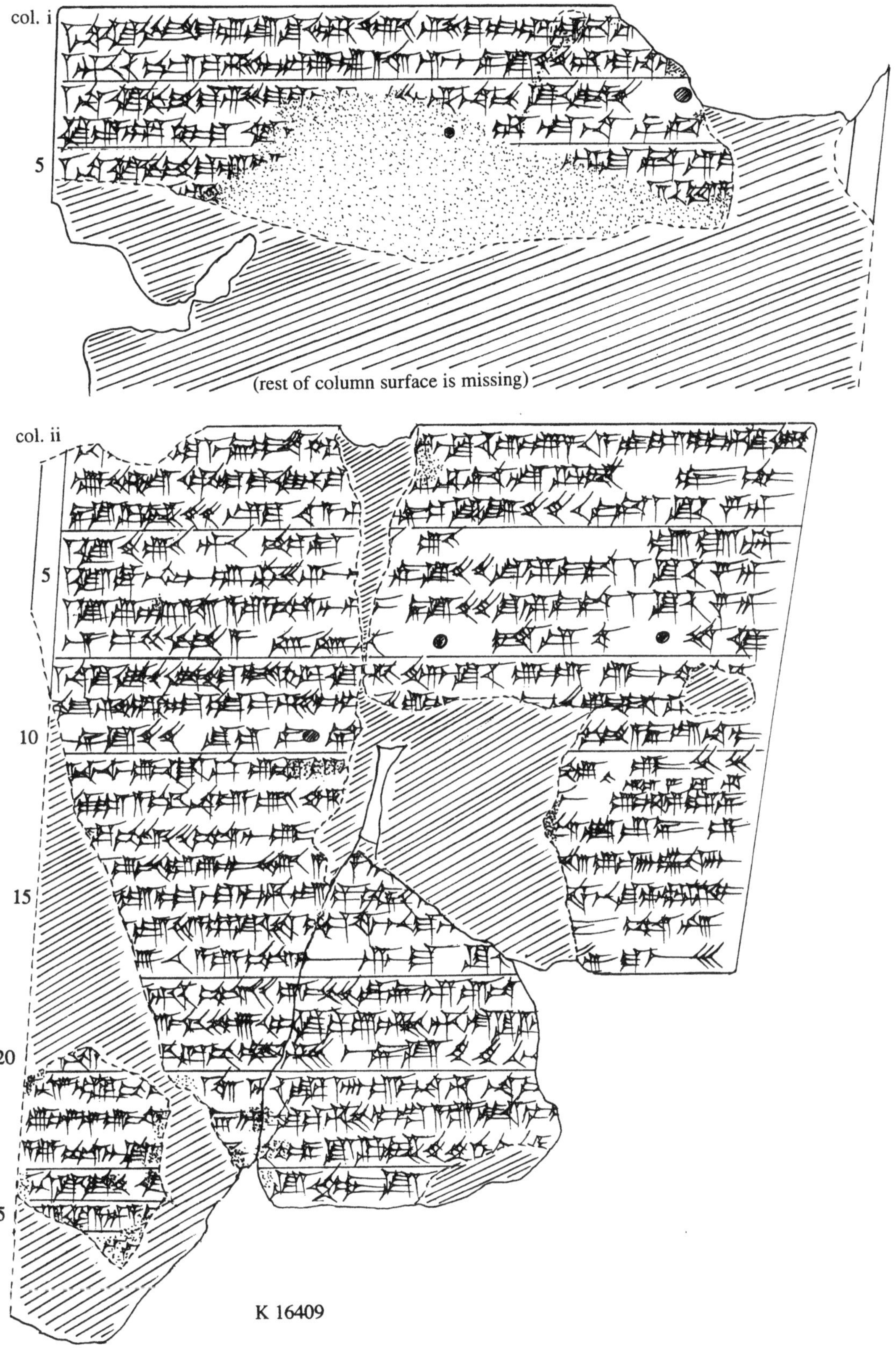

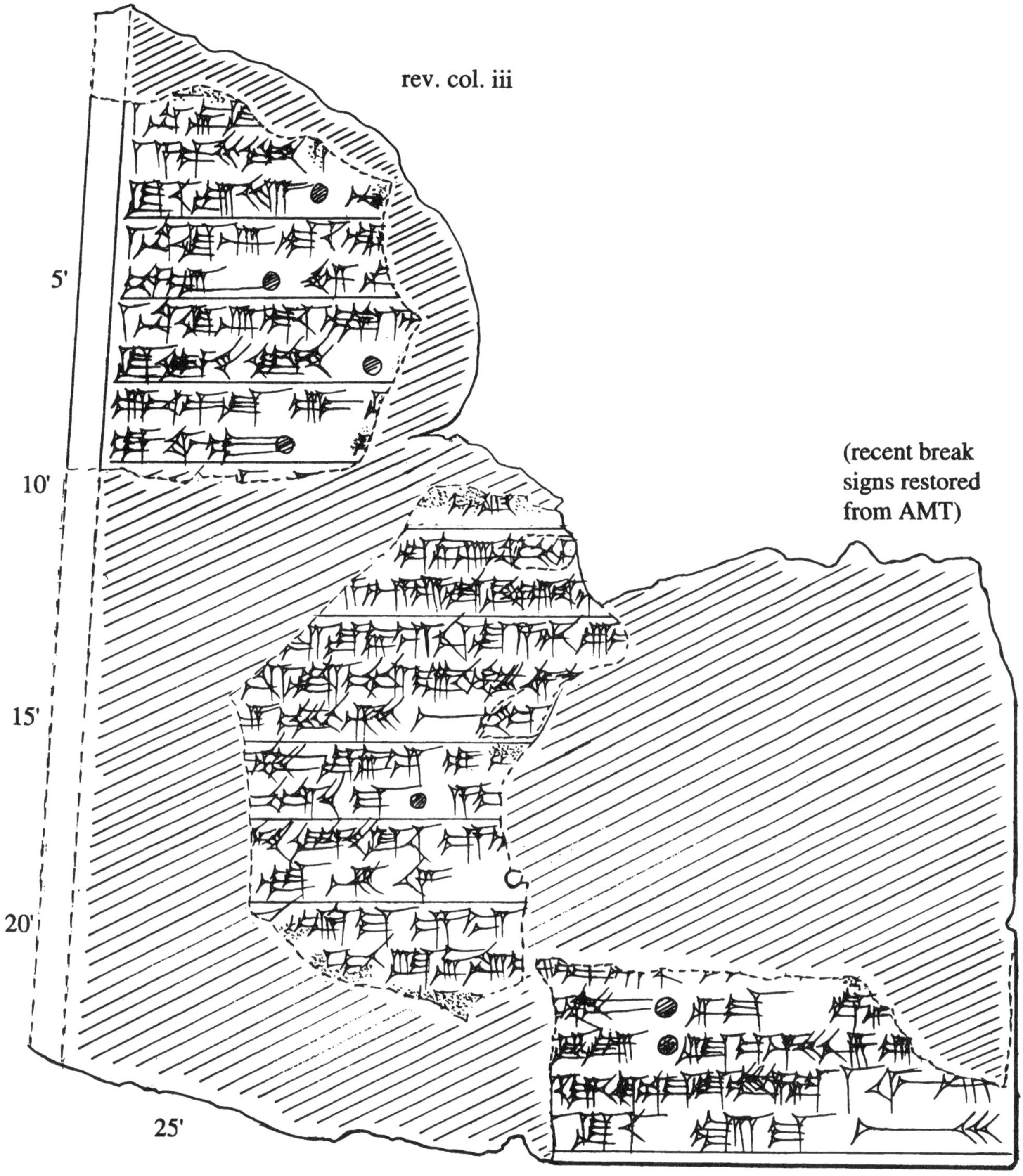
rev. col. iii
(recent break signs restored from AMT)

K 2433 + 3989 + 4019 + 7818 + 8172 + 14216 + 14772 + 15762
+ 16409 + S 357

rev. col. iv

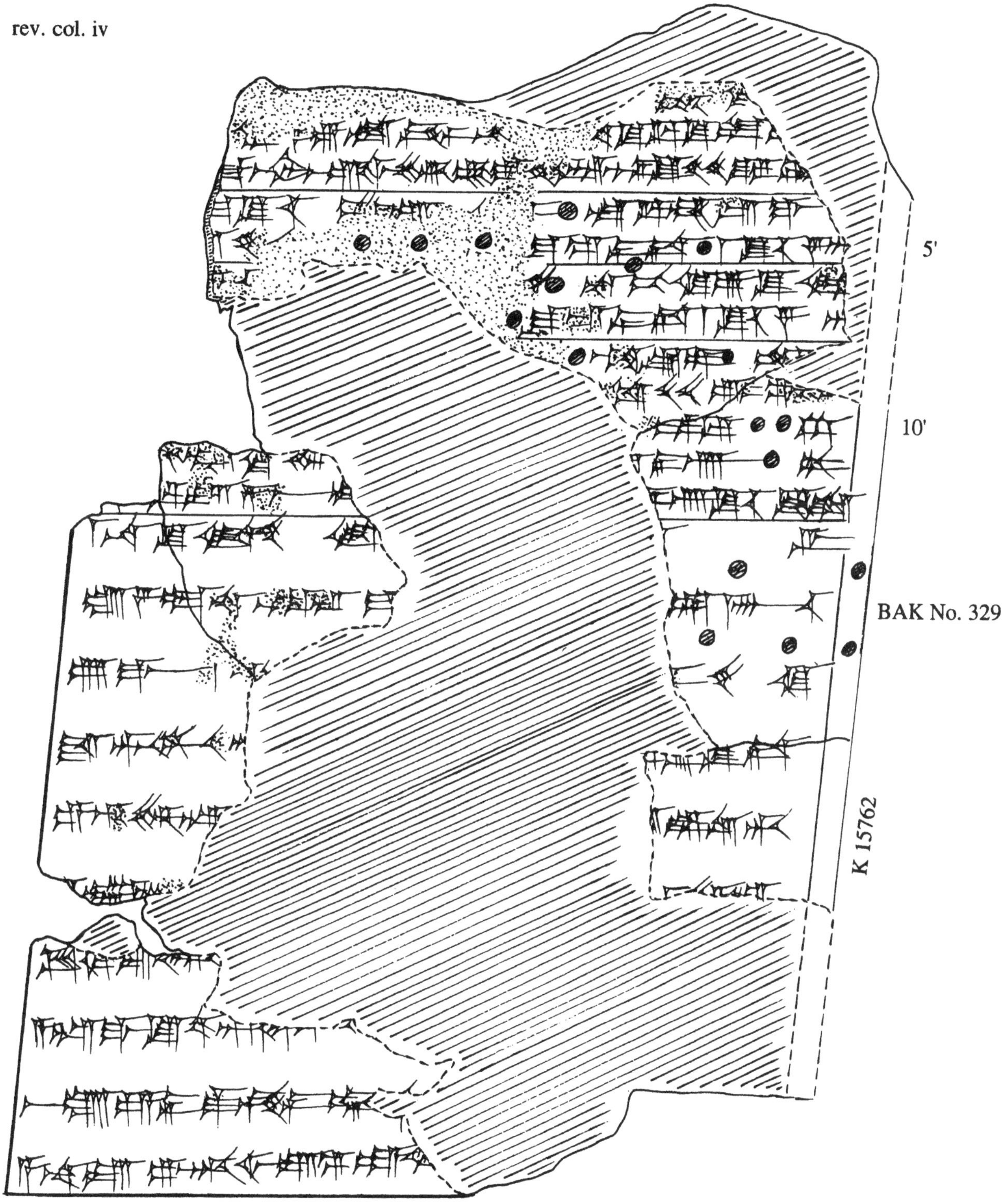

Ms. Y_2 S 1563 + 2061

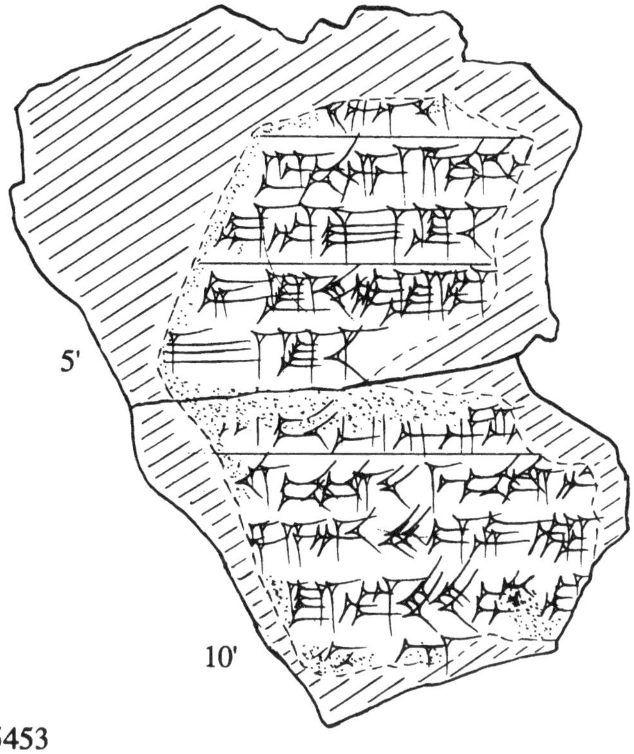

Ms. Y_3 K 15453

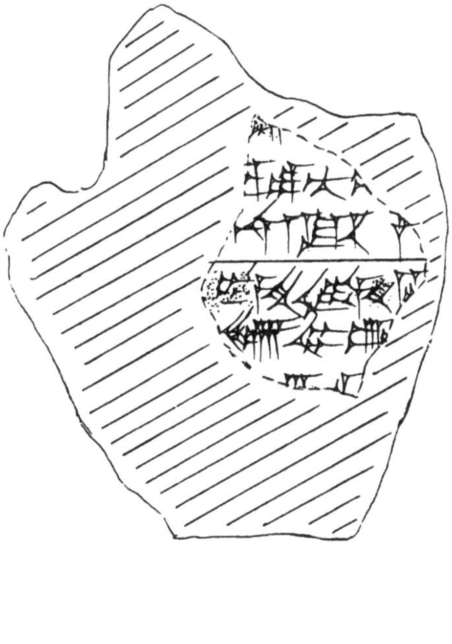

No. 30 Ms. dd
S 1283 + 1947

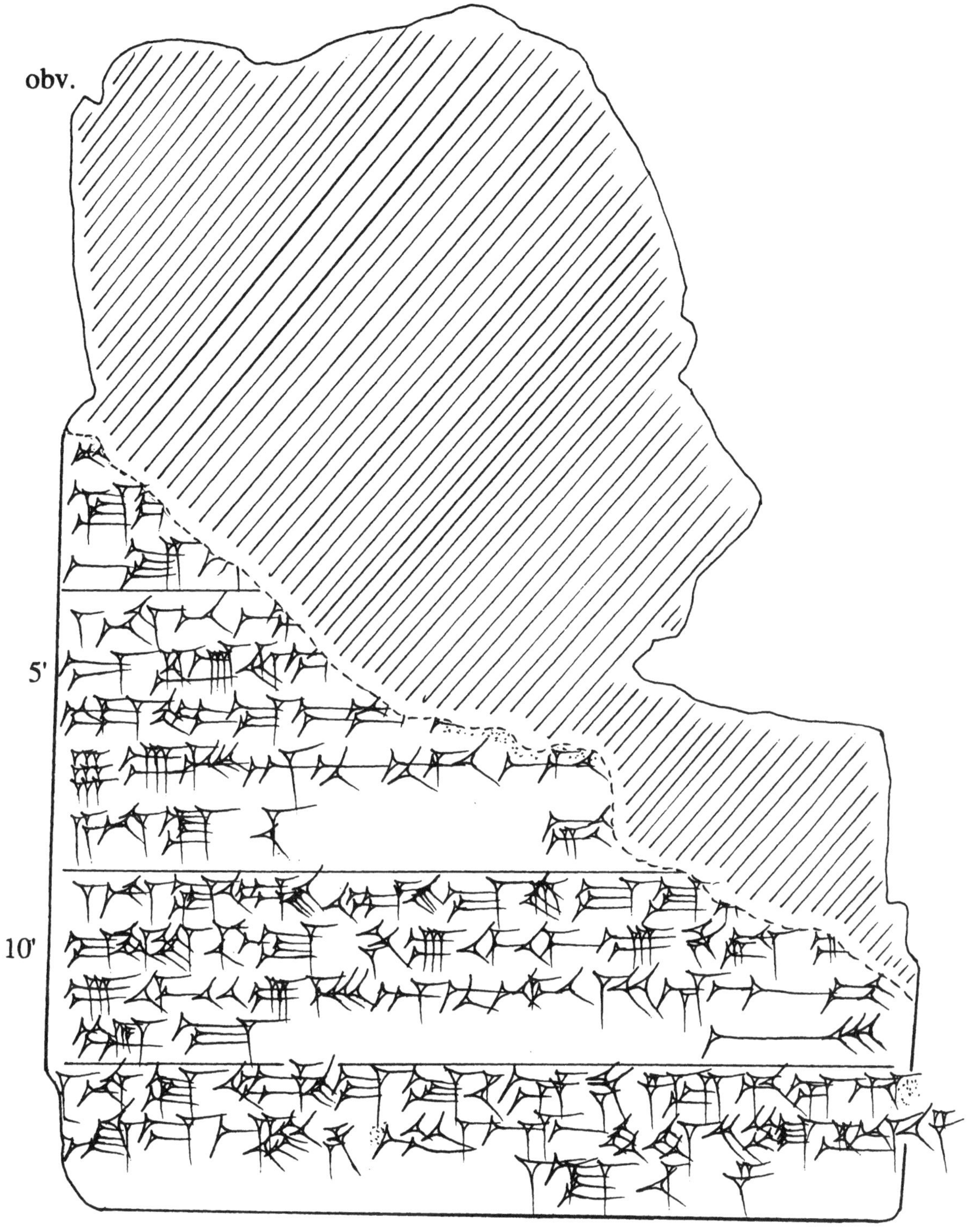

rev.

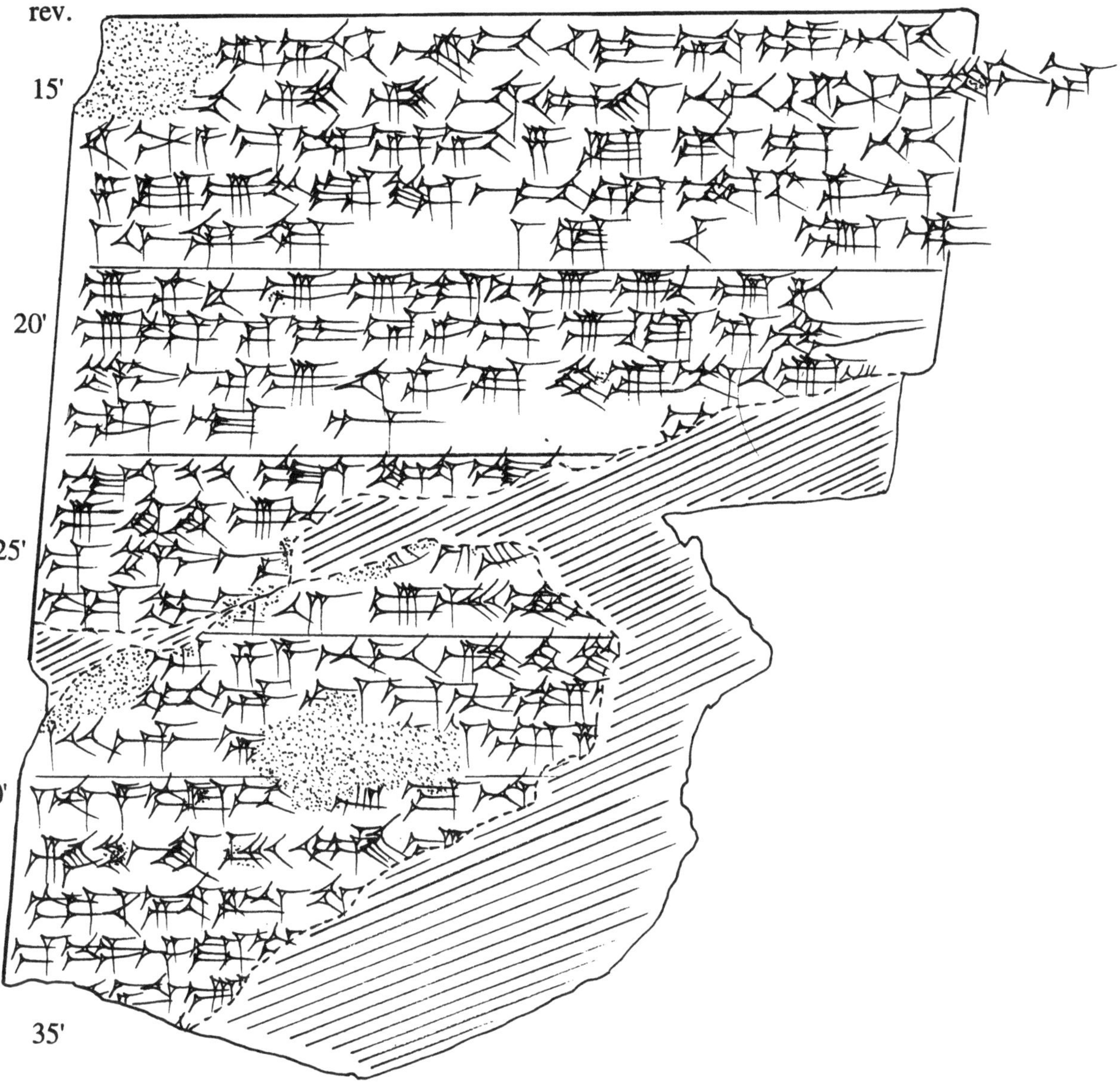

No. 37 Ms. KK
K 8182 + 11102 + 13404

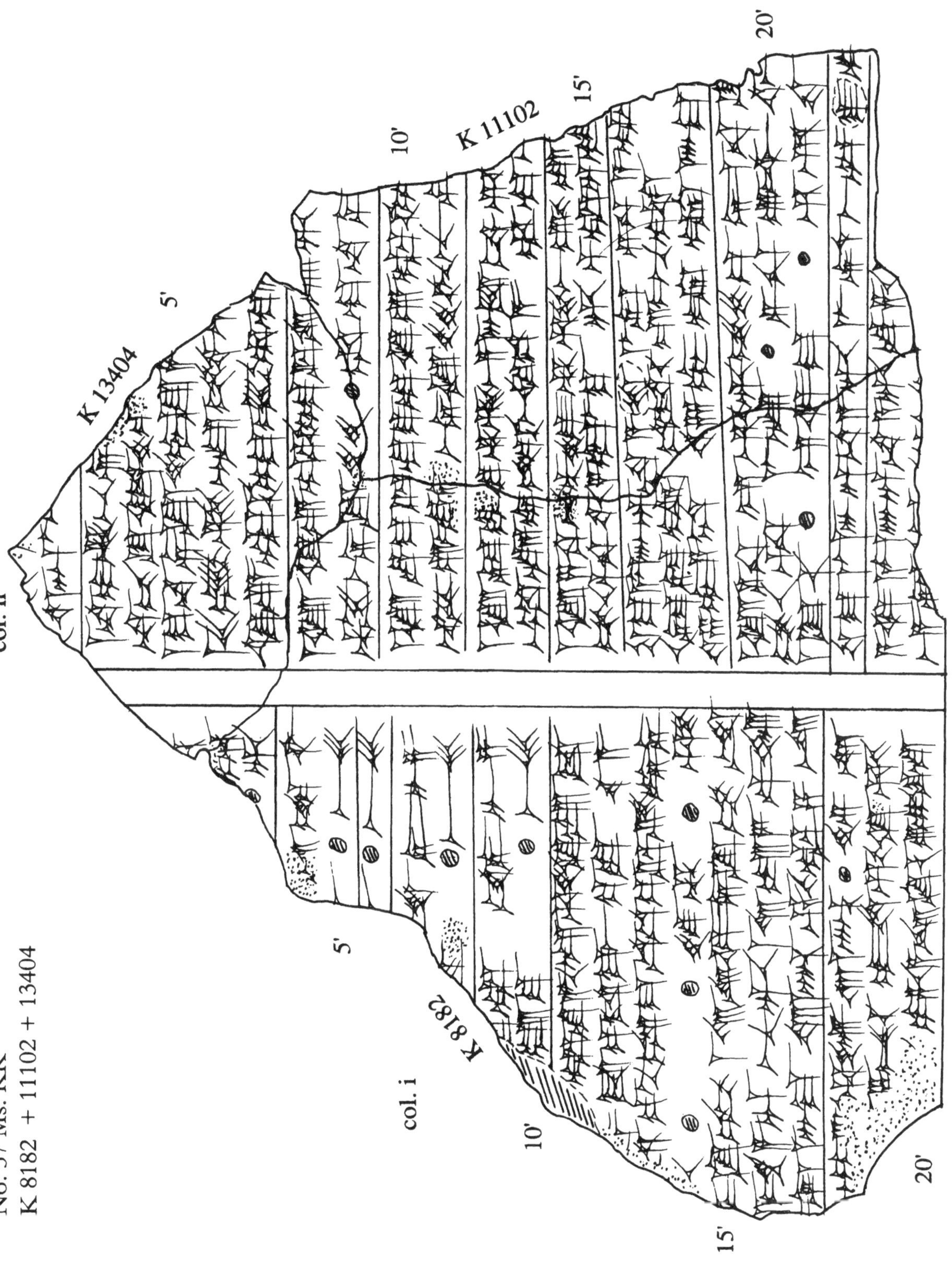

No. 44 Ms. rr
K 10567 + 13901

obv.

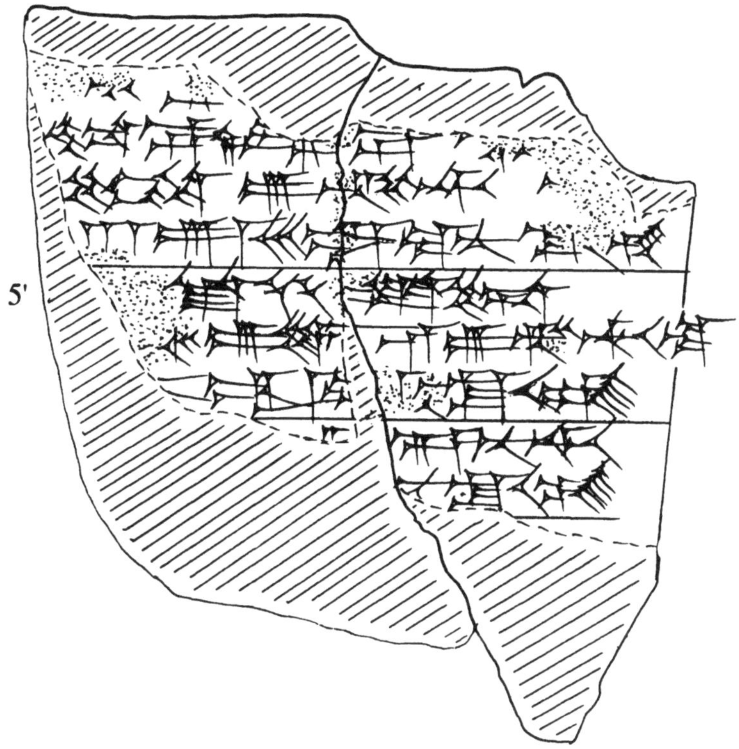

rev.

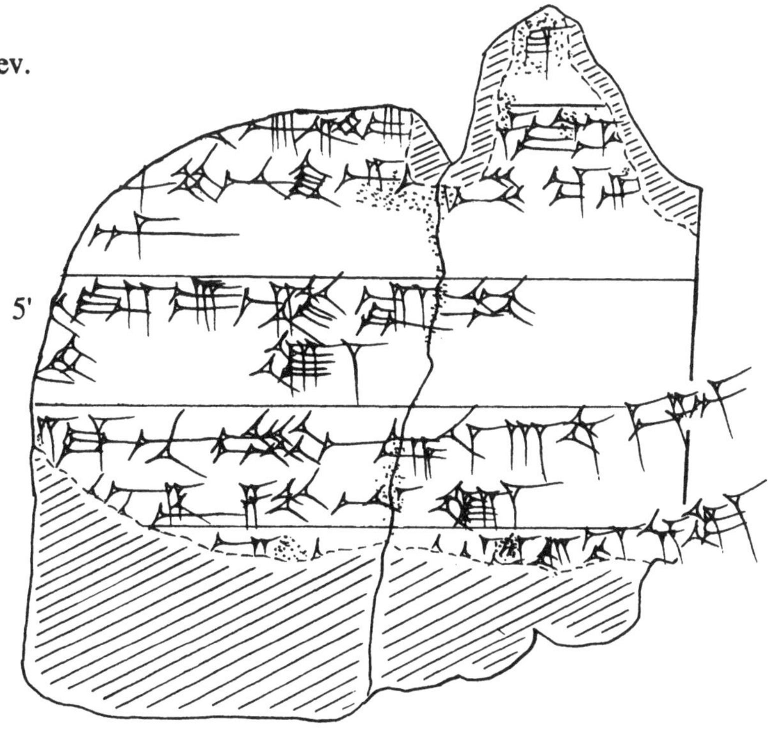

No. 45 Ms. SS
K 2428 + 2458 + 6728

obv.

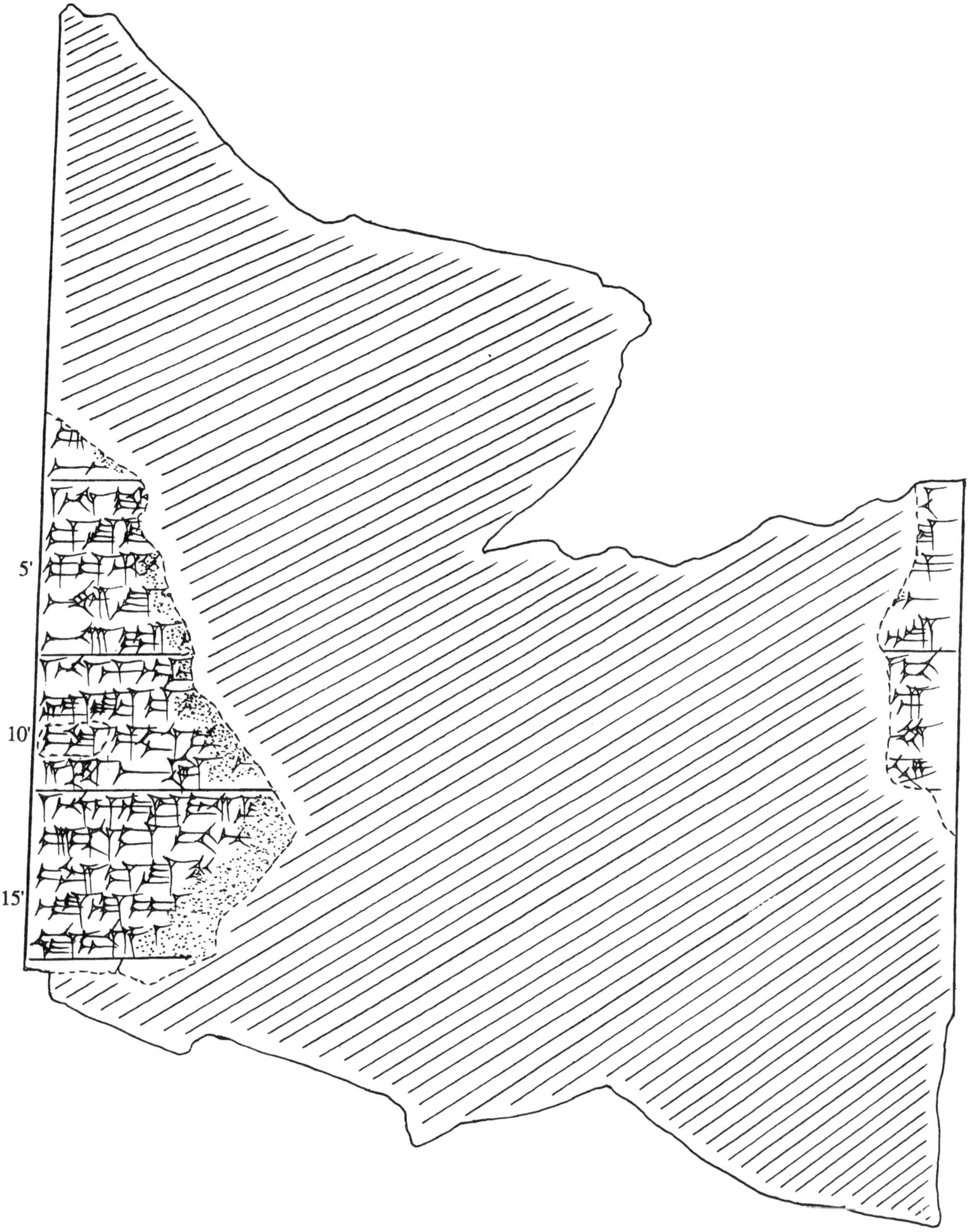

K 2428 + 2458 + 6728

rev.

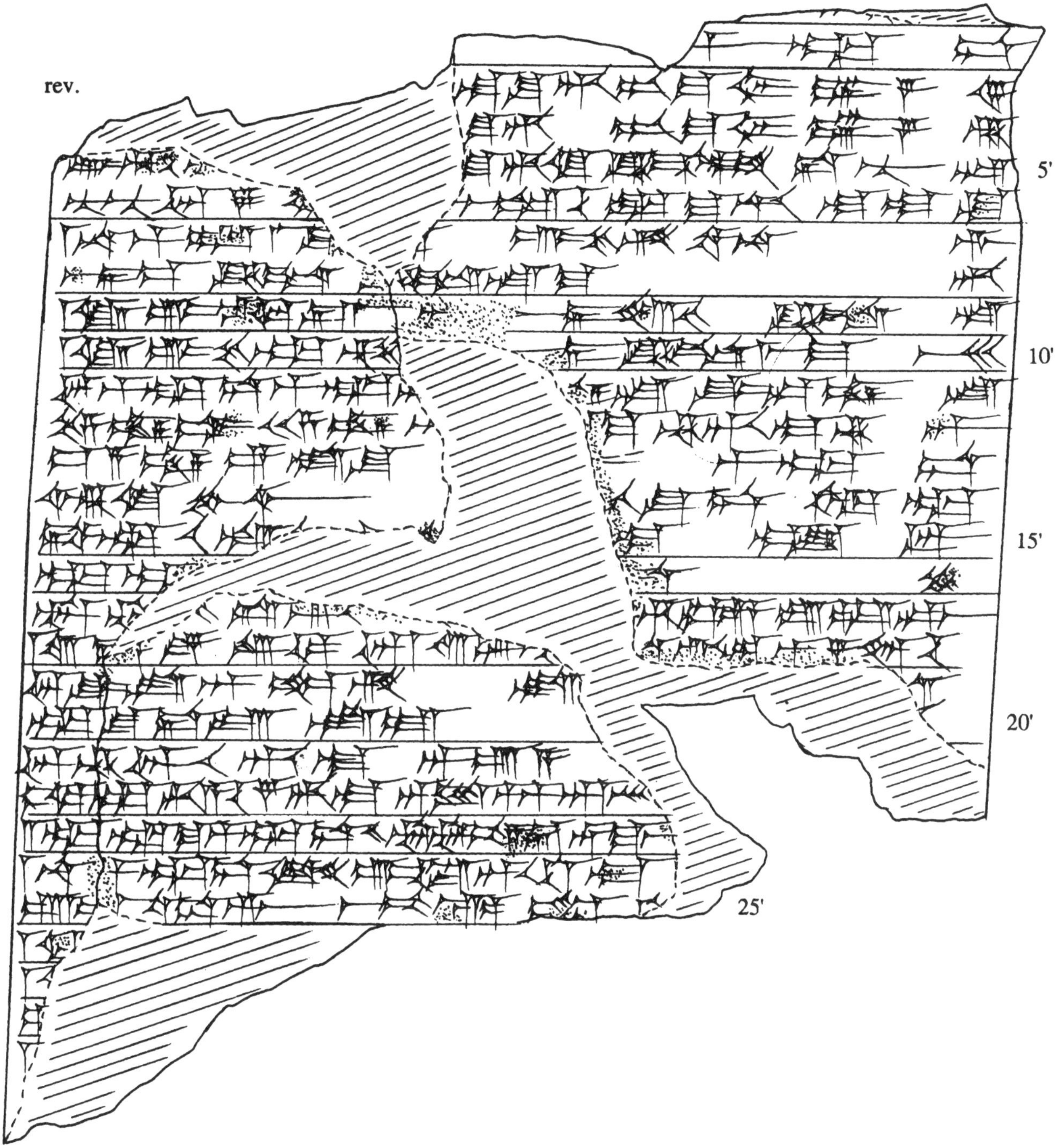

No. 49 Ms. ww
VAT 303 + 404 + 579 + 589 + 1751

obv.
col. i

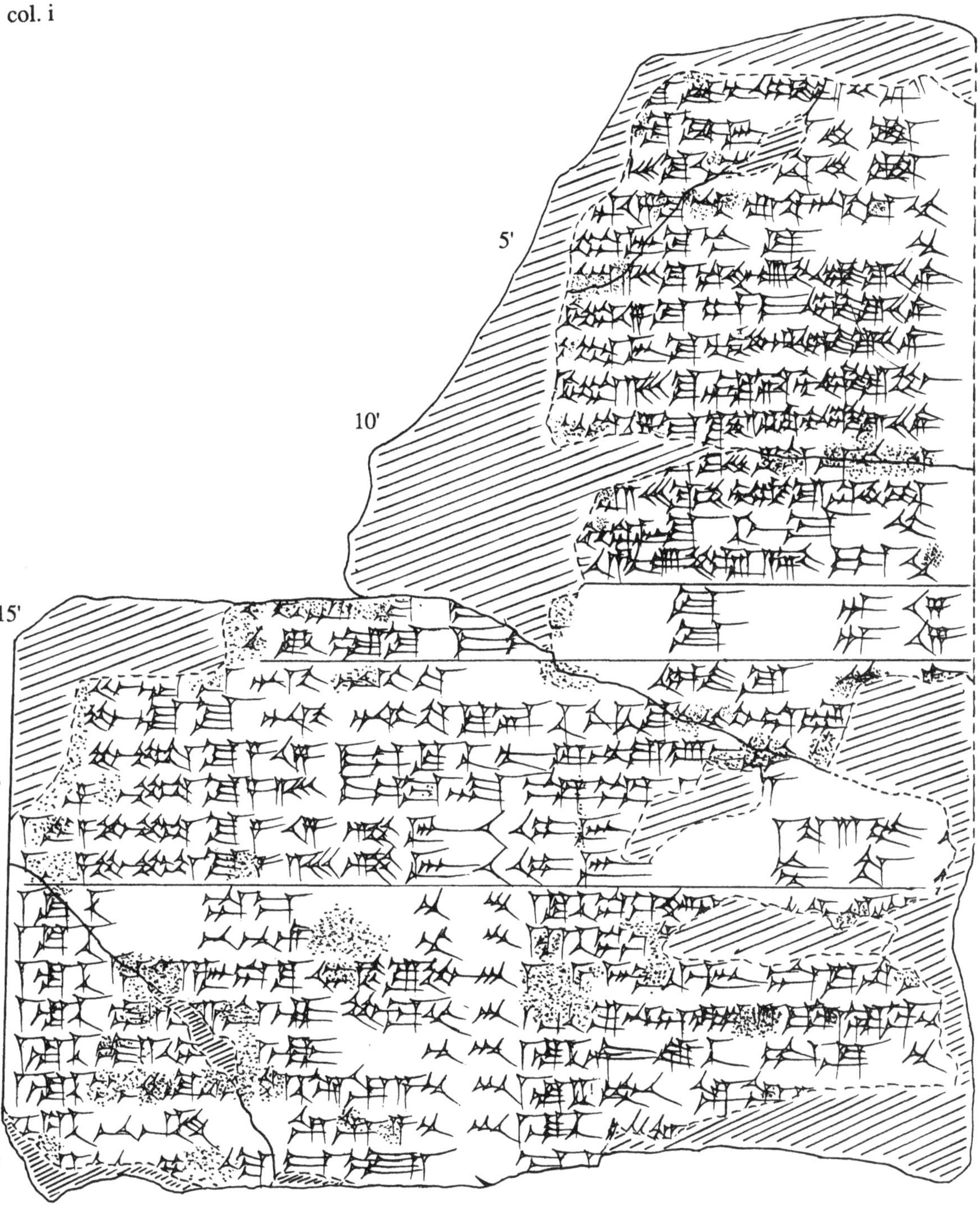

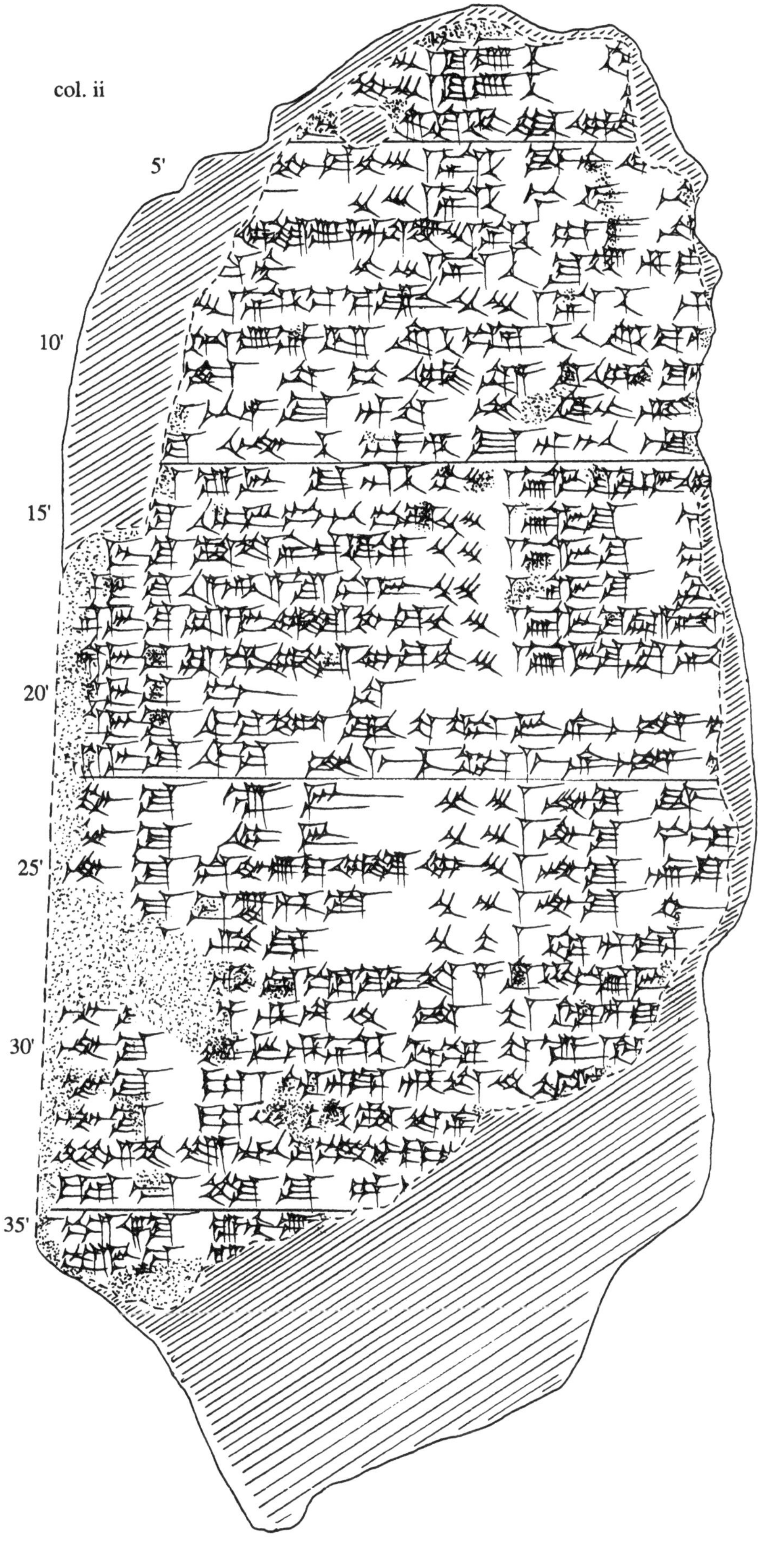
col. ii

rev. col. iii

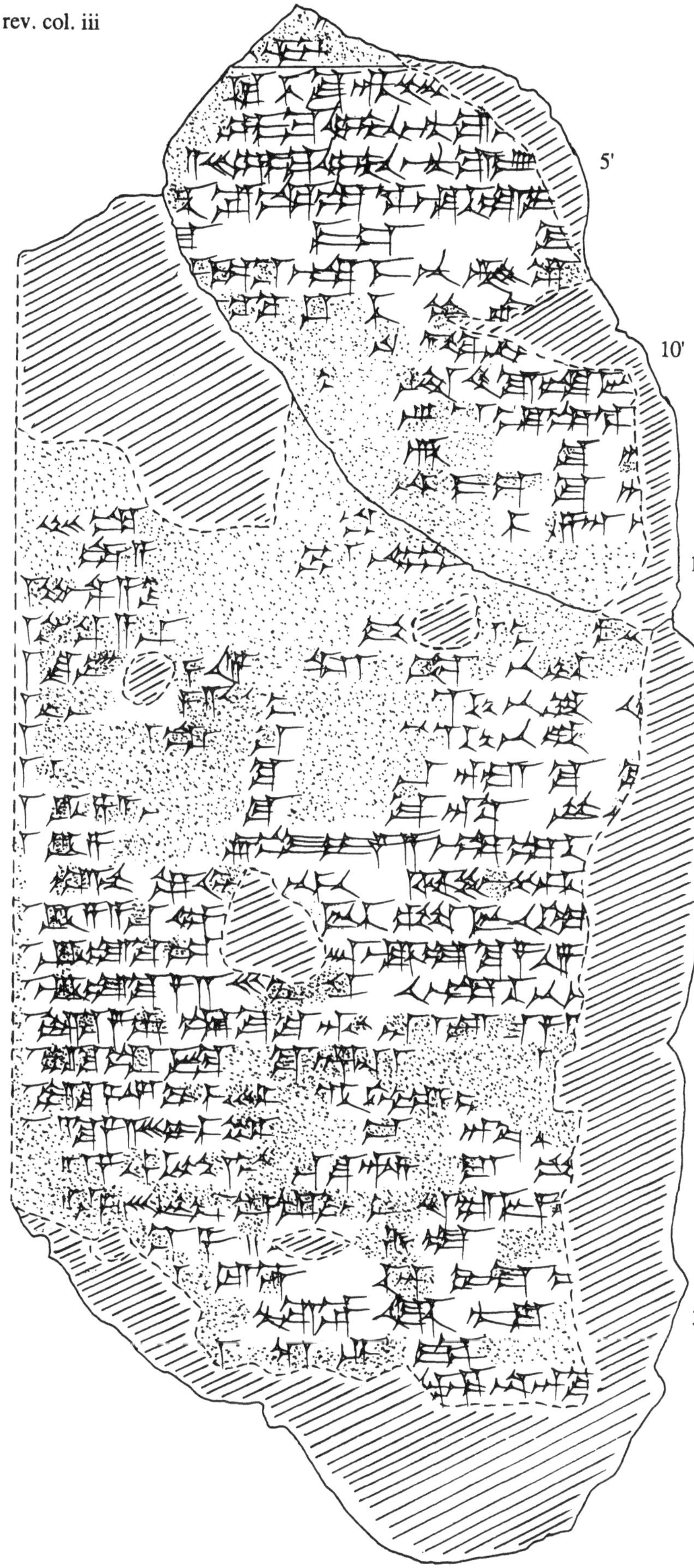

rev. col. iv

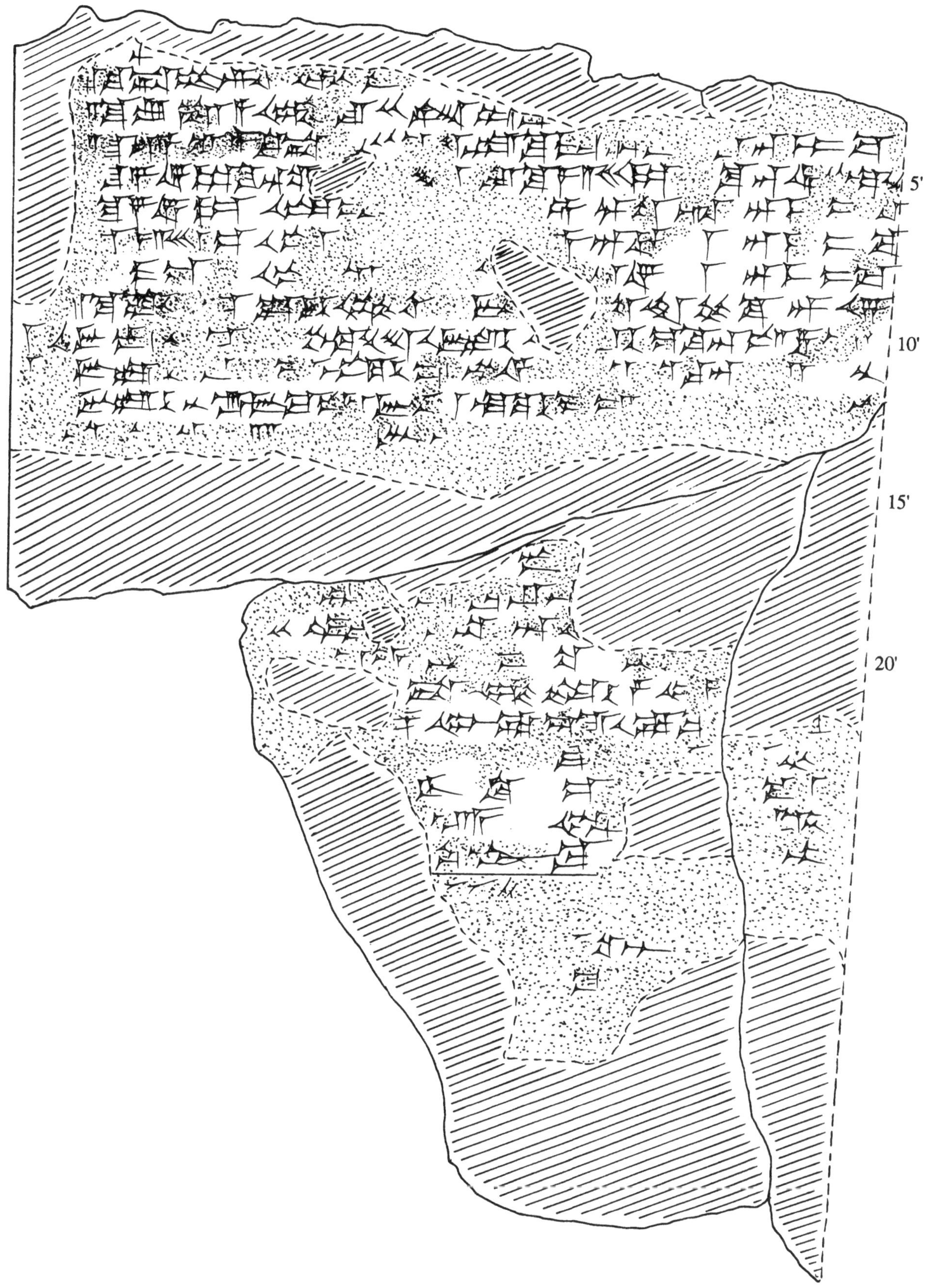

Ms. ww2
BM 38655

obv.

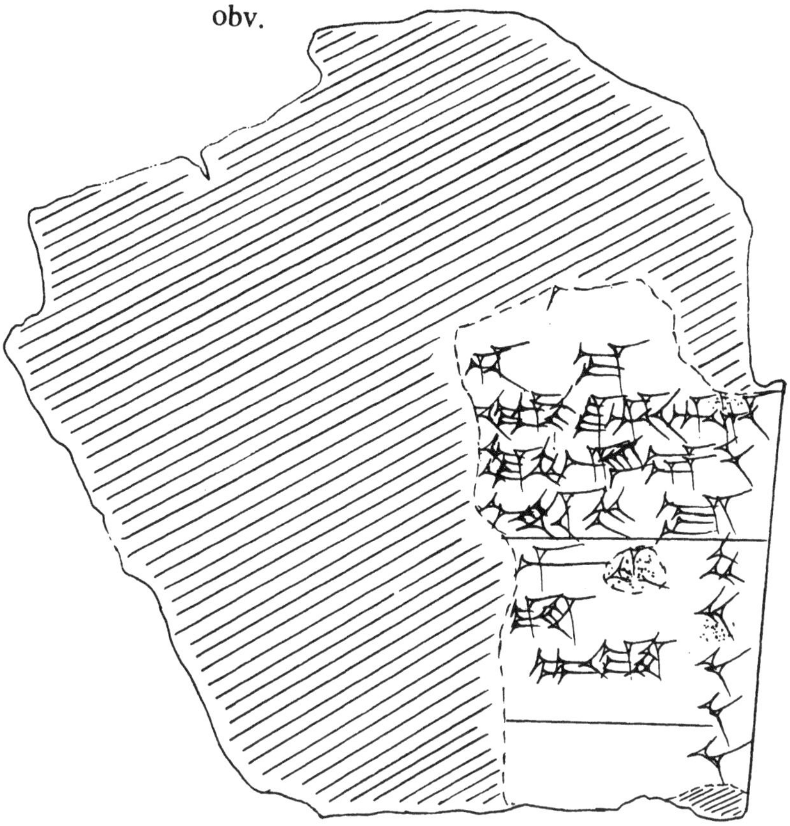

rev.

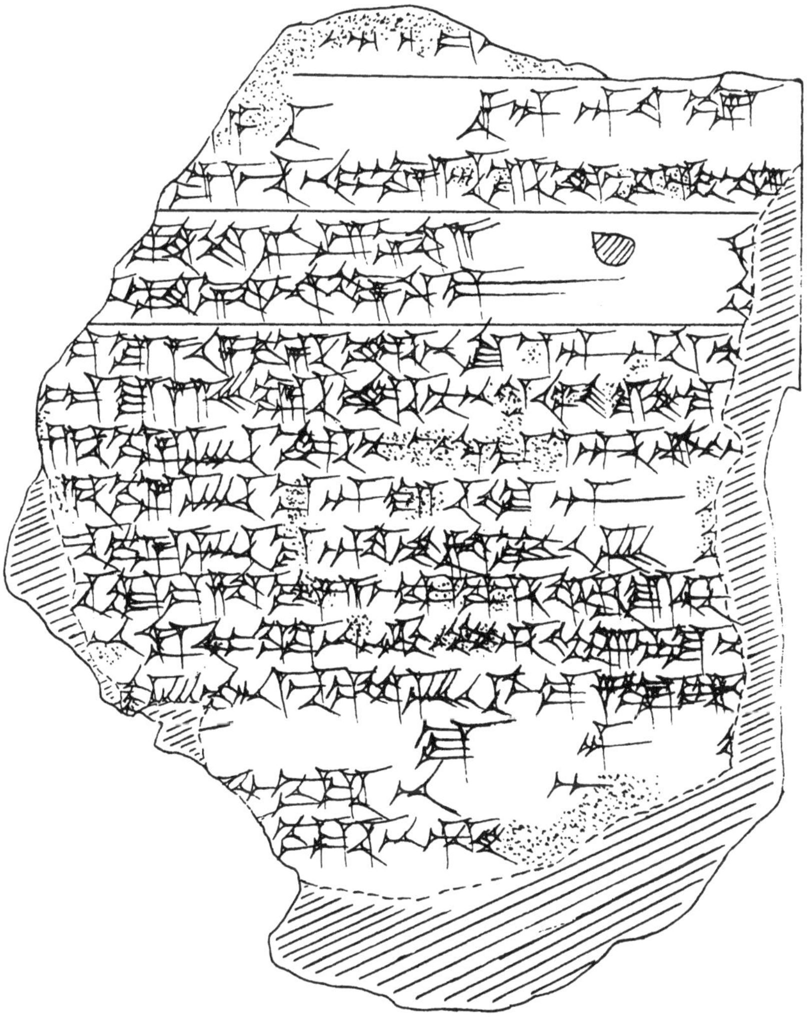

No. 51 Photo Bab. 2941
Excav. No. 47097

obv.

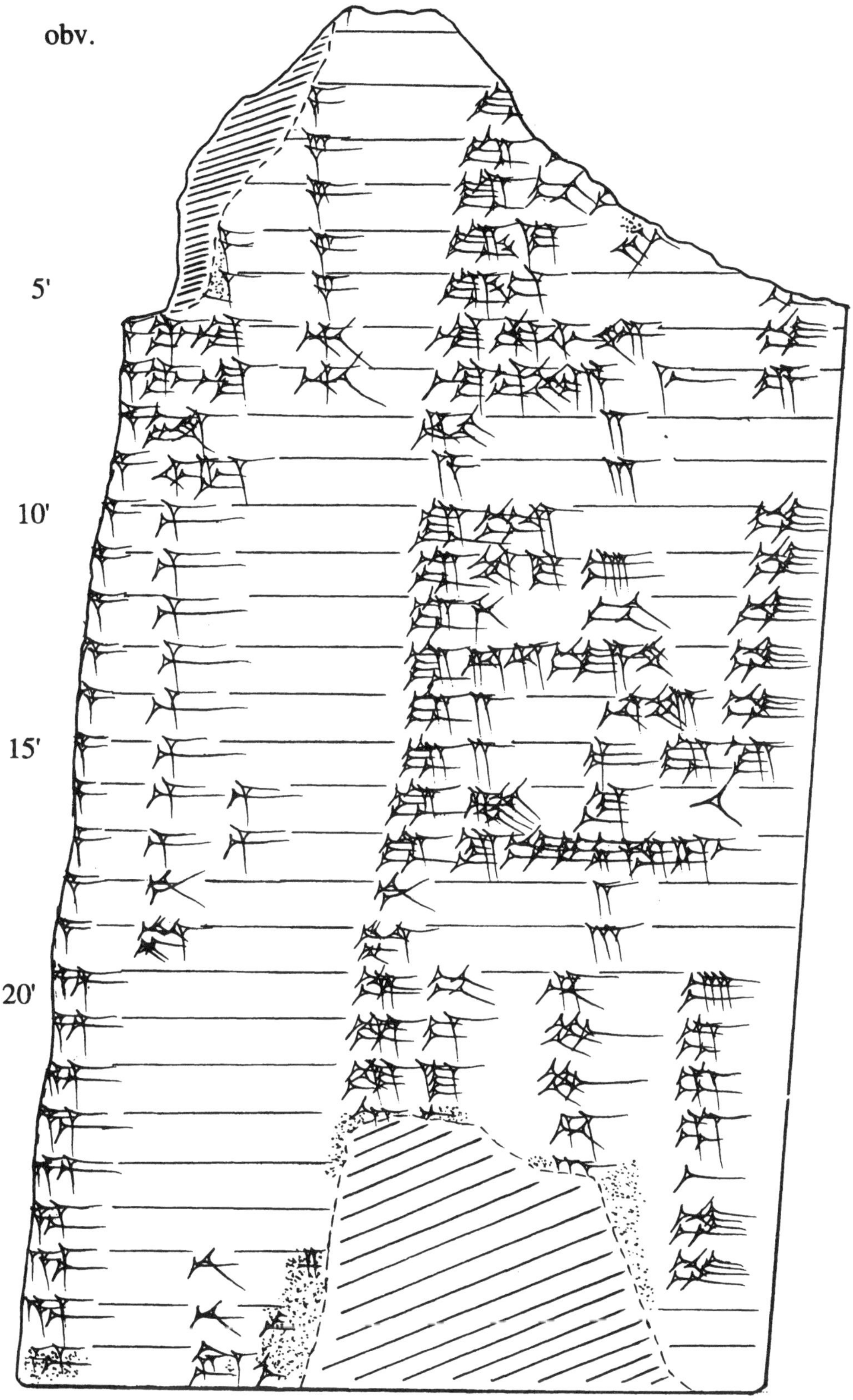

rev.

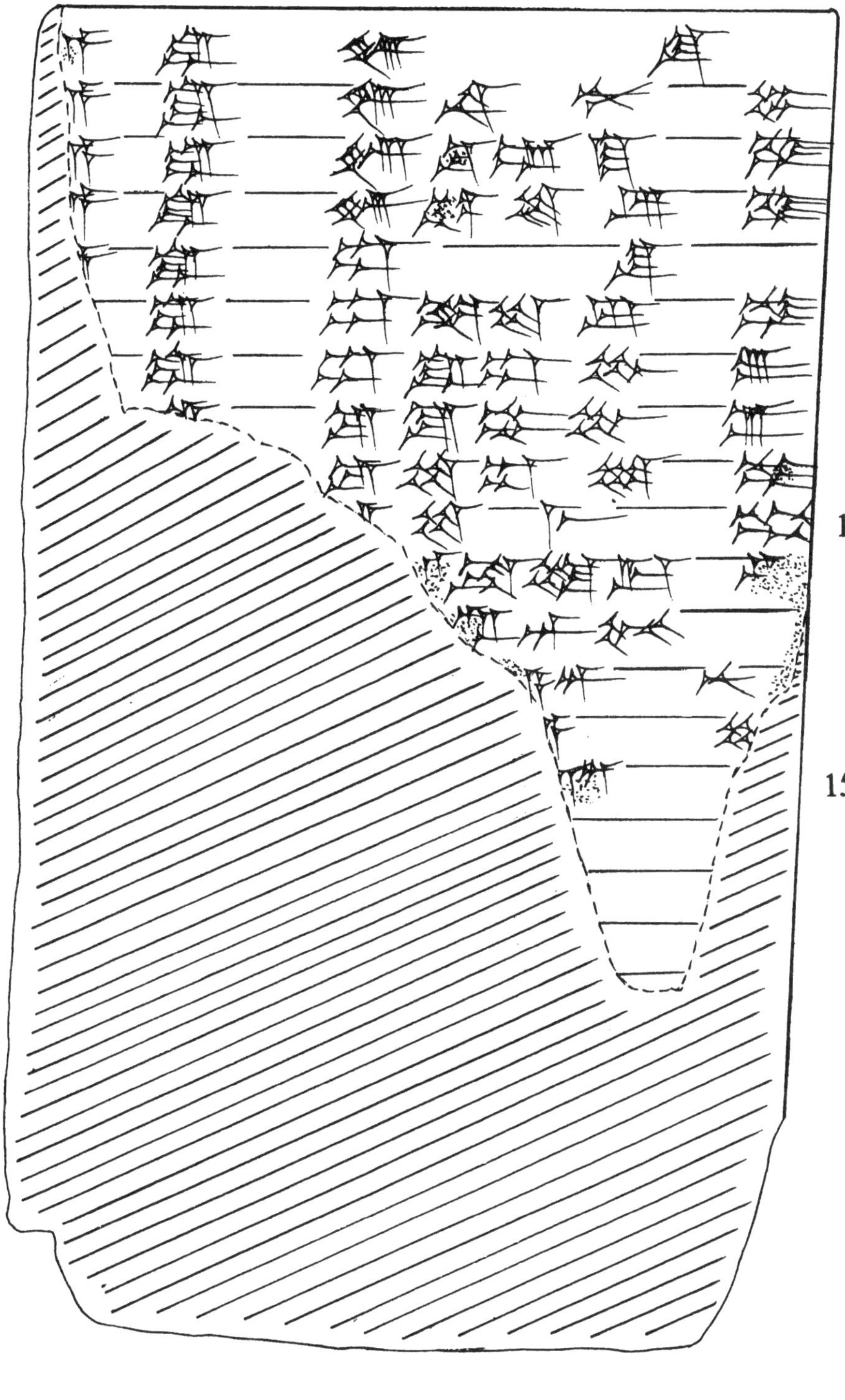

Bei Fragen zur Produktsicherheit wenden Sie sich bitte an:
If you have any questions regarding product safety,
please contact:

Walter de Gruyter GmbH
Genthiner Straße 13
10785 Berlin
productsafety@degruyterbrill.com